The

Self-Health Handbook

*Low-Cost, Easy-to-Use
Therapies from Around the World*

**Kenneth A. Dachman, Ph.D.
Joen Pritchard Kinnan**

Facts On File, Inc.

AN INFOBASE HOLDINGS COMPANY

The Self-Health Handbook: Low Cost, Easy-to-Use Therapies from Around the World

Copyright © 1996 by Kenneth A. Dachman, Ph.D., and Joen Pritchard Kinnan

Facts On File, Inc.
11 Penn Plaza
New York, NY 10001

Library of Congress Cataloging-in-Publication Data

Dachman, Ken.
    The self-health handbook : low-cost, easy-to-use therapies from
around the world / Kenneth A. Dachman, Joen Kinnan.
        p.   cm.
    Includes bibliographical references and index.
    ISBN 0-8160-3201-7 (hc). — ISBN 0-8160-3227-0 (pbk.)
    1. Self-care, Health. 2. Alternative medicine. I. Kinnan, Joen.
II. Title.
    RA776.95.D33   1996
    615.5—dc20   95-46516

Facts On File books are available at special discounts when purchased in bulk quantities for businesses, associations, institutions or sales promotions. Please call our Special Sales Department in New York at 212/967-8800 or 800/322-8755.

Cover design by Neuwirth & Associates

This book is printed on acid-free paper.

Printed in the United States of America

MP FOF 10 9 8 7 6 5 4 3 2 1

*For KLD, my one and only. And in loving memory of
Florence Waskin Snitovsky, one of a kind.—KAD*

*For Glynis and Jason with love. And to all the treaders on this
planet: May you treat it gently.—JPK*

CONTENTS

ACKNOWLEDGMENTS

My heartfelt gratitude to Dr. John Lyons of Northwestern University for his steadfast support and incomparable scholarship, to Dr. Marvin Surkin of the Union Institute for his wisdom and guidance, and to Chicago attorney Donald Leibsker for his invaluable counsel.—*KAD*

My grateful appreciation to librarian Hella Westbrook of the River Forest, Illinois, Public Library for her forbearance in allowing me to denude her shelves for an unconscionably long time and to the staff of the Oak Park, Illinois, Public Library for being similarly inclined.—*JPK*

INTRODUCTION

Want a hot conversational topic that's sure to spur controversy? Try healthcare. Debate about it spans borders, cuts across all economic levels, permeates political campaigns, and influences boardroom decisions. People everywhere are taking a new look at healthcare: what it means, what it costs, who should receive it, who should pay, and how it should be delivered. The way that governments, employers, and ordinary citizens answer these questions will have far reaching consequences.

As humankind has evolved, our concepts of what constitutes healthcare have changed dramatically. In the beginning, there was no healthcare except that provided by the individual through his or her wits and common sense. Yet people survived and even prospered. Gradually, systems of folk medicine developed in various communities that were often remarkably similar despite vast geographic separations. With the rise of civilizations came a corresponding increase in the scope and sophistication of medical care. Trained physicians now treated the sick and counseled the well. Though their practices might differ, almost all early healthcare systems were *holistic*; that is, practitioners believed that the mind and body were one and could not be treated separately. Physicians treated the person and not the disease, and most medications were derived from plants and other naturally occurring substances. With some modifications, physicians practiced this type of medicine for centuries. Eastern civilizations and native cultures never abandoned the naturalistic approach, but early in this century, Western medicine took a different course.

Spurred by technological advances and an emerging pharmaceutical industry, Western medicine opted for more aggressive tactics. Myriad powerful synthetic drugs (many based on compounds originally derived from plants) replaced herbal teas and homemade tonics in the treatment lexicon. Researchers developed sophisticated scientific equipment that could plumb the depths of the human body as never before. Progress in medicine came to be measured by the latest miracle drug and cutting-edge technology.

The "pill for an ill" philosophy shifted focus from the person to the disease and thus helped sever the mind-body connection that is the crux of holistic healing. Also, technological medicine made healthcare very complicated—and costly. Only trained physicians knew what was going on in this sophisticated, high-tech environment. The patient simply said, "Okay, doc," and swallowed the pill or underwent the treatment. Nevertheless, people had high hopes that Western medicine would lead to an unprecedented era of good health.

We're now well into the technological era, and things haven't gone exactly as planned. Western medicine *has* provided major breakthroughs in many areas, but technology and miracle drugs have done little to reduce the risk of major killers like cancer, heart disease, and stroke. People have discovered that potent drugs have potent side effects that can cause new health problems. The cost of high-tech medicine puts it out of reach of vast segments of the population with neither financial resources nor insurance. Those who do have insurance are often told where they can be treated, by whom, and for how long. There is talk of healthcare rationing where those who are too old, too young, or too sick may not be treated at all. These are disturbing problems, and most people feel powerless to move the entrenched bureaucracies that govern mainstream medical practice.

Couple this with the downside of our fast-paced modern existence. Labor-saving devices have allowed an appalling number of people in the industrialized world to become overweight, improperly fed, and inactive. Job insecurity, family tensions, and a host of other problems have vaulted stress to the top of the health-problems list. People are living longer, but are they living better?

Few dispute that modern medicine can do some things better than any other healing practice and some things the others can't do at all. But there is a growing belief that conventional medicine may not have the best answers for some of our most common problems. What about quality of life? Stress? Chronic pain? Yes, there are drugs that can lift your spirits, calm you down, and kill the pain, but people want to know: Isn't there something safer, more conservative? Fed up with the doctor-as-god concept, people everywhere are opting to find some of their own answers and to take responsibility for their own well-being. They're electing to become selective—and informed—healthcare consumers. Often this means investigating complementary therapies that may be outside the mainstream.

As people delve into Ayurveda or herbalism, they discover that millions have been using such therapies for thousands of years. (Would these methods still be around if they hadn't worked for people?) They find that most alternative treatments are gentle, safe (often much more so than drugs), and comparatively inexpensive. Natural treatments may take longer to work, but healing won't occur at the expense of unwanted side effects or dangerous complications.

People today want more than treatment for disease; they want to feel good in body *and* mind. They yearn for a return to holistic principles. Most alternative therapies fill this bill. Furthermore, alternative methods emphasize prevention—staying healthy—rather than cure. When a person does become ill, natural treatments bolster the body's ability to heal itself. Whereas conventional treatments typically override a body function that isn't working properly, alternative therapies try to restore the function.

Until fairly recently, a preponderance of the mainstream medical community viewed most alternative treatments with skepticism. (This despite the fact that, before the advent of synthetic drugs, their forebearers used many of these same treatments.) Now the pendulum is swinging the other way. Caught in the twin pincers of shrinking health-care dollars and mounting consumer demands, conventional physicians are reexamining alternative practices. Practices that promote wellness are gaining widespread acceptance, and most traditional doctors today accept the mind-body connection. There's also an acknowledgment that for common ailments, drugs are often a sledgehammer wielded to kill a gnat.

A study published in the *New England Journal of Medicine* in 1993 found that one in three U.S. adults had used some form of alternative therapy during 1990. In fact, as a group they made 87 million. *more* visits to alternative practitioners than to their primary-care physicians. However, 72 percent of those who visited alternative practitioners failed to mention the visits to their mainstream physicians, fearing they would disapprove. Now that physicians themselves are learning more about alternative treatments and integrating them into their practices, these barriers to communication may be crumbling. The outlook is hopeful that, in the future, alternative and orthodox treatments will be truly complementary.

HOW TO USE THE SELF-HEALTH HANDBOOK

All the therapies in *The Self-Health Handbook* are well-established. None is experimental, although some are practiced by millions throughout the world, while others have much smaller followings. Some have been used since the beginning of recorded history. Many are based on the healing traditions of indigenous peoples; others are derived from the results of modern-day research. We've provided a wide range of choices, all of which have two things in common: You can do them yourself, and they cost little or no money.

We don't expect that anyone will want to try *everything* in this book, and we make no claims that any specific therapy will work for you. There are no prescriptions here. Our goal is to provide the means for you to make informed choices and to give you an opportunity to try out various therapies to see what works. To find out what you'd like to try, you may want to read the book in its entirety—we hope you do—but that's not necessary. We've organized the book into nine broad categories to make it easier for you to find the therapies that might interest you. Each category is self-contained as is each therapy within the category.

The choice of categories and the therapies included within them is somewhat arbitrary. Yoga, for example, might have been placed in the "Mind as Healer" section or in "Exercising the Body." (It's in the latter.) There is no way to avoid this sort of overlap, especially when using a holistic approach, so if you don't find what you're looking for in one section, try another.

At the beginning of each category, there's a brief essay that gives an overview of the types of therapies included in that section. The therapies themselves are arranged alphabetically within the category. The discussion of all therapies throughout the book is structured the same way: **Definition** (what the therapy is); **Applications** (physical and/or psychological conditions for which the therapy can be used); **Collateral Cross Therapies** (other therapies in this book that might be used in conjunction with the therapy under discussion to enhance the beneficial effects); **Recommended Adjunct Activities and Behaviors** (activities that are not classified as therapies but that are nonetheless appropriate to do along with the therapy to heighten either the enjoyment or the effect); **Contraindications** (physical and/or psychological conditions that would prevent your using the particular therapy); **Equipment & Materials** (tools, clothing, materials, etc., that you will need to perform the therapy); **Origin & Background** (the history of the therapy); **Instructions** (how to perform the therapy); **Further Reading** (other books, magazines, audiotapes, and / or videotapes that provide more information about the therapy); and **Resource Groups** (professional or special interest groups related to the therapy that offer memberships, information, mail-order sources, referrals, and / or training or classes). Occasionally, one of these headings will be missing from a given therapy, indicating that the heading is not applicable for that particular therapy or that we have no information.

Before you decide which therapies to try, you should make a quick self-appraisal. Consider your age, general physical condition, specific health problems, current level of activity, likes and dislikes, time available, and any other relevant factors. Do you want to make wholesale lifestyle changes? Treat a specific physical condition? Solve some psychological problems? Have you got plenty of time to learn an exacting discipline or do you simply want some quick fixes? (Surprisingly, there are a lot of quick and easy techniques you can use to treat common, everyday problems like stress and headache.) Your answers to these questions will help you focus on the therapies that will work best for you.

Please read through the entire discussion of any therapy you're going to try before you begin. Pay particular attention to the listings under **Contraindications**. If you have one of the conditions listed, *don't try the therapy*. Because everyone is unique and we can't possibly anticipate all risks, we suggest checking with your healthcare practitioner to be sure any given therapy is safe for you. Another caveat: If you have a serious or life-threatening illness, do not rely on these therapies alone to treat your condition. Put yourself under the care of a licensed practitioner. By the same token, don't discontinue any treatments you're now taking without consulting your practitioner. When a particular therapy cites "cancer," "heart disease," or another major illness in the list of applications, it doesn't mean that the therapy will cure the disease. It simply means that the therapy has benefited some people with that disease in some way. It might be control of pain, relief of symptoms, or a calmer mind. These are important benefits, but they are not cures.

Because of space limitations, no book of this type can cover all topics in depth. We've anticipated that you'll want to learn more, and we're particularly proud of our **Further Readings** and **Resource Groups** listings. There we've given you the tools to really delve into any therapy that interests you. We list lots of books, where to find referrals to professional practitioners of the therapy, and much more. Plus we suggest audio- and videotapes that you can rent or buy to use as you practice the appropriate therapies.

Finally, once you've familiarized yourself with *The Self-Health Handbook* you'll want to keep it handy as a first-aid reference for common ailments that are not serious enough to warrant consulting a practitioner.

There are dozens of stress reducers, headache remedies, treatments for cuts and bruises, and helps for other everyday problems. Many use simple techniques or products you may already have on hand.

The pursuit of good health and well-being is a lifelong journey. The *Self-Health Handbook* offers many alternative routes, but you must choose the itinerary. Have a good trip!

FLOWERS, PLANTS, AND HERBS

Flowers and plants delight the eye with their beauty, the nose with their scent, and the palate with their flavor. Most people already like plants, so it's very agreeable to think that they have a place in maintaining and restoring health. The remedies in this section—aromatherapy, the Bach Flower Remedies, and herbalism—all have long and intriguing histories. They're fun to read about and they're delightful to use. With few exceptions, they have no unpleasant effects whether or not they work for you, so you can experiment to your heart's content.

These therapies have nothing in common with our conventional notions of taking care of our health. They're more like the kind of pampering one would get at a luxurious spa. Can treatments so pleasant really work? Millions of people worldwide think they do. Some of the remedies date back to the dawn of history, so one would think that people must be impossibly slow learners not to have discarded them by this time if they're ineffective. But judge for yourself. You'll discover some fascinating lore about flowers and plants, you'll have a good time doing it, and you may find at least a few remedies that work for you.

AROMATHERAPY

DEFINITION

Aromatherapy treats the body and mind using the essential oils of flowers, herbs, and plants. The oils may be inhaled (either directly or with steam), added to baths, used with massage, used as perfume, or taken internally as medicines. (Internal use is not covered here.)

APPLICATIONS

Physiological (topical application): Wounds and bruises, scars, inflammation, antibacterial uses, antiseptic uses, body odor, sensitive or dry skin, seborrhea, dry scalp and and hair, fatigued muscles, pain, aching (see chart for others)

Physiological (inhalation): Colds, poor memory, overweight, headache, premenstrual stress, menstrual cramps (see chart for others)

Psychological: Anxiety, insomnia, stress, depression, lethargy, sexual lassitude (see chart for others)

COLLATERAL CROSS-THERAPIES

Meditation, relaxation, music therapy, visualization

RECOMMENDED ADJUNCT ACTIVITIES AND BEHAVIORS

When using aromatherapy in conjunction with massage or a tub soak, you can enhance your enjoyment with other sensory experiences, such as candlelight or soft lighting, and music. (Be sure to keep the radio away from the tub. Aromatherapy doesn't cure electrocution.)

CONTRAINDICATIONS

As with all products applied to the skin, you should do a patch test to check for possible allergic reactions if you are going to apply the oils to your body. (To do the patch test, apply a little of the oil to your wrist or forearm and wait 24 hours. If a rash develops, do not use the oil.) Some individuals with allergies may also have reactions to inhalation.

EQUIPMENT & MATERIALS

You will need to purchase one or a variety of essential oils. For inhalation, you can use a container for natural evaporation (unglazed pottery is wonderful because it absorbs some of the oil and releases it over time), a cold steam vaporizer, or a device that diffuses aromas through heat. If you use steam inhalation, you'll need a towel to put over your head to keep the vapors from dissipating in the air.

ORIGIN & BACKGROUND

Nearly 3,000 years before the birth of Cleopatra, the ancient Egyptians used flowers, herbs, and other plants for their aromatic effects in embalming, medicines, religious celebrations, and cosmetics. That makes the origins of aromatherapy about 5,000 years old. Before long, Romans, Greeks, and other Mediterranean inhabitants began exploring the therapeutic properties of fragrant botanicals.

During their conquest of the then-civilized world, Roman soldiers carried lavender with them to use as a disinfectant. This practice later spread to Europe and continued into the Middle Ages. (Today we know how on-target these folks were. Lavender contains numerous biologically active compounds, some of which kill bacteria and viruses, including those that cause typhoid, diphtheria, strep throat, and staph infection.)

The Bible mentions healing with aromatics, and they were commonly used as medicines in the fifteenth century. During the Great Plague of the Middle Ages, fearful citizens built fires upon which they heaped fragrant resins to purify the air.

Although aromatherapy was known to the ancient world, distillation of the essential oils of plants was not. It wasn't until the tenth century that an extraordinary Arab philosopher and physician, Avicenna, developed the distillation process for extracting essential oils. Avicenna was a highly regarded authority who had become a physician at the age of seventeen. He wrote treatises on almost every scientific subject, and his works were published both in Europe and the Orient, so knowledge of his accomplishments spread throughout much of the world.

The Role of Lavender: Lavender plays a starring role in the history of aromatherapy. Victorian women scented their handkerchiefs with lavender oil, not only for its pleasing scent, but also to revive them when they felt faint—a common condition among young ladies attempting to achieve hour-glass figures with overtight corsets.

The man who is credited with coining the name *aromatherapy*, French chemist René Gattefossé, owed his interest in the subject to an experience he had with lavender oil. Gattefossé discovered its benefits quite literally by accident. When he burned his hand badly in the laboratory, Gattefossé instinctively thrust it into a nearby container of lavender oil to relieve the pain. The soothing oil did ease the pain, but Gattefossé later noted in some astonishment that the burn healed more quickly than he would have expected. Intrigued, Gattefossé began looking into the healing properties of lavender and other essential oils. When he wrote about his findings in the 1930s, he called his book *Aromatherapy*, and the name stuck.

Gattefossé's work revived interest in fragrant botanicals, which had flagged during the 1800s when scientists began to make synthetic compounds that mimicked the active ingredients in plants.

During World War II, French physician Jean Valnet took aromatherapy to the battlefield, treating war injuries with essential oils. His book, *The Practice of Aromatherapy*, was published in English in 1977.

Aromatherapy Today: Today aromatherapy is among the fastest-growing of the natural healing arts. In the United States, aromatherapy is still viewed skeptically by a high percentage of the traditional medical community. However, in Britain, an aromatherapist's client is called a patient, and he or she receives a blood test and a physical examination before treatment with essential oils begins. Germany and France go one step further. There, holistic spa visits—which may include aromatherapy treatments—are covered by health insurance. Although aromatherapy does not yet enjoy the same status in this country, acceptance is growing among traditional healthcare practitioners.

Although scientific studies of aromatherapy are sparse, researchers have proved that inhaled or topically applied essential oils do enter the body, either through the respiratory system or the bloodstream. Researchers have noted traces of the oils in the exhaled breaths of study subjects. Most members of the scientific community readily accept that some essential oils have a calming and relaxing effect; their dispute is with the claims that oils have therapeutic effects on specific diseases. Indeed, anyone who has a serious disease should certainly consult a health practitioner before trying aromatherapy to treat the problem; however, everyone can enjoy the restorative effects of essential oils in a relaxing bath or massage or get a mood lift from inhaling the aromatic vapors.

Aromatherapy and Other Healing Systems: Aromatherapy has similarities to components of many of the oriental healing systems, which often combine use of essential plant oils for massage or inhalation with diet, exercise, mental control, and breathing techniques. Aromatherapy also has ties to herbalism. However, herbalism uses plants in many forms, whereas in aromatherapy, only the essential oils are used.

INSTRUCTIONS

Technically, aromatherapy involves the use of inhaled, ingested, or externally applied essential oils for therapeutic or mood-altering purposes. However, due to their potency, no one should take essential oils internally without the advice of a health practitioner, so we have not included any internal applications in this book.

Aromatherapy is principally a self-help system. You can use it for enjoyment and relaxation without knowing very much about it, but if you learn more, you'll find that essential oils are extremely complex substances that can have various effects, especially when several are used in combination. Some are stimulants, while others promote relaxation. Still others regulate bodily functions, and some produce a euphoric effect.

Essential oils can be:

- used in conjunction with massage or a rubdown,
- inhaled either directly or with steam, or
- added to the bath.

Essential oils are highly concentrated. For example, it takes more than a ton of rose petals to produce a single pound of essential oil, so a few drops go a long way.

Massage: Because of the concentration, essential oils used for massage are always diluted with vegetable oil to avoid irritating the skin. Essential oil-containing massage oils are available commercially, but you can make your own by adding approximately twenty drops of essential oil to each ounce of vegetable oil. Peach kernel, almond, grapeseed, or sunflower oil make good carriers. You can also buy unscented massage oil and add the therapeutic essential oil to that.

Essential oils massaged into the skin may aid in cell regeneration and healing. For maximum effectiveness:

- Use firm strokes to warm the skin and help the oils penetrate.
- Perform the massage for at least ten minutes and for as long as an hour if you like.

Massage by itself improves blood circulation and stimulates the lymphatic system to remove toxins and lactic acid that have built up in the muscles. When you add essential oils, you may find other benefits, depending upon the oil you choose.

Try a peppermint foot massage to perk up your feet after a hard day's work or a long walk. Massage each toe, move to the ball of the foot, then the instep, the heel, and finally the ankle. Then massage the whole foot with long, firm strokes. Feel the tingle.

Inhalation: Some people put essential oils in unglazed pots or boil them in water on the stovetop. These methods will diffuse your house with lovely scents, but they probably will not have major therapeutic benefits because of the low concentration of vapors. To get maximum benefit from inhalation:

- Fill a bowl (or your bathroom sink) with boiling water.
- Add a few drops of essential oil.
- Put a towel over your head and inhale the vapors for five minutes.

(*Don't* try this with the boiling-water, top-of-the-stove method. You're likely to be burned, scalded, or set yourself on fire.)

For a nighttime treat, give your face a peppermint facial (using the above inhalation method) followed by a massage with wheatgerm oil (lots of vitamin B) to which you have added a few drops of lavender and rose massage oils, not the full-strength essences. Unless you fancy the hound-dog look, always massage your face upward and outward.

You can also put some oil on a tissue, press it to your nose, and inhale deeply. Or you can use a commercially available cold- or hot-steam vaporizer. Health-food stores and herbal shops sell special appliances made for aromatherapy diffusion.

Baths: A warm aromatic bath after a long day is sheer bliss to most of us. To relieve stress, soak in a warm tub to which you've added lavender, marjoram, orange blossom, sandalwood, or chamomile oil. If your spirits need a lift, choose the oil of clary sage, rose, grapefruit, jasmine, ylang-ylang, or bergamot. Ylang-ylang is an antiseborrheic (it relieves oily secretions), so it's particularly helpful if you have problems with oily skin. Use rosemary oil for dry skin and chamomile oil for sensitive skin.

You can, of course, combine oils. Experiment until you find the prescription that's personalized just for you (or consult an aromatherapist). A couple caveats: Don't soak too long and don't make the water too hot. Fifteen minutes is long enough for the bath to work its wonders. Water temperature should be around 100° F or slightly warmer. Hotter water is a shock to the system and will cause the muscles to contract, not relax.

The chart below lists some essential oils, their purported benefits, and the usual methods of application. Remember to consult a health practitioner if you want to use an oil to treat a serious condition. Aromatherapy treatments won't hurt you (unless you're one of the few with allergic reactions), but you may need other types of treatment as well.

This list is by no means all-inclusive. If you want to know more about aromatherapy, consult a professional aromatherapist or one of the organizations listed under *Resource Groups*. Check your local bookstore or healthfood store for books on aromatheraphy.

ESSENTIAL OIL	PROBLEMS TREATED	METHOD OF USE
Arnica	Bruises; wounds; swellings	Bath
Bergamot	Anxiety; depression; eczema; skin rashes	Bath; inhalation; massage
Chamomile	Anger; stress; mentrual problems; menopausal symptoms	Bath; inhalation; massage
Cistus	Insomnia	Bath; inhalation; massage
Clary Sage	Depression; menstrual cramps; PMS	Bath; inhalaton; massage
Cypress	Fatigue; lethargy	Bath; massage
Eucalyptus	Arthritis; colds; flu; infections; muscular pain; bronchitis	Inhalation; massage
Frankincense	Nightmares; fears; rheumatoid arthritis	Bath; inhalation; massage
Geranium	Fatigue; lethargy; stomach ulcers; diarrhea; moodiness	Bath; massage

Grapefruit	Depression; unexpressed anger	Bath; inhalation; massage
Jasmine	Depression; sexual impotence/frigidity; low self-esteem	Bath; inhalation; massage
Lavender	Burns; anxiety; insomnia; eczema; insect bites; dermatitis; stress; scars	Bath; inhalation; massage
Lemon	Fatigue; lethargy	Bath; massage
Lemon Balm	Aches and pains; fatigue	Massage
Marjoram	Stress; tension; insomnia	Bath; inhalation; massage
Neroli	Insomnia	Bath; massage
Orange Blossom	Stress; anxiety; premature aging; insomnia	Bath; massage; inhalation
Peppermint (or Spearmint)	Muscle and joint fatigue and pain; mental fatigue; lethargy; low concentration	Bath; inhalation; massage
Rose	Anxiety; stress; depression	Bath; inhalation; massage
Rosemary	Arthritus; muscle pain; poor memory; mental fatigue; headache; PMS; dry skin	Bath; inhalation; massage
Sage	Fatigue; lethargy	Bath; inhalation; massage
Sandalwood	Fear; stress; low self-esteem; sexual inertia	Bath; inhalation; massage
Tangerine	Insomnia	Bath; inhalation; massage
Ylang-ylang	Anger; depression; sexual lethargy; hypertension	Bath; inhalation; massage

Many essential oils have antibacterial; antifungal; antiseptic, and cleansing properties. Arnica, for example, is an antibacterial agent. Lavender has antiseptic properties. Chamomile's excellent cleansing and conditioning properties make it a desirable hair-care ingredient. Eucalyptus oil is a deodorant, an antiseptic, and an antibacterial agent. Look for these oils in cosmetics, shampoos, and soaps made by companies such as Aveda and The Body Shop. Many mainstream skin-care and cosmetic companies now also include essential oils in their products.
Essential Oils as Perfume: The majority of essential oils can also be used as perfumes. If you like the scent, wear it and reap the extra benefit

of giving yourself a spirit lift or a mood change. Or do as the Victorians did and sniff a lavender-scented handkerchief during that next brutal staff meeting. People will wonder why you're so calm.

FURTHER READING

Lewis, Angelo John. "The Art of Aromatherapy: Healing with Essential Oils," *East/West*, October 1988.

National Association for Holistic Aromatherapy. *Aromatherapy and Essential Oils*. Boulder, Colo.

Pounds, Laraine. "Holistic Aromatherapy," *Beginnings*, March 1992.

Tisserand, Robert B. *The Art of Aromatherapy*. Rochester, Vt.: Destiny Books, 1977.

Valnet, Jean. *The Practice of Aromatherapy*. Saffron Walden, Essex, England: C.W. Daniel, 1977.

RESOURCE GROUPS

American Society for Phytotherapy & Aromatherapy International
PO Box 3679
South Pasadena, CA 91031
Phone: 818/457-1742

Aromatherapy Institute of Research
PO Box 2354
Fair Oaks, CA 95628
Phone: 916/965-7546

Flower Essence Society
PO Box 459
Nevada City, CA 95959
Phone: 916/265-9163 or 800/548-0075

National Association for Holistic Aromatherapy
PO Box 17622
Boulder, CO 80308-7622
Phone: 303/444-0533

Pacific Institute of Aromatherapy
PO Box 606

San Raphael, CA 94915
Phone: 415/459-3998

BACH FLOWER REMEDIES

DEFINITION

The Bach Flower Remedies consist of thirty-eight different flower-based formulas for the treatment of various emotional problems. Each remedy contains the diluted essence of a particular flower that has been distilled and then preserved in unflavored brandy. The remedies are purported to cure such things as fear, vicious temper, resentment, shyness, and loneliness.

APPLICATIONS

Physiological: None directly
Psychological: There are one or more remedies for a wide variety of psychology problems. See the chart later on in this section for specific problems and their remedies.

COLLATERAL CROSS-THERAPIES

Affirmations, meditations, self-hypnosis, yoga, zen, chakra balancing, jin shin jyutsu

RECOMMENDED ADJUNCT ACTIVITIES AND BEHAVIORS

If you're interested, you can learn how to coordinate the Bach Flower Remedies with your astrological chart. The *Flower Remedies Handbook* by Donna Cunningham, which is listed in the *Further Reading* section, tells you how to do this.

CONTRAINDICATIONS

Those who entirely avoid alcohol should be aware that the essences are preserved in a 27-percent alcohol base. (However, the remedies can be diluted to the point where the alcohol content is minuscule, and there are companies that make alcohol-free remedies similar to Bach's.) Some people with allergies could have reactions. People who are addicted to drugs or alcohol or those who are taking potent tranquilizers sometimes don't do well on the remedies, and people who are totally resistant to change will probably find that the remedies do little or nothing for them.

EQUIPMENT & MATERIALS

Remedies come in "stock" bottles and/or "dosage" bottles. In most cases, remedies can be taken directly from the stock bottle (which contains the full-strength essence), but if you want to make your own dosage bottles (containing more diluted essences), you will need one-ounce dropper bottles, which are available from most pharmacies or through Ellon USA Inc. (See address in *Resource Groups*.)

ORIGIN & BACKGROUND

Flowers have been important to people throughout history. Although they have always been admired for their beauty, in many cultures both ancient and modern, flowers have also had symbolic meaning. We still say, "He extended the olive branch," when we mean that someone tried to patch up a quarrel. That cliche dates from ancient Greece, where the olive branch was a symbol of peace. The forget-me-not is so called because long ago people gave the dainty blue flowers to others as a token of enduring friendship.

Another symbol of remembrance, rosemary, figures prominently in Christian tradition. Brides wove it into their bouquets to signify fidelity, and when a person died, mourners placed rosemary sprigs in the grave as pledges that the deceased would not be forgotten.

The Language of Flowers: During the Middle Ages, the "language of flowers" enjoyed quite a vogue among the nobility. Brought to Europe from the Orient, the custom derived from the notion that each flower conveyed a different personal message. A mixed bouquet was a real challenge, as many a young lady discovered when she attempted to decipher the true meaning of her lover's gift. In France, the language of flowers was such a rage that suitors often sent their ladies bouquet after bouquet, each with a different message.

Clearly in earlier times people had a much more symbiotic relationship with plants than most of us do today. One rather bizarre tradition held that favorite plants had to be told of the death of a family member. Survivors festooned the plant with black crepe as a mark of respect in the hope that the plant would not fade and die of grief.

Throughout recorded history, people have used flowers for magical, medicinal, and religious purposes. The lotus figures prominently in several oriental religious and healing practices, among them yoga. In Incan Peru, the sunflower symbolized their sun god, and priestesses adorned themselves with hammered-gold blossoms worth a king's ransom.

Healing Power of Flower: With flowers playing such important roles in people's lives, it is little wonder that people believed strongly in their healing powers. Centuries ago, the aboriginal peoples of Australia used a form of flower remedies as did the Indians and the Chinese. In the 1500s, the controversial Swiss physician and alchemist, Paracelsus, experimented with the properties of the dew on flowers. Because it bloomed in winter, Paracelsus felt that the Christmas rose could be used to restore health to people in the "winter" of their lives, and he prescribed it for elderly patients to extend longevity. Modern scientists have now discovered that *Hellebores niger*—the Christmas rose—contains compounds useful in treating atherosclerosis, a major killer of older people. Flower remedies as we know them today are a modern development, however.

Dr. Bach's Discoveries: In the early 1930s, Dr. Edward Bach, a highly regarded British physician, noticed that many of his patients displayed psychological and emotional symptoms such as fear, depression, boredom, and worry before they developed physical illness. He also observed that patients with these problems were less able to resist disease or to recover from it. Bach left his lucrative Harley Street practice and moved to the English countryside, where he began studying the relationship between disease and state of mind. (Today we know that there are close ties, but this was a rather revolutionary concept in Bach's day.)

Traditional medicine focussed on treating specific physical symptoms, but Bach became convinced that disease could be warded off and better cured by addressing underlying emotional causes. Bach wanted to avoid the harsh effects of chemical drugs and their side effects, so he turned to nature for a safer, gentler healing method.

Bach's search led him to wildflowers and plants, and here he made an interesting observation. He noted that when he drank the dew from flowers that had been in the sun, each flower gave him a different emotional feeling. He began treating patients with flower essences and noting their responses. Over the next few years, Bach conducted many trial-and-error experiments and eventually developed the thirty-eight treatments (and a "Rescue Remedy") that are now known as the Bach Flower Essences. (The number is thirty-eight because Bach felt that there were thirty-eight principal negative states of mind from which people suffer.)

After his death, the Bach Centre in England carried on his work, investigating and documenting case histories, so that by now, the remedies have been studied for over sixty years. In England and continental Europe, the remedies are well known and widely accepted. They are not as popular in the U.S. yet, but their use is growing.

Studies of the Bach Remedies: The Bach remedies have been studied by others besides the Bach Centre, but most have not been double-blind studies. (In plain English, double-blind means that subjects take either a remedy or a placebo [harmless substitute], but they don't know which they're taking and neither does the researcher. This precaution ensures a fair and unbiased test result.) However, one such study by Michael Weisglas was reported in *The Flower Essence Journal*.[1] Weisglas gave three groups of students a psychological test to determine their emotional states. He then gave one group a placebo. Another group received four remedies mixed together, and the third a seven-remedy mix. After taking the preparations for several weeks, the groups took the psychological test again. The group taking the placebo experienced no changes, while the group receiving four remedies had very positive changes. Apparently, seven remedies were too many. People in this group had fewer positive changes, and several dropped out of the study.

Other evidence, much of it documented, confirms that a person's emotional state is closely related to the physical state of the body. Many mainstream medical studies now show that a person with a healthy emotional state has a better chance of fighting off disease than one whose emotional outlook is poor.

Bach Remedies Differ from Other Natural Treatments: The Bach Flower Remedies do *not* treat specific physical illnesses, but users say a person's physical condition often improves as emotional and psychological problems are stripped away. Neither are the remedies traditional homeopathic treatments, although the difference is subtle. One difference is the degree of dilution. Homeopathic remedies are many times more diluted than the Bach Flower Essences.

Flower remedies also differ from herbalism. For example, you might relax with a cup of chamomile tea (an herbal remedy) after a stressful day, but you would take the flower remedy Chamomile over time to relieve the emotional problems that produced the stress in the first place.

INSTRUCTIONS

Theoretically, the Bach Flower Remedies work on energy frequencies. Flowers are picked at dawn when they are most vital and then put in water in sunlight for several hours to transfer the energy from the flower to the water and intensify the essence. The liquid is enhanced, diluted, and strengthened. After the essences are distilled, they are preserved in unflavored brandy to prevent spoilage.

Using the Remedies: If you want to use the remedies, you should first determine which ones are appropriate. A complete list of the remedies and the emotional states that they address is available wherever the remedies are sold, or you can order it from Ellon USA Inc. (The address is listed in the **Resource Groups** section.)

The Ellon™ Bach remedies are sold in stock (concentrate) bottles. For immediate relief of a stressful situation or passing negative mood, people usually place a few drops from the concentrate bottle under the

---

[1] *The Flower Essence Journal*: 1(1): pp 11–14, 1980.

tongue or mix a few drops in a quarter glass of water or juice and sip it until the feeling passes.

For long-term use, prepare a "dosage" solution:

- Put two to four drops of concentrated oil from a stock bottle into a one-ounce dropper bottle.
- Add a teaspoon of brandy or apple cider vinegar as a preservative.
- Fill with filtered or spring water (not carbonated or distilled water).

Take four to six drops at a time, four times a day. Take it when you get up, between meals during the day, and at bedtime. (It is safe to use as often as every ten or fifteen minutes if it is really necessary.)

If you are alcohol-sensitive, you can further dilute the dosage in hot water. Want to avoid internal use altogether? You can apply the concentrate directly to your temples, wrists, behind your ears, or under your arms.

Combining Remedies: You can mix several remedies in one dosage bottle, but to maximize effectiveness, limit the number to six. Fewer is better. Resist the temptation to try a lot of remedies at the same time to "get well" immediately. Instead make a priority list and start with no more than the first six issues. As problems resolve and you stop taking one remedy, you can add another on the list.

How quickly will it work? Because the remedies have unique and personal effects upon each person using them, there are no certainties as to how long you will need to take a specific remedy or even exactly what effect it will have on you. Experts say most people can solve the problem they're treating within one to three weeks, but it may take several months. (The remedies are neither toxic nor addictive, so you can take them for as long as you need to.)

If the remedy is working, you should notice some effects within a few weeks, but don't expect instant changes. Unlike many chemical drugs that often deliver an instant wallop, the flower remedies are subtle. You may not even be aware that positive changes are occurring until you view your situation in retrospect.

Many people keep a journal to record their changing emotions as they use the remedies over time. As you read back through your journal, you may discover that you've changed more than you realized. (See Journaling in Healing "Arts.")

When to Reassess: When changes don't come after a reasonable period, it's time to reassess. You may (subconsciously) be stubbornly clinging to old feelings or you may be taking an inappropriate remedy. Ellon USA offers free Self-Help Questionnaires that can help you resolve the issue. If the remedy is right, you may just need more time. If it's the wrong one, you can switch to one that works better. (Of course, it's possible that the remedies just aren't the right type of therapy for you.)

Peeling Effect: Often, people experience what is known as the "peeling" effect. The peeling effect occurs when a person gets rid of one emotional problem only to discover that there is another previously undiscovered problem underlying it. In that case, a different remedy is usually in order to address the new situation.

Flower remedies aim to restore balance to the system; therefore, they're self-adjusting. Once the remedy starts working, the idea is to take less and less of it until finally you stop taking it altogether. There is no benefit to continuing the remedy once the problem has been solved.

Side-Effects: Usually there are no unpleasant side effects with Flower Remedies. Rarely, a person may experience a minor rash, mild diarrhea, or an accentuation of the emotion under treatment. These reactions can be part of the process of confronting feelings, or they may be associated with resistance to change. The remedies are nontoxic, but if you experience a reaction, you may want to discontinue the remedy in question. If the symptoms persist, consult a healthcare practitioner. Your symptoms could be coincidental to the taking of the remedy, and you may need treatment for another condition.

You may use other self-help healing techniques like transcendental meditation and affirmations to help speed up the process of changing undesirable negative feelings. The remedies are not incompatible with other healthcare practices, traditional or otherwise, so if you need to see a healthcare practitioner for a specific disease, by all means do so. If you're already working on self-improvement through a therapist or support group, you may find that the remedies enhance your ability to work through problems and clear out unwanted emotional baggage.

Choosing the Right Remedies: How do you choose which remedies to use? Admittedly, this can be difficult, since there is often more than one remedy for a particular problem. You can, of course, consult a professional practitioner. A knowledgeable person at the store where you purchase the remedies might also be helpful, and you can send for the Self-Help Questionnaire. You can try visualization or meditation to see which remedies seem right. There are also a number of helpful books (see *Further Reading*). If all else fails, experiment. The remedies won't hurt you; the worst they can do is fail to help.

Who Should Use the Remedies?   The Bach remedies can be used by people of any age, including children. Parents report that the remedies work well for temper tantrums, sibling rivalries, fussiness, and shyness in children. Teens respond well to remedies that develop coping mechanisms during personal crises.

Gardeners report that ten to fifteen drops of the right remedy added to a small watering can or plant mister can revitalize drooping houseplants or

those shocked by the effects of transplanting. Ellon USA has free literature on using the remedies with plants and pets too.

Below is a partial list of the remedies and the conditions they're designed
to treat.

BACH REMEDY	INITIAL NEGATIVE EMOTIONS	POSITIVE REPLACEMENTS
Agrimony	Cheereful on the outside; tortured on the inside. Good for those who abuse substances to cover pain.	Exhibits true feelings; genuine cheerfulness; sense of optimism; humor
Aspen	Unknown fears; apprehension; foreboding	Fearlessness; ability to face events
Beech	Arrogance; intolerance; judgmental of self/others; hypercriticism	Tolerance; acceptance
Centaury	Submissiveness; tendency to be taken advantage of; inability to say no; exaggerated desire to please	Self-determination; individuality; ability to set limits
Cherry Plum	Fear of losing control, going crazy, or hurting one-self or others; outburst of rage; self-destructive habits	Ability to control oneself even under pressure
Chicory	Selfishness; possessiveness; desire for even negative attention	Concern for others
Clematis	Escapism; inattention; indifference	Renewed interest in real events/feelings
Crab Apple	Shame; self-disgust; unclean feeling (body or mind)	Broadmindedness; self-acceptance
Elm	Temporary inability to cope with responsibilities	Self-confidence, assurance; ability to cope
Gentian	Discouragement; dejection; pessimism	Perseverance despite setbacks; optimism
Gorse	Despair; pessimism; hopelessness; negativity	Positivity; hope; belief that difficulties can be overcome
Heather	Self-centeredness; overtalkativeness; inability to listen; dread of being alone	Ability to share conversation; selflessness; helpfulness

Holly	Envy; jealousy; self-hatred; hatred of others; spite; resentment; suspicion	Affection; tolerance; generosity
Honeysuckle	Inability to let go of the past; homesickness; wish to live life over	Ability to appreciate and learn from the past but not live in it.
Hornbeam	Fatigue and tiredness often due to boredom or procrastination	Renewed mental energy; ability to tackle problems and self-start
Impatiens	Impatience with others' slowness; hastiness	Tolerance; understanding
Larch	Feelings of inferiority; fear of failure; unwillingness to try	Faith in own ability; perseverance
Mimulus	Specific fears, e.g., of the dark, water, heights	Ability to face the particular fear
Mustard	Melancholia; deep gloom for no apparent reason	Inner serenity; stability; joy
Oak	Workaholism and neglect of self and family	Renewed hope, courage, ability to fight problems
Pine	Guilt; self-reproach; tendency to blame oneself for the mistakes of others	Appropriate sense of responsibility; refusal to dwell on past mistakes
Red Chestnut	Exaggerated fear that something will befall others	Rational concern for others
Rescue Remedy*	Physical or emotional crisis	This is a mixture of remedies designed for immediate help in a crisis
Rock Rose	Panic attacks; terrifying situations	Calmness; ability to face situation coolly
Scleranthus	Indecision; uncertainty; inability to make choices; shifting moods	Balance; poise; ability to make choices and take action; determination
Star of Bethlehem	Shock; trauma; significant sorrow; reaction to terrifying experience; emotional numbness	Release of tensions and residual trauma

Sweet Chestnut	Anguish; desolation; feeling that problems are beyond endurance (*not* suicidal feeling)	Faith; belief that dark times will pass
Vervain	Fanaticism; outrage at injustice	Self-control; open-mindedness; calmness
Vine	Dominance; overambition; desire for power	Enlightened leadership; understanding
Wild Rose	Apathy; passivity; chronic boredom; belief that circumstances can't be changed; "nothing matters"	Vitality; renewed interest in all things
Willow	Bitterness; brooding; tendency to collect injustices	Optimism

* The Ellon USA equivalent is called Calming Essence.

Other Flower Remedies: Bach is the acknowledged father of emotional therapy using flower essences, and his remedies are certainly the best known and most widely distributed. However, today there are a number of companies around the world that make high-quality flower essences. Bach developed his Flower Remedies during a time of worldwide economic depression, and many of his remedies are keyed to problems like despair and loss of hope, which were major concerns of the day. Some of the newer companies make essences that address these traditional problems and more contemporary ones as well.

Probably the best known of the recent introductions is the line developed by Flower Essence Services (FES) of California, which is based on North American plant species. The FES essences include Quince to foster the positive power of love, Basil to resolve conflicts between spirituality and sexuality, and Bleeding Heart for releasing painful emotional attachments.

Another U.S. company that uses essences made from native plants is the Alaskan Flower Essence Project. Their remedies include Sticky Geranium for removing blocks that prevent further growth, Sitka Burnet to help reach closure over past issues, and Shooting Star for alienation.

Combination Remedies: If you are inexperienced with flower remedies, you might want to look into the combination remedies that are available from many companies. The combination formulas take the guesswork out of determining which individual remedies work well together. One company that sells both individual essences and combinations is Running Fox Farm. A few of their combinations are Creative Flow, Pre-Trauma (to prepare for upcoming stresses), Motivation, and Relaxation. Running Fox Farm also has boxed kits of essences for situations like childbirth and trauma, and you can special-order the company's essences in a vinegar base if you want to avoid all alcohol.

These are but a few of the companies that make flower essences. Your health-food store or herbal shop will undoubtedly carry many others. Mention in this book is not an endorsement of any product or company. Except for the Bach Remedies, we chose the ones we did randomly from among the long list of reputable companies that make high-quality essences.

FURTHER READING

Bach, Edward, M.D., and F.J. Wheeler, M.D., *The Bach Flower Remedies*. New Canaan, Conn.: Keats, 1979.

Barnard, Julian, and Martine Barnard. *The Healing Herbs of Edward Bach: an Illustrated Guide to the Flower Remedies*. Hereford, England: The Bach Educational Programme, 1988.

Chancellor, Philip M. (ed.). *Illustrated Handbook of the Bach Flower Remedies*. Saffron Walden, Essex, England: C.W. Daniel, 1971.

Cunningham, Donna. *Flower Remedies Handbook*. New York: Sterling Publishing Co., Inc., 1992.

Ewart, Neil. *The Lore of Flowers*. Dorset, England: Blandford Press, 1982.

Flower Essence Society. *The Flower Essence Repertory*. Nevada City, Calif.: The Flower Essence Society, 1987.

Hyne Jones, T.W. *Dictionary of the Bach Flower Remedies: Positive and Negative Aspects*. Saffron Walden, Essex, England: C.W. Daniel, 1976.

Pickles, Sheila, ed. *The Language of Flowers*. New York: Harmony House, 1990.

Rotella, Alexis. *The Essence of Flowers: New Age Wisdom*. Mountain Lakes, N.J.: Jade Mountain Press, 1990.

Vlamis, Gregory. *Flowers to the Rescue: The Healing Vision of Dr. Edward Bach*. Rochester, Vt.: Healing Arts Press, 1988.

Weeks, Nora. *The Medical Discoveries of Edward Bach*. New Canaan, Conn.: Keats Publishing, 1979.

Wright, Machaelle Small. *Flower Essences*. Warrenton, Va.: Perelandra Ltd., 1988.

RESOURCE GROUPS

Alaskan Flower Essence Project
PO Box 1369
Homer, AK 99603-1369
Phone: 907/235-2188

Information and catalog

Bach Flower Remedies Ltd.
The Bach Centre
Mt. Vernon
Sotwell Wallingford, Oxon OX10 0PZ, U.K.

The manufacturer accepts mail orders (but you should be able to buy either single bottles or complete kits from your local health-food store or herbalist)

Ellon USA Inc.
644 Merrick Rd.
Lynbrook, NY 11563
    For literature: Department IN-02
PO Box 320
Woodmere, NY 11598
Phone: 800 4BE-CALM; 516/593-2206

Mail orders; free literature on how others use flower remedies and how to use remedies for animals and plants; free Self-Help Questionnaire.

Flower Essence Services (FES)
Box 176
Nevada City, CA 95959
Phone: 916/265-0258

Illustrated brochure describes essences; catalog includes flower remedies, aromatic oils, books, and flower photographs

Flower Essence Society, The (same address as for FES, above)
Phone: 916/265-9163
Publishes *The Flower Essence Journal*

Running Fox Farm
PO Box 381
Worthington, MA 01098-0381
Phone: 413/238-429; Fax: 413/238-5575

Individual essences, combinations and kits; vinegar-based (no alcohol) essences available by special order

HERBALISM
(BOTANICAL MEDICINE, HERBAL MEDICINE)

DEFINITION

Herbalism is the practice of using some part of a flower, plant, shrub, or tree for therapeutic benefit to the body and/or mind.

APPLICATIONS

Physiological: Colds, immune-system deficiencies, indigestion, headache, fever, and many others (See *Instructions* and the chart for other applications.)

Psychological: Stress, tension, and others. (See the chart for other applications.)

COLLATERAL CROSS-THERAPIES

None specifically, but herbalism is compatible with other therapies of all types. Herbalism and gardening are an obvious combination. Even if you have no outdoor garden space, you can grow pots of herbs on a sunny windowsill.

RECOMMENDED ADJUNCT ACTIVITIES AND BEHAVIORS

If you find yourself frequently needing remedies for stress and headache, you may want to take a close look at your life to see if you can make some changes to get rid of underlying tensions.

CONTRAINDICATIONS

When properly used, herbal remedies are safe for nearly everyone. However, some people with allergies could have reactions. Herbal preparations contain active ingredients, and no one should use unfamiliar herbs without knowing the expected effects, the proper dosage, and the correct method of preparation (including which part of the plant to use).

EQUIPMENT & MATERIALS

The usual kitchen equipment will do fine for preparing herbal concoctions. A tea ball and a mortar and pestle are quite handy, but you can improvise if you don't have them.

ORIGIN & BACKGROUND

When humans first began to try to cure what ailed them, they used herbs. Herbalism predates any other form of medical practice by thousands of years. Prehistoric peoples depended upon their surroundings—and the plant and animal life within—for all their necessities, including healing. Early humans attributed catastrophic events to supernatural powers because they had no other way to explain them. A person who fell ill had obviously angered some temperamental god out there, and the tribal healer needed a magic potion to effect a cure. The shamans of the day thought that herbs possessed magical properties, so they used them as part of their healing rituals.

Early healers were the first research scientists, and their laboratory was the whole natural world. They were remarkably intuitive in their ability to find plants that worked "magic" for various diseases, but a great deal of what they learned came through trial and error. In the beginning, of course, the only available herbs were those that were native to the area.

At least 5,000 years ago, Egypt, India, and China had well-developed systems of medicine that relied, in large measure, on medicinal herbs. As healers experimented with various plants, they recorded what they learned in books called *herbals*. One Chinese herbal from that period lists herbs that are still used today, among them aconite, poppy, and rhubarb. Much of what we know about herbs comes from those ancient volumes, and even today we turn to them to determine which plants can properly be called herbs. Ancient records from Babylon, Sumeria, and Crete also describe herbal cures for various diseases.

Herbalism in Egypt: The earliest physician mentioned by name in ancient records was an Egyptian named Sekhet'enanch, who lived around 3,000 B.C. He apparently cured the king of a "disease of the nostrils" and thus earned a place in history. A few hundred years later, another physician—Imhotep—was worshipped as a virtual demigod by the Egyptians.

By 2,000 B.C., there were at least 2,000 Egyptian physicians versed in herbal medicine. The Ebers Papyrus, a sort of medical encyclopedia of the period, lists remedies for many diseases, including arthritis, conjunctivitis, and tumor. The papyrus reveals that early Egyptians knew and used nearly one third of the medicinal plants known today. This is amazing, considering the limits of the ancient world. One remedy of the time was the poppy, which was used to soothe crying infants; another was castor oil, which was used then as now as a laxative. To prevent disease, Egyptians consumed vast quantities of onions, garlic, and radish. They also used herbs as antibiotics and antiseptics. Recently scientists have discovered that the Mediterranean sea onion, which was used by Egyptians for heart problems, is an extremely potent cardiac stimulant.

Traders introduced many medicinal herbs to Egypt. From Crete they got henna, saffron, and sage. Travelers brought myrrh, olibanum, and sandalwood from other parts of Africa, and those who ventured as far as China brought back cinnamon, ginger, and pomegranates.

Herbalism in China: The tradition of herbal medicine is as ancient in China as it is in Egypt. The emperor Shen-nung is said to have written one of the earliest Chinese herbals, the *Pen-ts'ao*. Legend has it that Shen-nung had a transparent abdomen, a handy feature for observing the effects of the hundreds of herbal concoctions he prepared and swallowed.

Huang-ti, who succeeded Shen-nung as emperor, wrote one of the most famous of all medical texts: the *Nei-Ching*, also called *The Yellow Emperor's Classic of Internal Medicine*. The book was really a review of the state of medicine in China, but it included information on the use of herbs.

Around 2000 B.C., Chinese physicians etched "oracle bones" with the names of plants and the diseases they treated. Ginseng—probably the most widely used medicinal herb in the world—was first mentioned in a Chinese herbal dating from around 2800 B.C. The Taoists later contributed the concept that disease could be prevented by moderation in all things, and the Chinese began to use a combination of acupuncture, herbs, massage, diet, and gentle exercises to correct the body's imbalances. These practices still form the basis of Chinese medicine today.

Herbalism in India: Most of our knowledge of early Indian medicine comes from the *Vedas*, the ancient scriptures of the Hindus. The *Vedas* are purported to date back to 10,000 B.C., but no records remain from that period. We know that by 1000 B.C., the Indians had a highly developed medical system. An Indian medical text, the *Charaka Samhita,* was passed on orally for many generations before it was finally written down in the first century A.D. In it is a list of 500 herbal medications. Another Indian text, the *Rigveda*, records twice that many medicinal plants along with a list of the physicians who knew their secrets.

Ancient Greek Healing Practices: The Egyptians strongly influenced Greek healing practices. The Greeks developed two types of medicine: temple medicine and rational medicine. All over Greece there were temples dedicated to various gods. The sick went to temples dedicated to Asklepios, the god of medicine. Temple healing was a bit like going to a modern-day spa with a few barbaric touches thrown in. The temple itself was usually set on a hillside and surrounded by lush gardens and sacred trees. In this restful environment, the ailing received special diets, herbs, and massage. Treatment also included sacrifice and prayers to Asklepios to intervene and make the person well. Customarily, the patient would sleep before the altar of the god and receive, in a dream, the knowledge necessary to recover health.

After a while, the temple priests noticed that some types of illnesses were likely to be cured by this regimen, while others were not. They began turning away people with diseases likely to have poor outcomes, their cure rate soared, and the fame of temple medicine spread far and wide.

Hippocrates: Many people who were turned away were too sick to go home, so they were cared for nearby by lay people trained in medicine called Asclepidæ. Hippocrates, who was one of the Asclepidæ, became the great spokesperson of rational medicine. He and his followers believed that everything in nature had a rational basis, and therefore, the physician's role was to look for the causes of disease in natural law, not in superstition or supernatural intervention. Hippocrates' views laid the foundation for modern medicine.

Hippocrates recognized the healing power of nature itself, and he used many herbs in his treatments, including mint, verbena, and mugwort. His influence was so widespread that it affected the course of western medicine down to the present time, and his admonition to physicians, "You shall first do no harm," is an oath still taken by doctors today.

Other Greeks who contributed to the advancement of herbalism were Aristotle, who is said to have had a garden of more than 300 medicinal herbs, Galen, and Theophrastus.

Roman Contributions to Herbalism: The Romans soon picked up a knowledge of herbs from the Greeks, and references to their use appeared in the works of Pliny the Elder, Vergil, and Homer. Dioscorides, a Greek physician who traveled with the Roman army, wrote a very extensive herbal catalog called *De Materia Medica* around the time of Christ's birth.

As the Roman Empire spread, so did the lore of herbs. The conquerors planted many herbs on foreign soil that were later used by the native people. By the same token, Roman legions returned home with new healing plants to add to their pharmacopeia.

Christianity and Herbalism: We know from the many references to herbs in the Bible that early Christians knew and used herbs for medicinal purposes. Medieval European medicine was dominated by the Catholic Church, so it is not surprising that any root shaped like a cross was thought to have curative powers.

In the Dark Ages, it was the monks in Christian monasteries who kept herbal healing traditions alive, both in writing and in experimentation. Oddly, although they often illustrated their works, the drawings rarely bore any resemblance to the actual plants described.

During the Renaissance, formal herb gardens became very popular for their ornamental value. In the fifteenth century, the first true-to-life botanical illustrations of herbs appeared, and about a hundred years later, an Englishman named John Gerard published an herbal that is still used today, *Gerard's Herball*.

The "Signatures" of Herbs: Some time later Nicholas Culpeper wrote a treatise that connected herbs with their "signatures" and also with astrology. According to the theory of the signatures (which did not originate with Culpeper), one could determine the appropriate use of the plant by some element of its appearance. Thus garlic's hollow stalk indicated that it should be used to treat windpipe ailments. Plants shaped roughly like certain organs were to be used for diseases of those organs. Weeds that ran rampant were good for nearly everything; that was why they were so common. The astrological connection may have been based on the fact that farmers often planted according to the phases of the moon.

Herbs in America: When colonists first came to America, they brought their herbs with them, but they found that Native Americans were already using nearly every indigenous plant for one purpose or another. For example, they used willow bark to treat headache pain. Today we know that willow bark contains salicin, which is the natural form of salicylic acid, the active ingredient in aspirin.

When they weren't sneaking up on each other with murderous intent, natives and immigrants swapped plant lore. Before long there were many books on native cures, and the first arboretum in America was established to study the medicinal plants used by Native Americans.

Patent Medicines: In the early 1800s, a self-taught physician named Samuel Thompson patented a few of his most useful plant remedies for common, easily diagnosed diseases. The remedies sold well, and the patent-medicine business took off. Herbs were in such great demand that gatherers couldn't supply enough and professional growers stepped in, among them the religious community popularly known as the Shakers. The Shakers stayed in the herb business until well into the twentieth century, and even today individual Shaker communities still sell herbal products.

The patent-medicine era was a boon to herb growers, but it definitely had a down side. Hucksters who cared more about the health of their wallets than of sick people put most anything in a bottle and sold it as a miracle cure for everything from low virility to cancer. Thompson himself spent most of the rest of his life fending off the medical establishment in court. Ironically, although Thompson had patented his own cures to make sure that people got the right formulas, he unintentionally set the stage for just what he feared: an era of flagrant quackery.

The Parting of the Ways: At the turn of the century, herbal medicine and traditional medicine coexisted rather amiably, and mainstream physicians often prescribed herbal teas, tinctures, and tonics for a wide variety of ailments. However, with the rise of the pharmaceutical industry, things changed. Physicians turned more and more to manufactured drugs (which were often based on substances originally found in plants). Herbalism continued to have its adherents, but few were traditionally trained physicians.

Today there is a renewed interest in herbalism in the United States. In the rest of the world, it has never flagged. Nearly three fourths of the world's population relies upon it as a principal source of healthcare.

Herbalism's increasing popularity in this country stems from several sources, among them a greater acceptance of Oriental medicine, movement back toward the use of all things natural, the rise of holistic medicine, and the individual's desire to take charge of his or her own healthcare.

Scientific Research: Research scientists too are taking another look at herbalism. Right now there is tremendous medicinal-plant research going on in the Amazon rain forests and other remote places. It is worthwhile to note that more than 40 percent of the prescription drugs now available are based on ingredients found in plants and other natural substances. The angina remedy digitalis, for example, was first made from the powdered leaves of the foxglove.

A small but increasing number of mainstream doctors is rediscovering the value of ancient plant remedies. As one physician put it, "If it's safe and it does the trick, why should I turn to a prescription drug. I look at some of the more established herbal treatments this way: Would people have continued to take them for 5,000 years if they didn't work?"

INSTRUCTIONS

We run into an immediate problem when we begin to talk about how to use herbs. Exactly what is an herb? Most of us expect to find plants like sage, thyme, and rosemary in an herb garden, but a poplar tree? Yet poplar is an ancient herbal cure. For our purposes, the best definition of an herb seems to be: "a plant or plant part valued for its medicinal, savory, or aromatic qualities." That definition allows us to include trees and shrubs as well as herbaceous plants.

Clues from Names: The names of herbs sometimes give us some clue as to their uses. A plant whose name includes the word *officionale* is one that has been known as an official medicinal plant. "Wort" as part of a plant's name also indicates that it is used for healing. Some plant names tell us specifically what they're used for. Fleabane and cancer-root, for example, don't leave much to the imagination.

Experimenting Can Be Dangerous: Just because you know what a plant is used for doesn't mean you should brew up a pot of tea from its leaves or stew the roots. Medicinal plants can be toxic if they're used improperly or in the wrong doses. Some plants have beneficial leaves and toxic roots or vice versa. You need to know what you're doing before you start concocting your own herbal treatments. Consult a good herbal manual, a professional herbalist, or a healthcare professional familiar with plant remedies. If you have a serious condition, you should always consult a healthcare professional before you start any treatment, herbal or otherwise.

Preparing Herbs: Medicinal herbs are prepared in nearly every imaginable way, depending on their use. You can make a poultice, squeeze the juice, make a paste of various parts, boil them, soak them, make a tea, and grind them into powder. You can also add other ingredients to make essences, tinctures, salves, liniments, wines, and syrups.

The practice of herbalism differs from one culture to another. The Chinese and Ayurvedic (Indian) systems are very old, and over the millennia, they have evolved into elaborate systems of diagnosis and treatment. When it began in Greece and Rome, Western herbalism was headed in the same direction, but it stopped developing after the Middle Ages. Western herbalism as it is practiced today comes basically from the folk-medicine tradition.

Traditional Chinese Herbalism: At the core of Chinese herbalism is the Taoist theory of *yin* and *yang*, which represent opposites in nature: dark and light, hot and cold, positive and negative, masculine and feminine, and so forth. Taoists believe that one must balance yin and yang to achieve good health. Harmony in all things is the watchword.

The system is very complex, but basically, Chinese herbalists use combinations of yin herbs (rarely a single herb) to treat yang diseases and vice versa. Salty, sour, bitter, cold, cool, heavy, strong, or very fragrant herbs are yin; yang herbs are bland, sweet, hot, warm, sharp, light, or lightly scented. There are also herbs that contain both yin and yang characteristics.

Yin herbs are often used to treat more serious or chronic diseases. A minor condition like a cold is treated with yang herbs. Other herbs are chosen because they have a particularly beneficial effect upon a specific organ.

Some herbs can be taken almost indefinitely with no unpleasant side effects. These herbs are called superior herbs, and they are used for tonics and maintenance of good health. Ginseng is this kind of herb. Others, called general herbs, are used to treat diseases. When the disease is cured, the person stops taking the herb. Still others, called inferior herbs, would be toxic if taken in large amounts or over a long period. They are used very sparingly in some medicinal herbal formulas.

We should note that, in Chinese medicine, the words "inferior" and "superior" have nothing to do with good and bad. The idea that one thing is good and another bad is Western thinking. To the Chinese, everything—whether it is a ginseng root or a ball of dust—has its own inherent qualities and therefore is neither good nor bad. It simply is what it is, and it cannot be any more or less than that.

An attractive feature of Chinese herbalism is its emphasis on not getting sick in the first place. The Chinese use tonics to strengthen the whole body and particularly the immune system. The principle of harmonious balance is always at work. If you have too many yang characteristics (which include activity, excitement, and stimulation), you take a yin preparation. If you are too cold, passive, or inactive (yin characteristics), you take a yang preparation. (A mainstream physician might give you a tranquilizer or a mood elevator for these conditions.)

This explanation is very simplified and does not do justice to the subtleties of Chinese herbalism. At present, the Chinese pharmacopoeia contains nearly 6,000 entries (not all of which are herbal). Practitioners can choose from about 500 herbal formulas, but there are about 200 that are in common use. One must also remember that herbalism is only one part of the Chinese medical system.

Although treatment for serious conditions should be left to the professional practitioner, you may want to explore the use of Chinese herbal medicines for health maintenance and treatment of minor problems. Already-prepared formulas can be purchased at herbal shops and health-food stores.

For example, if you have a cold, you might like to try a formula called Yin Chiao Chieh Tu Pien. (You might like to try it, but could you *pronounce* it to get what you want? No problem. Just say "yin-chow-chee-due-pee-in.") This formula contains both forsythia and honeysuckle, which the Chinese believe act on the respiratory tract to counteract excess "heat" and "wind." As with most other cold remedies, Yin Chiao Chieh Tu Pien works best if taken at the first sniffle, before the cold is full-blown.

There are a number of self-help books available. Several are mentioned in the *Further Reading* section, and you can find others in the bookstore, library, or the place where you buy herbs.

(For information on Indian herbalism, see AYURVEDA.)

Western Herbalism: Western herbalism has its roots in the theories of Hippocrates. Like the Orientals, Hippocrates believed that disease should be treated by balancing the cause against its opposite, but his classification of opposites was according to the Four Humours (blood, phlegm, yellow bile, and black bile) and the Four Seasons. He also assigned qualities like hot, dry, cold, and wet to herbs.

Modern herbalists consider the effects plants have on the body, but there are still practicing herbalists who define herbs according to their "qualities." Thus, an herb might be called either a "diuretic" or a "dry" herb, depending upon the orientation of the herbalist.

Treating serious diseases with herbs is a sophisticated undertaking that depends upon accurate diagnosis among other things, so that should be left to the professional. However, there are many herbs that can safely be taken by the do-it-yourselfer as overall body strengtheners, nutritive supplements, or treatments for minor ailments, stress, and the like. Herbs that strengthen the body are called "alternatives" because they provide a nutritional boost for many different conditions.

Western herbalists often use a single herb for its effects, although combinations are becoming more popular as our lives grow more complex. Single herbs that have wide-ranging uses include aloe vera, garlic, and ginseng.

Aloe Vera: Nearly everybody knows that the juice from the aloe vera plant can soothe burns, but aloe vera has other uses too. The juice can also be applied to stings, fly bites, abrasions, and muscular aches. In liquid form, it is good for sore throats (used as a gargle), upset or acid stomach, flatulence, and diarrhea. Some people have found it an aid to overcoming impotency. One physician prescribes it for gastrointestinal problems, including gastritis, diverticulosis, and duodenal ulcers. His patients take one or two tablespoonsful every two or three hours. Aloe vera is very safe, has no adverse side effects, and contains no aluminum, which is a component of commercial antacids.

Aloe vera plants are very easy to grow as houseplants, so you can have a supply of the juice on hand whenever you need it. You can purchase the liquid form from a health-food store or herbal shop.

Garlic: Garlic has been used since antiquity as a culinary herb, a medicine, and a vegetable. Nearly every culture all over the world does something with garlic. New England colonists even put garlic in a child's shoes to cure whooping cough. (Needless to say, this is not a popular remedy today!)

Medicinally, garlic is an expectorant (loosens phlegm so it can be spit out), a diuretic (increases the flow of urine), a diaphoretic (increases sweating), an antibiotic, and a stimulant. Right there you can see it has a lot of possibilities.

Garlic syrup is used for bronchitis, coughs, colds, and sore throats. To prepare it, steep a pound of sliced garlic cloves in a quart of boiling water for half a day. Add enough sugar to make a syrup and some vinegar and honey if you want. You might also wish to add a sweet-tasting herb (perhaps anise) for better flavor. You can make a simpler syrup for coughs by mixing raw garlic juice with sugar or honey. Take either syrup by the tablespoonful as needed.

Some herbalists recommend taking a tablespoon or two of garlic syrup nightly for three nights for rheumatism. Or you might try just rubbing your aching joint with garlic cloves.

Russian physicians prescribe garlic for their hypertensive patients to help open up the blood vessels, and they use it so often as an antibiotic, it has acquired the nickname "Russian penicillin." In fact, the active ingredient responsible for the antibiotic action is allicin, a relative of penicillin. Allicin also gives garlic its pungent aroma.

Use garlic poultices to treat snakebite, insect stings, and whooping cough. Some soothe a toothache by applying a raw garlic clove to the gum. A mixture of honey and garlic browned in butter is supposed to be good for kidney and bladder problems. Garlic is also used to treat arthritis, sciatica, sinus infections, and intestinal parasites in both animals and humans. For parasites, use raw garlic juice or milk boiled with garlic.

Try a garlic spray to banish garden pests. One recipe uses chopped garlic steeped in a little mineral oil, a bit of liquid soap, and water. Another uses just garlic and water whipped in a blender. Strain and dilute with more water if necessary. It won't hurt your plants, and it's safe to use around animals and children. (Some think that eating raw garlic keeps mosquitoes at bay too.)

Perhaps the most powerful reason to look into garlic is its apparent anticancer effects. Recent scientific studies from both China and Italy found that people who ate at least one or two garlic cloves a day had a reduced risk of getting stomach cancer. The more garlic they ate, the lower the risk. Preliminary studies also indicate that garlic may help prevent breast, prostate, colon, rectal, and skin cancers too.

If eating lots of garlic sounds like good preventive medicine but social disaster, you can cleanse your breath with parsley. Or take one of the nearly odorless garlic pills available in stores. Be aware, though, that garlic in pill form does not always contain all the same compounds found in raw garlic. Capsules containing aged garlic extract, for example, contain only about five percent of the active ingredients in raw garlic.

Ginseng: Ginseng is the most widely used herb in the world. It is even more fabled than garlic for its curative powers. Part of the mystique about ginseng is its shape. Some roots have almost human form; the more a root looks like a man, the more highly prized it is. Really exotically shaped roots can fetch up to $10,000 an ounce at market. Ginseng is native to both North America and China. Wild Asian ginseng costs more than American ginseng, but even U.S.-grown roots sell for around $90 a pound.

The Chinese have used ginseng for centuries as a general tonic, strength-builder, and aphrodisiac, but until recently American scientists were skeptical of the health-promoting properties of ginseng. Some still are, but recent studies show that ginseng has complex chemical properties that could account for its healing reputation. Ginseng contains a host of vitamins and minerals and a few other substances that are unique to the plant. These chemicals may have a beneficial effect on the cardiovascular system, the circulatory system, and the endocrine system.

The raw root probably contains more active properties than the dried, but roots that are steamed and then slow-dried (red ginseng) or sun-dried are supposed to retain nearly all their potency. Roots are sold whole, sliced, or powdered. You can also buy ginseng in liquid and capsule form.

People use ginseng to promote longevity, increase the appetite, improve digestion, and increase virility, but most of all, to fight stress and stress-related diseases like high-blood pressure, fatigue, and anxiety. Scientists have done a lot of research on ginseng and have made some startling discoveries. For example, ginseng seems to behave like the hormones that the adrenal cortex naturally produces in response to stress. In other words, ginseng supplements the body's own stress-fighters.

From its legendary reputation, one might assume that ginseng has an intriguing, exotic flavor. One would be wrong. Ginseng will never win any prizes for taste. In fact, ginseng tea has a rather unpleasant flavor. One herbalist likens it to the taste of boiled dirt. Still, it's not the flavor you're after, so grit your teeth and boil up this concoction: Put one slice of ginseng root per half cup of boiling water into a pan. Boil until the water is reduced by about one fourth. Strain. Sweeten to taste with sugar or honey.

Herbs act more slowly than synthetic medicines, so don't expect to feel like Superperson after one cup of ginseng tea. The effect is gradual, but people who use ginseng regularly say it gives them a real energy boost.

Many healing herbs are also kitchen herbs, and you may already grow them in your garden. The chart below lists herbal remedies for some common ailments. You can use either fresh or dried herbs. To make an infusion or tea, the usual amount is one ounce of dried herb to a pint of water. Use more if you're using fresh herbs. Add lemon and/or honey to the teas if you like.

COMMON/ BOTANICAL NAME	METHOD OF PREPARATION	USE
Angelica (*Angelica atropurpurea*)	Tonic (usually made from root but leaves and seeds are also usable)	Colds; menstrual problems; general immunity against diseases; stimulant to digestion; general stimulant
Anise (*Pimpinella anisum*)	Hot infusion (tea)	Indigestion
Arnica (*Arnica montana*)	Ointment	Bruises
Barberry (*Berberis vulgaris*)	Tonic	Diarrhea; yeast infections
Chamomile (*Anthemis nobilis*)	Hot infusion made from blossoms (tea)	Insomnia; nervousness; nightmares
Caraway (*Carum Carvi*)	Chew seeds	Flatulence; indigestion

Cranberry	Juice (unsweetened); cooked berries	Bladder infections
Elderflow (Sambucus canadensis)	Hot infusion made from dried flowers (tea)	Fever; insomnia; colds (rubbing bruised leaves on the skin may also keep flies away)
Feverfew (Chrysanthemum parthenium)	Tincture	Repel gnats; mosquitos and bees
Golden Seal (Hydrastis canadensis)	Tonic (with baking soda, mouthwash)	Catarrh; stomach problems; constipation
Lemon balm (Melissa officinalis)	Hot infusion (tea)	Headache; fever; said to promote longevity
Marjoram (Origanum vulgare)	Oil Hot infusion of leaves (tea)	Toothache; muscular aches Nervous headache
Parsley (Petroselinum hortense)	Chew leaves Infusion (chill for use) Compress (crush leaves)	Bad breath Arthritis; as a diuretic Insect bites
Peppermint (Mentha piperita)	Chew leaves; hot infusion (tea)	Colic; cramps; muscle spasms; indigestion
Rosemary (Rosmarinus officinalis)	Hot infusion (tea) Oil	Headache; insomnia Muscular aches
Thyme (Thymus vulgaris)	Tincture (gargle)	Sore throat
Valerian (Valeriana officinalis); also known as heliotrope	Infusion of powdered root mixed with other herbs*	Use in small doses as sedative, tranquilizer

* Try 1 part each valerian, skullcap, and mistletoe or 1 part each valerian, ginger, and lobelia plus 2 parts pleurisy root. Take one tablespoon two to four times daily. (Any valerian concoction should be used sparingly. Too much or too frequent use can cause headaches and possibly even hallucinations.)

FURTHER READING

Dwyer, James, and David Rattray (sr. eds.). *Magic and Medicine of Plants.* Pleasantville, N.Y.: The Reader's Digest Association, Inc., 1986.

Griggs, Barbara. *Green Pharmacy: A History of Herbal Medicine.* New York: The Viking Press, 1981.

Health Center for Better Living. *A Useful Guide to Herbal Health Care.* Naples, Fla.

Hsu, Hong-yen. *How to Treat Yourself with Chinese Herbs*. Los Angeles: Oriental Healing Arts Institute, 1980.

Hyatt, Richard. *Chinese Herbal Medicine*. New York: Schocken Books, 1978.

Kowalchick, Claire, and William H. Hylton (eds.) *Rodale's Illustrated Encyclopedia of Herbs*. Emmaus, Pa.: Rodale Press, Inc., 1987.

Le Strange, Richard. *A History of Herbal Plants*. New York: Arco Publishing Co., Inc., 1977.

Reid, Daniel P. *Chinese Herbal Medicine*. Boston: Shambuhala, 1987.

Shar, Douglas. *Thirty Plants That Can Save Your Life!* Washington, D.C. Elliott & Clark Publishing, 1993.

Tierra, Michael. *Planetary Herbology*. Santa Fe: Lotus Press, 1988.

Weiss, Gaea, and Shandor Weiss. *Growing and Using Healing Herbs*. Emmaus, Pa.: Rodale Press, Inc., 1985.

RESOURCE GROUPS

American Botanical Council
PO Box 201660
Austin, TX 78720
Phone: 800/373-7105 or 512/331-8868

American Herbalists Guild
PO Box 1863
Soquel, CA 95073-1863
Phone: 408/1700

American Herb Association
PO Box 1673
Nevada City, CA 95959
Phone: 916/265-9552

Herb Research Foundation
1007 Pearl St., Ste. 200
Boulder, CO 80302
Phone: 303/449-2265

Herb Society of America
9019 Kirtland Chardon Rd.
Mentor, OH 44060
Phone: 216/256-0514

HEALING THROUGH NATURE'S ELEMENTS

In this section, you'll find some tried-and-true remedies that you probably already use—putting ice on a swelling, for example—but you'll also find therapies that may be new to you. If you're a pragmatic, down-to-earth, no-nonsense person, you may be skeptical about healing with color, crystals, or magnets or wonder how chakra balancing could really help.

We don't claim that *any* therapy in this book will work for everybody, so of course, we don't know whether these will do anything for you, but they've all worked for somebody—actually a lot of somebodies—or they wouldn't be listed here.

Don't try these out-of-the-mainstream therapies if you don't want to; they probably wouldn't do you much good anyway if you didn't believe in their merits, but *do* try to have an open mind when you read about them. You may find the principles behind them more logical and/or scientific than you had imagined (or you may not). Nearly all the therapies in this section have been practiced in some form for thousands of years, but that doesn't mean you'll find them appealing. Give them your best open-minded read, and then if you're still doubtful, go take a nice warm bath. We're pretty sure you'll find some therapeutic benefit in that.

CHAKRA BALANCING

DEFINITION

Ancient Sanskrit texts tell us that the body has seven major energy centers called *chakras*. Chakra balancing refers to keeping these energy centers in harmony through the use of meditation, color therapy, crystal therapy, and/or visualization.

APPLICATIONS

Physiological: Any problems or diseases of the major systems of the body
Psychological: Stress, anxiety, tension, depression

COLLATERAL CROSS-THERAPIES

Light therapy, color therapy, crystal therapy, yoga, visualization, meditation, Ayurveda

RECOMMENDED ADJUNCT ACTIVITIES AND BEHAVIORS

None

CONTRAINDICATIONS

None

EQUIPMENT & MATERIALS

The materials that you will need depend upon the method you use to balance the chakras. If you use crystal therapy, you'll need crystals and gemstones. For color therapy, you might use colored lights, colored clothing, tinted glasses, or colored dish- and glassware. If you use meditation or visualization, you won't need any equipment.

ORIGIN

Chakra balancing has its roots in the ancient lore of India. It is one of the methods used in ayurvedic healing, and it is also part of the theory and practice of yoga. Although chakra balancing is considered a method of healing in itself, it uses other forms of alternative therapy to accomplish this purpose.

   According to yogic theory, human beings are just one part of a universal continuum of energy and consciousness. Energy and consciousness are continuously exchanged among people and the rest of the universe. People themselves are composed of three bodies: a *physical* (material) body, an *astral* (conscious) body, and a *causal* (absolute) body. These bodies can be roughly likened to the Western concepts of body, mind/emotions, and spirit.

The Three Bodies: The physical body we are familiar with. The astral body contains all desires and emotions. Both the physical and astral bodies possess duality; characteristics can be positive or negative, attractive or repulsive. Through a connecting system of energy called the *etheric double*, energy and information passes between the physical and astral bodies. Our awareness of the astral body comes through intuition, dreams, memory, and the like.

The causal body is the highest part of our being. The causal body is individual, but it is also absolute; therefore, there can be no duality. All elements required for existence are combined in the causal body in perfect equilibrium. The causal body is pure life energy.

At birth, we know only the physical body. Gradually we become aware of (and learn to control) the astral body, but we must develop our consciousness to the fullest to comprehend the causal body.

Yogis believe that the three bodies are interconnected through the seven chakras, which exist at the same time in both the astral and causal bodies. In Sanskrit, the ancient language of India, *chakra* means "wheel" or "vortex," and chakras are often depicted as spinning wheels of energy or light.

The chakras supply energy to the various bodies through channels known as *nadi*. Interestingly, the nadis appear to correspond closely to the Chinese system of meridians, although the two models were probably developed independently. Both nadis and meridians also have counterparts in western medicine, where they are known as the "systems" of the body.

The Chakras: The central axis of the chakras corresponds to the spinal cord in the physical body. The lowest chakra is found at the base of the spine, the highest at the crown of the head. Each chakra controls the physiological function of a particular biological system, but each is also associated with mental, emotional, and spiritual characteristics. In the mental and spiritual realms, each higher chakra represents a greater understanding and harmony with the universe as a whole.

The first (root) chakra is the *muladhara*. The muladhara purportedly houses a potent form of energy called *kundalini*, which can be roughly characterized as the primal force. The kundalini is largely dormant, but when awakened, it is very powerful. Yogic theory holds that the original state of kundalini lies in the Absolute.

The second chakra, the *swadhistana*, governs the sexual and elimination functions of the body. It is also associated with the deep, instinctive drives of the unconscious.

The third chakra is the *manipura*. The manipura governs the digestive functions of the physical body. In the astral plane, it is associated with the emotions and rudimentary extrasensory perception (ESP) and clairvoyance.

The fourth chakra, the *anahata*, governs the heart and circulatory system. When fully developed, this chakra is the first one that has a truly spiritual connotation. The anahata is associated with selfless love and compassion.

The fifth chakra is called the *visshuda*. Physically, the visshuda controls the respiratory system. Mentally and spiritually, it relates to a deeper ability to communicate, higher intelligence, and greater under-standing.

The sixth chakra, the *ajna*, is often called the "third eye" because it is situated between the eyes behind the brows. It is associated physically with the autonomic nervous system and the pituitary gland. On the other planes, the ajna relates to intuition, perception, higher functions of the mind, and the concept of Self.

The highest chakra, the *sahasrara*, is found at the crown of the head, in the cerebral cortex. Physiologically, the sahasrara is the coordinator of all the body's functions. On the astral and causal planes, it represents the highest union of all the bodies. One whose sahasrara is fully devel-oped has an understanding of the Cosmic or Universal Self.

Until so-called "New Age" therapies became popular, most people in the United States had probably never heard of chakras. Now the term is well known among alternative healers, and chakra balancing is practiced throughout the country.

INSTRUCTIONS

Proponents say that chakra balancing becomes necessary when blocks impede the free flow of energy throughout the body. These blocks can originate within the body or they can come from external sources. Physical and emotional trauma can block energy too.

A blocked or imbalanced chakra can cause illness or malfunction in that part of the body to which it relates. A person can also have mental or emotional problems related to that chakra. For example, blockage in the third chakra, the manipura, could cause digestive problems and/or emotional instability.

Some people who practice chakra balancing concentrate on the af-fected chakra, while others believe that all the chakras should be treated to keep them in harmony.

Each chakra is associated with a color, so practitioners often use color therapy to clear the chakras. The following chart gives a thumbnail sketch of the chakras and their related colors.

CHAKRA	COLOR	ASTRAL & CASUAL ASPECTS	PHYSIOLOGICAL SYSTEM
Sahasrara (crown)	Violet	Imagination; Universal Self	Cerebral cortex; nervous system; pineal gland; coordinates entire physiolgocial system
Ajna (brow)	Indigo	Intuition; intellect; Individual Self	Autonomic nervous system; pituitary gland

Visshuda (throat)	Blue	Conceptualization; communication	Respiratory system; thyroid gland
Anahata (heart)	Green	Love; compassion; intuitive understanding	Heart; circulatory system
Manipura (solar plexus)	Yellow	Desire for power; anger; dreams; simple ESP; clairvoyance	Digestive system; adrenal glands
Swadhistana (spleen)	Orange	Sex instinct; desire; hatred; jeolousy	No system as such; houses the kundalini (life force)
Muladhara (base of spine)	Red	Physical sensations; survival instinct	Genitourinary system; reproductive system

Using Color to Treat the Chakras: Color can be used in various ways to treat the chakras. You can wear clothing in the appropriate color, use that-colored dishes and glassware, wear tinted glasses, or use colored lights. One method that many people use is to fill a colored glass pitcher with water and expose it to the sunlight. Theoretically, the water will take on the properties of that particular wavelength of light (color), so the water will have a therapeutic effect when you drink it.

Food of a certain color may also affect the chakra of the corresponding color. In his book, *Spiritual Nutrition and the Rainbow Diet*, Dr. Gabriel Cousens suggests that nature tells us how to heal our chakras by color-coding the food to match the chakra. To nourish the total being, eat a "rainbow" diet of foods in all colors (vegetarian only, no meat). For breakfast, try red, orange and yellow foods; for lunch, Dr. Cousens recommends yellow, green and blue foods, and for dinner, blue, indigo and violet foods. (If you're stumped on blue, indigo and violet, think Concord grapes, eggplants and plums, to name just a few.) White foods (cauliflower, potatoes, tofu, etc.) go with any meal because they're full-spectrum. (The reason that Dr. Cousens recommends eating foods in this order is that it corresponds to the progression of light throughout the day, so your chakras will be in rhythm with the rest of nature.)

Crystal therapy is another method of balancing the chakras. You can place the gem or crystal on the body directly above the site of the chakra you wish to address. (See CRYSTAL THERAPY, page 47.)

Still another method is visualization. To do this, form a mental picture of the chakra and "see" the energy flowing freely without any obstruction.

If you'd like to know more about chakra balancing, consult a professional or read one of the many books available. Many health-food stores and herbal shops carry books on alternative therapies, including chakra balancing. Also check your local library.

FURTHER READING

Bohm, Warner. *Chakras: Roots of Power*. York Beach, Me.: Samuel Weiser, 1991.

Breaux, Charles. *Journey into Consciousness*. York Beach, Me.: Nicolas-Hays, 1989.

Bruyere, Rosalyn L. *Wheels of Light—Chakras, Auras, and the Healing Energy of the Body*. New York: Fireside Books, 1994.

Cousens, Gabriel. *Spiritual Nutrition and the Rainbow Diet*. Boulder, Colo.: Cassandra Press, 1986.

Judith, Anodea. *Wheels of Life: A User's Guide to the Chakra System*. St. Paul: Llewellyn Publications, 1987.

Judith, Anodea, and Selene Vega, *The Seven-Fold Journey*. Freedom, Calif.: Crossing Press, 1993.

Motoyama, Hiroshi. *Theories of the Chakras*. Wheaton, Ill.: Theosophical Publishing House, 1981.

Selby, John. *Kundalini Awakening*. New York: Bantam Books, 1992.

Thomas, James M. *The 7 Steps to Personal Power*. Deerfield Beach, Fla.: Health Communications, 1992.

Weinman, Ric A. *Your Hands Can Heal: Learn to Channel Healing Energy*. New York: Dutton, 1988.

Willis, Pauline, and Theo Gimbel. *16 Steps to Health and Energy*. St. Paul: Llewellyn Publications, 1992.

RESOURCE GROUPS

Lifespan Associates
70 Sable Ct.
Winter Springs, FL 32708
Phone: 407/699-672

Resource for crystal therapy; audiotapes, videotapes, workbooks, *Psychic Research Newsletter*; crystals; also referrals to crystal therapists

Dinshah Health Society
100 Dinshah Drive
Malaga, NJ 08328
Phone: 609/692-4686

Resource for color therapy; membership: $3; newsletter, *Breath Forecast* (light calculations based upon the new moon); books, pamphlets

COLOR THERAPY (COLOR HEALING)

DEFINITION

Color therapy is the use of color for physical, mental, and emotional healing. In some forms, color therapy is closely akin to light therapy but with the addition of specific colors.

APPLICATIONS

Physiological: Chronic pain, skin diseases, muscle aches, neuralgia, rheumatism, arthritis, migraine headache, jaundice, overweight, vision problems
Psychological: Stress, agitation, depression, lethargy, overeating, violent behavior

COLLATERAL CROSS-THERAPIES

Light therapy, chakra balancing, Ayurveda

CONTRAINDICATIONS

There are no contraindications to using colored paints, clothing, or ordinary lights with color filters to alter your mood or treat ordinary illnesses, such as headache.

EQUIPMENT & MATERIALS

Colored paints, light fixtures with colored filters, or clothing in particular colors

ORIGIN

We know that color therapy dates back at least as far as the ancient Egyptians. In Egypt, priests built healing temples that contained separate rooms, each painted in one of the seven colors of the rainbow: red, orange, yellow, green, blue, indigo, and violet. A patient was placed in one of these rooms to heal; which room depended upon the nature of the illness or injury.

The Greeks also built light temples that made use of color for healing. Pythagoras, the great Greek mathematician, was an early proponent of the therapeutic use of color. In the East, color was a component of health and healing in both the Chinese and ayurvedic traditions.

People probably first noted the effects of color in the day and night cycles of their lives and in the changing seasons. The "day" colors red, orange, and yellow seemed energizing, while the "night" colors blue, indigo, and violet were calming and restorative.
Where Does Color Come From? Color comes from light. We need to know something about light to understand color. Light is one form of radiant energy; microwaves, x-rays, and ultraviolet rays are other forms

of radiation. All forms of radiant energy are closely related. Each is produced by electromagnetic waves. The various forms of radiant energy differ only in the length of the waves. We need special equipment to "tune in" certain kinds of waves, like radio waves. Waves of other lengths are visible to us. We see these waves as color. All the colors that we can see make up what is called the *visible spectrum*. The color violet has the shortest wavelength in the visible spectrum, red the longest. (Other forms of energy that have longer or shorter wavelengths are part of the spectrum too, but not the visible spectrum.)

Most of our modern ideas about color arose from a discovery in 1666 by Sir Isaac Newton, who is most famous for a discovery of another sort: gravity. While trying to build a better telescope, Newton noticed that a beam of sunlight shining through a prism formed a band of color like a rainbow. This observation led to Newton's theory that sunlight contains all colors and that the prism merely separated them.

Newton arranged the colors (red, orange, yellow, green, blue, indigo, and violet) into a circle. He explained his theory of colors in sunlight by saying that light contained tiny spinning particles that moved in a straight line. The particles of red were large, while the particles of violet were small. Later another scientist named Robert Hook suggested that light traveled in waves. Scientists argued Newton's theory against Hook's for over 150 years. In the end, it turned out that both were right.

Nature's most showy display of the visible spectrum can be found in a rainbow and in the aurora borealis and aurora australis, the so-called polar lights.

Scientists agree that the invisible wavelengths of ultraviolet rays, microwaves, and x-rays affect the human body, but there is still controversy over whether the visible rays that we know as colors have any effect.

Color in Everyday Life: Scientific disagreement aside, people certainly associate color with behavior and well-being. When they feel good, folks say they're "in the pink" or "looking at the world through rose-colored glasses." On the other hand, there's "blue Monday," and we either have the "blues" or we sing them. A novice at a particular task is said to be "green," while a coward is "yellow." Get angry? You see "red." A "black" day is one on which something catastrophic happened. And so on.

Some colors soothe and relax us while others stimulate energy and creativity. Still others can depress us or even make us feel ill. Red, orange, and yellow excite the nervous system; blue and green calm us down; and black is universally thought to be depressing.

One graphic proof of the power of color is the famous Blackfriars Bridge in London. With its black ironwork, it was a dark and depressing sight, made all the more so by its long history of suicides. The authorities decided to repaint the bridge green, and the incidence of suicide dropped by more than a third.

The color of foods has an effect upon whether we find them appetizing or not. Many foods today are artificially colored in order to give them a more healthful appearance. Not everyone finds the addition of color an improvement upon nature, but the practice is widespread.

Color and the Life Process: We perceive color when light enters our eyes and moves through neurological pathways to the brain. The cortex of the brain, the most "educated" part, knows the names of the colors, differentiates one from another, and reacts aesthetically to color. However, our more primitive midbrain also reacts to color instinctively and reflexively. The midbrain's reaction to color suggests that at some level color is involved in the whole life process.

Through animal studies, scientists have found that certain regions of the brain respond differently to different wavelengths of light (colors). This means that we may be able to influence various functions of the endocrine system with colored lights.

Ancient writings in Sanskrit tell us that long ago Indian scholars were aware of this possibility. According to their theory, the body is composed of seven major energy centers known as chakras. (See CHAKRA BALANCING, page 33.) Each chakra is located at the site of major endocrine glands. The chakras correspond to particular states of consciousness, and each is governed by a color.

Today most scientists accept that colors can have psychological effects on human beings, but there is more controversy over the physiological effects of color. A number of scientific studies support the premise that color can affect heart rate, blood pressure, and respiration rate. One study found that yellow light caused the greatest increase in these rates and black light the greatest decrease.

Color and Healing: Modern practitioners use blue light to treat neonatal jaundice and arthritis pain. Blinking red light has been found to be effective for treating many patients with migraine headaches. Other physicians use blue light for the same problem. Experts have found that bubble-gum pink is a color that calms and alleviates aggressive tendencies, so this color is used to paint the walls of jail cells, juvenile reformatories, mental institutions, and other locations where aggressive behavior is a problem. Because it has such a calming effect, bubble-gum pink (also called Baker-Miller pink) can also reduce the nervous tendency to snack in overeaters.

Red and blue lights may affect athletic performance. One study found that viewing red light gave athletes quick bursts of energy, whereas blue light produced a steadier level of energy.

INSTRUCTIONS

Color therapy is of two types: the use of pigments or dyes (as in wall colorings or clothing) and the use of colored lights. For do-it-yourselfers, the use of colored lights should be confined to regular light bulbs with colored filters.

Want to change the way you feel through the colors of the clothing you wear? The chart below can help you choose the right color to create a certain mood:

COLOR	CHARACTERISTIC ELICITED
Red	Strength; dynamism; courage
Yellow	Happiness; carefree attitude; ability to communicate
Green	Stability; feeling of abundance
Blue	Calm; inner peace
Orange	Vibrancy; sexuality; self-esteem
Purple	Connection with higher purpose
Black	Self-effacement (some people say that black absorbs negativity and keeps it from touching the person)
White	Clarity; focus

If you want to use color in your home to advantage, try bright colors in rooms where you want to be stimulated and alert. Use shades of blue or green for the bedroom. Orange is said to stimulate the appetite, so you might want to put a little orange into your dining room and kitchen. Very dark colors are generally depressing, so you may want to stay away from dark brown, gray, and black.

Some people believe that the benefits of colors can be absorbed by water. If you want to try water treated in this way, fill a red glass pitcher with water and put it in a window where the sun strikes the glass. (The longer you leave the pitcher in the sun, the more of the red light is absorbed, according to proponents.) To get a greater boost in energy, use this water to make your morning beverage. You can do the same thing with a blue glass pitcher to prepare water for a calming effect. Use water treated with a blue light for a soothing drink before bed. Some healthcare practitioners report that they have successfully treated ulcers with water exposed to green light and constipation with yellow-charged light.

You can also use colored lights for healing. A plain lamp with various colored filters that can be changed is probably the easiest to use. The chart below lists some uses for various colored lights.

COLOR	EFFECTS/CONDITIONS
Red	Urticaria; eczema; circulation; vitality; energy; anemia; muscle contractions; rheumatism; arthritis
Orange	Asthma; respiratory disorders; cramps and spasms; digestion; general body normalizer; hiccups
Yellow	Constipation; arthritis; promotes wakefulness
Green	General healing; balance; congestion
Blue-green	Stress; fever; inflammation
Turquoise	Headache; swelling; sunburn; itching; burns; skin toning
Blue	Fever; stress; high blood pressure; sore throat; insomnia; baldness
Indigo	Ear problems; eyestrain; insomnia
Violet (this is violet-colored light, not ultraviolet light)	Cramps; high blood pressure; bladder problems; neuralgia
Magenta	General stimulant; diuretic

FURTHER READING

Bassano, Mary. *Healing with Music and Color*. York Beach, Me.: Samuel Weiser, 1992.

Clark, Linda. *The Ancient Art of Color Therapy*. Old Greenwich, Conn.: The Devin-Adair Co., 1975.

Gimbel, Theo. *Form, Sound, Colour and Healing*. Saffron Walden, Essex, England: C.W. Daniel, 1987.

———. *Healing with Color and Light*. New York: Simon & Schuster, 1994.

MacIvor, Virginia, and Sandra La Forest. *Vibrations: Healing Through Color, Homeopathy and Radionics*. York Beach, Me.: Samuel Weiser, Inc.

Perrigoue-Messer, Terri. *Color Vision*. Diamond Springs, Calif., 1991.

Wood, Betty. *The Healing Power of Color*. Rochester, Vt.: Destiny, 1992.

RESOURCE GROUPS

Dinshah Health Society
100 Dinshah Drive

Malaga, NJ 08328
Phone: 609/692-4686

Membership: $3; newsletter, *Breath Forecast* (light calculations based upon the new moon); books; pamphlets

CRYOTHERAPY (ICE THERAPY, COLD THERAPY)

DEFINITION

Cryotherapy is the use of ice, cold water, or freezer packs to aid in healing.

APPLICATIONS

Physiological: Burns, fever, heat exhaustion, sprains, swelling, inflammation, arthritis, back pain, athletic injuries, dermatitis, hamstring injuries, hemorrhoids, headache, nosebleed, bruises, contusions, insect bites and stings, joint stiffness, muscle spasm, chronic pain, poison ivy, tendinitis, itching, toothache; acts as local anesthetic
Psychological: None

COLLATERAL CROSS-THERAPIES

Heat therapy, hydrotherapy

RECOMMENDED ADJUNCT ACTIVITIES AND BEHAVIORS

None

CONTRAINDICATIONS

Pregnant women, the elderly, and people with heart conditions or diabetes should not subject their bodies to extremes in temperature without first consulting their healthcare practitioners.

EQUIPMENT & MATERIALS

Ice water, ice cubes, crushed ice and/or frozen gel packs; chilled cloths

ORIGIN

Cold water has probably been used for healing since humans first trod the earth. We know that the ancient Greek physician Hippocrates, who lived in the fifth century B.C., recommended cold-water baths for a variety of ailments. In the days of the powerful Greek city-states, the people of Sparta were known for their great courage and rigorous lifestyles. (The word *spartan* eventually came to mean anyone undaunted by pain or danger.) Spartan babies literally got a cold reception when they entered the world: a dunk in frigid water. Spartans thought this toughened their newborns and kept them immune from diseases.

Some Like It Hot . . . And Cold: The Romans loved bathing and built palatial bathhouses where they soaked and swam while catching up on the latest gossip with their neighbors. To the Romans, the bathhouse was a community center with water. In their luxurious spas—the grandest was the Baths of Caracalla, which covered nearly thirty acres—they had small pools of very hot water, very cold water, and warm water. These quick-plunge pools were in anterooms away from the main bathing pool. The idea was to jump into an icy pool and then immediately into a hot one. The more faint of heart could slip a quick trip to the warm pool in between to lessen the shock.

The Scandinavian belief in the therapeutic value of alternating heat and cold dates back at least to medieval times. The first sauna treatments were apparently very much like they are today: sit naked in a small very hot room for as long as you can stand it, and then make a mad dash for the nearest snowbank or icy pool and plunge in.

Using cold water to treat illness has always been a part of folk medicine in nearly every culture. Native Americans used a treatment similar to the sauna. Healers put their patients in "sweat houses," which were just what they sound like—plenty hot—then took them outside for a dip in a cold stream.

Victorian ladies and gentlemen flocked to the English seacoast whenever they could. There they indulged in hot and cold seawater baths to restore their health. The practice fell out of favor for a while, but it has become popular again.

Healing Baths: Around the turn of the century, physicians in the United States prescribed baths for all sorts of ailments. One household medical guide of the day, *The Family Physician*, listed no fewer than seventeen different kinds of baths, and that's not counting hot, cold, and warm! Water treatments in this era were called *hydropathy*, and the author of *The Family Physician* highly recommended them. One cold-water treatment that he advocated was the "nose bath." (To accomplish the nose bath, a person inhaled cold water through the nostrils and then spit it out by mouth.) The nose bath was recommended for head colds, inflammation and ulceration of the nasal passages, and nosebleed, but principally to cure snuff addiction. "Take cold water often instead of the abominable weed," admonished the author.

In earlier times, people could only use ice, snow, and cold water when nature provided it, but with the advent of refrigeration, cryotherapy became as close as your kitchen.

INSTRUCTIONS

There are many minor household injuries and ailments that can effectively be treated by cold water or ice. Cold constricts the blood vessels, thus reducing the flow of blood to an injured body part. Because ice has a numbing effect, it also acts as a local anesthetic. You probably always have ice in your kitchen, but you might want to keep a gel pack or two in the freezer as well. Gel packs stay cold for a long time, and they're less messy than melting ice.

Use ice or a frozen gel pack for:

- Burns (Ice not only reduces the pain by numbing, it also lowers the temperature to stop any further burning action.)
- Sprains
- Nosebleeds (Crushed ice in a small plastic bag can be held comfortably on the nose.)
- Headache
- Bruises
- Insect stings and bites
- Muscle spasms
- Sunburn
- Swelling (Prompt application of ice can keep swelling to a minimum and help preserve range of motion.)
- Inflammation

You can use cold cloths or immersion in cold (or cool) water to reduce the effects of fever or heat exhaustion, but if you're doing this to someone else, be sure the water isn't too cold in an immersion bath. It might be best to start with cool water and gradually lower the temperature. (Consult your healthcare practitioner first for very high fever, extreme heat exhaustion, or pre-existing health problems.)

Although heat and cold have apparently opposite effects, they're often used together, especially when increased circulation would produce a desirable effect. Here's how the combination works: Heat causes the blood vessels to dilate and then constrict as a person cools off. Cold first constricts blood vessels; then they dilate as the person warms up. When used alternately, heat and cold act like an auxiliary pump to push more blood through the system. Increased circulation helps heal by bringing in more oxygen and taking away waste products and toxins.

For pain or stiffness caused by arthritis, rheumatism, sports injuries, or even just sitting too long at your desk, try alternately submerging your sore area in warm water for five minutes, then cold water for one or two minutes. Repeat at least five times. During the warm-water phase, gently exercise the injured part to facilitate range of motion.

Ice or cold water is inexpensive, easy to use, and it's nearly always handy. These factors make it an important self-care treatment that even children can safely use for minor burns, stings, and scrapes.

FURTHER READING

Michlovitz, Susan L., and Steven L. Wolf. *Thermal Agents in Rehabilitation.* Philadelphia: Davis, 1986.

Dail, Clarence W., and Charles S. Thomas. *Simple Remedies for the Home.* Banning, Calif.: Preventive Healthcare and Education Center, 1985.

Kovaler, Lucy. *Cold Against Disease.* New York: John Day Co., 1971.

Licht, Sidney Herman, and Herman L. Kamenetz. *Therapeutic Heat and Cold.* New Haven, Ct.: E. Licht, 1965.

CRYSTAL THERAPY (GEM THERAPY)

DEFINITION

Crystal therapy is the use of gemstones and quartz crystals to promote health and healing.

APPLICATIONS

Physiological: Headache, eye and ear problems, glandular disturbances, digestion, respiratory conditions

Psychological: Stress, anxiety, low self-esteem, anger, pessimism, sadness, lack of concentration, insomnia, poor memory

COLLATERAL CROSS-THERAPIES

Light therapy, color therapy, chakra balancing

RECOMMENDED ADJUNCT ACTIVITIES AND BEHAVIORS

If you want to use crystals in conjunction with meditation, you may wish to set a mood with soft lights and possibly low background music.

CONTRAINDICATIONS

None

EQUIPMENT

Crystals and gemstones

ORIGIN

From earliest times, people have been drawn to the beauty and sparkle of various rocks, stones, and gems. Precious gems have always been symbols of wealth and power, with the rarest being the most coveted. In many cultures, both ancient and modern, people have believed that gems have mystical and mysterious powers apart from their monetary value.

Nearly all the great religions refer to gems in their scriptures. In the Old Testament in the book of Exodus, there is a description of a religious breastplate worn by Aaron, the first High Priest of Israel. The breastplate was said to have fours rows of three gigantic gems. On each gem was written the name of one of the twelve tribes of Israel, and each had mysterious powers that the priests could call upon for healing and for matters of law, religion, and war. The principal stone in the breastplate is believed to have been a ruby, but we know very little about what the other stones might have been.

The ancient Egyptians used gems in religious rituals, and they used them for healing as well. Cleopatra is said to have dissolved a priceless pearl in her wine to achieve immortality. (At that time, pearls were thought to possess that attribute.)

The belief in the medicinal powers of pearls persisted down through the years. In the sixteenth century, Pope Clement VII spent a fortune on powdered pearls and other gems to restore his health. Apothecaries continued to stock pearls for use in powders, syrups, and tinctures until well into the eighteenth century.

The Koran, the Talmud, and the religious writings of Hindus and Buddhists contain references to the mysterious powers of jewels. Many native American tribes used crystals for healing.

Some of the ancients believed that jewels were powerful magnets. When a person was compatible with a certain stone, he or she would derive health and a sense of well-being from being in direct contact with it, but if the stone and the person were incompatible, the person would sicken. Certain metals were also thought to be endowed with healing powers, among them gold and silver. Therefore, the goldsmith and the silversmith were part of the healing community, just as were those who dispensed herbal medicines.

Our ancestors often wore jewels to prevent specific diseases. If a person were prone to a queasy stomach, he or she might wear a jasper around the neck to ward off the problem. People thought opals could prevent blindness, and emeralds were said to protect children against attacks of epilepsy. Garnets prevented "bad blood."

During the Black Plague in Europe in the fourteenth century, some survivors felt they owed their lives to the fact that they never took off their gems, which included rubies, opals, and sapphires, throughout the plague.

Ayurvedic physicians prepare some of their medicines from powdered gems or the ashes of gems that have been burned. In India, one can buy the powdered ashes of gems in ayurvedic pharmacies. Some ayurvedic practitioners liken gems treated this way to the modern isotope.

Burning or crushing precious stones is obviously an expensive way to prepare medicines, so some practitioners use an alternative, and cheaper, method of using the properties of gems. A good-quality gem is placed in a jar filled with a diluted drinkable alcohol solution. The container is kept in a dark place for a week to allow the vibrations from the gem to permeate the solution. The jewel is then removed and kept for future use. The alcohol mixture is given orally as a medicine, sometimes in combination with solutions made from other gems. Distilled water can be used instead of alcohol, if a person so chooses.

What is it that supposedly gives gems their healing power? Believers insist that stones have electromagnetic energy and that they emit vibrations and frequencies that can affect not only the body, but the mind and spirit as well. The healing power of gems is also associated with the planets and with chakra balancing and color therapy.

The clairvoyant Edgar Cayce believed in the vibrational qualities of gems, but he felt that the same gem might have different effects on separate individuals. If the gem was not right for a person, he or she would receive no benefit. Crystal therapists generally support this contention.

During the 1980s, interest in the healing powers of crystals reached new heights in the United States. People all over the country began wearing and using crystals and gems in their daily lives. Some stones are worn while others are placed about the house to evoke certain emotions. For example, rose quartz is a stone that is supposed to correspond to the heart area of the body. Placed In the home, it is purported to contribute to an atmosphere of nurturing.

Do crystals really work? There's almost no scientific evidence in the western world that they do, but there are plenty of anecdotal stories that support healing with crystals. In any event, there are no reports on record that crystals do any harm. People who don't actually ascribe any particular powers to crystals say that just the sight of the beautiful gems gives them a sense of calm and well-being.

INSTRUCTIONS

If you want to try crystal therapy, how do you know which stones can help you? You can consult a crystal therapist if you want to, but most people study the properties of various stones and then use the trial-and-error method. If a certain stone seems to help, then you may want to stick with it. Otherwise try another.

You can use crystals in various ways. You can wear them as jewelry, carry them in your pockets, sew them in the hems of your clothes, place loose crystals on your body while sitting or lying down, or use them as ornaments in your home or office. Some people place the crystals on various parts of their body (usually corresponding to the location of a particular chakra) and repeat a meditation associated with the healing power of the crystal at that particular location.

Practitioners of crystal therapy believe that crystals must be "cleared" before use to eliminate any imprints and bad vibrations from people who have previously handled them. To clear a crystal, you can wash it in sea water (salt water will do in a pinch), pack it in sea salt, bury it underground for a time, hold it under running water, or pass it through a flame or smoke. Stores that sell crystals also sell incense-like "smudge sticks" that you can burn to clear your crystals.

Below is a listing of some of the most commonly used crystals and the characteristics that they affect.

CRYSTAL/GEMSTONE	METAPHYSICAL USE
Adventurine	Balances emotions
Amber	Helps express emotions
Amethyst	Purifying and clarifying thoughts
Aquamarine	Peace of mind; relief of anxiety
Azurite	Mind clearing
Bloodstone	Physical healing
Boji stones	Healing; balance
Carnelian	Regeneration; overcoming inertia
Citrine	Anti-depressant
Clear quartz	Focusing; clearing
Fluorite	Mental clearing
Garnet	Invigoration
Hematite	Stress release; earth's energy
Jade	Cleansing; nurturing; problem-solving
Kunzite	Opens the heart

Lapis lazuli	Calming; strengthening; courage
Lepidolite	Tranquility
Malachite	Balancing; love; patience; self-control
Moldavite	Brain stimulation
Moonstone	Psychic awareness
Obsidian	Grounding
Onyx	Absorbing negative energy; gathering information
Orange coral	Protection
Peridot	Releasing anger; spirtual awareness
Rhodonite	Self-expression
Selenite	Concentration
Smoky quartz	Dreams; transformation
Sodalite	Metabolic balance
Sugilite	Spiritual awareness
Tiger's-eye	Decision making; concentration
Turquoise	Protection; imagination; creativity

FURTHER READING

Bravo, Brett. *Crystal Healing Secrets*. New York: Warner Books, 1988.

Chocron, Daya Sarai. *Healing with Crystals and Gemstones*. York Beach, Me.: Samuel Weiser, Inc., 1983.

Gardner, Joy. *Color and Crystals: A Journey Through the Chakras*. Freedom, Calif.: Crossing Press, 1988.

Hunt, Roland. *The Seven Keys to Color Healing*. San Francisco: Harper & Row, 1971.

Raphaell, Katrina. *Crystal Enlightenment*. Santa Fe: Aurora Press, 1985.

———. *Crystal Healing* Santa Fe: Aurora Press, 1987.

Silbey, Uma. *The Complete Crystal Guidebook*. San Francisco: U-Read Publications, 1986.

RESOURCE GROUPS

Lifespan Associates
70 Sable Ct.

Winter Springs, FL 32708
Phone: 407/699-1672

Audiotapes, videotapes, workbooks, *Psychic Research Newsletter*, crystals; also referrals to crystal therapists

HEAT THERAPY (THERMAL THERAPY)

DEFINITION

Heat therapy is the application of heat in any form for healing. It is often used in conjunction with cryotherapy (cold therapy) for certain problems.

APPLICATIONS

Physiological: Acid indigestion, arthritis, athletic injuries, colds, flu, boils, infections, joint stiffness, menstrual cramps, muscle pain, chronic pain, sore throat, stomach ache, wounds
Psychological: None

COLLATERAL CROSS-THERAPIES

Cryotherapy, hydrotherapy, light therapy

RECOMMENDED ADJUNCT ACTIVITIES AND BEHAVIORS

None

CONTRAINDICATIONS

The temperature of hot water in a bath or hot tub should not exceed 104° F. unless you have your health practitioner's okay. If you're using a hot water bottle or heating pad, don't place it on bare flesh. Either wrap the device in a layer of cloth or put it on top of your clothing. Pregnant women, the elderly, infants and very young children, and people with heart conditions, high blood pressure, circulation problems, nerve impairment, or diabetes should not subject themselves to extremes in temperature without first consulting a healthcare practitioner. Asthmatics and those with other breathing problems should get a professional okay first.

EQUIPMENT & MATERIALS

Hot water, hot water bottle, heating pad, hot cloths, heat lamp, hot tub, sauna, steam, warm water pool

ORIGIN

The sun produces an enormous amount of life-giving heat that sustains our earth. Heat and light from the sun are essential to life on our planet. If the sun should cool, all earthly life would disappear, and the earth would become a cold, dead mass like the moon.

Early on, humans discovered the healing powers of heat. Probably the first "heat treatment" occurred when prehistoric man rubbed an aching limb to make it feel better. (Friction from rubbing two surfaces against each other produces heat.)

Healing with Heat through the Ages: Physicians in the ancient civilizations of Greece, Rome, Egypt, and Babylonia all used heat for therapeutic purposes, and it is part of the healing tradition in Chinese and Ayurvedic medicine as well. In China, heat is sometimes used instead of (or in combination with) a needle to stimulate an acupuncture point. This process is called *moxibustion*. It is named for *moxa*, the leaf of the Chinese wormwood tree. When lit, moxa smolders without burning, so it can be placed on the body where its heat will stimulate the acupuncture point. Sometimes a ball of moxa is placed on the acupuncture needle, but moxibustion is also often used by itself. Today commercially prepared moxa sticks are available.

We can't think of heat therapy without thinking of water. All the ancient civilizations used therapeutic hot baths. The Romans, in particular, made a ritual of bathing, and their bathhouses would be the envy of a modern-day health club: hot baths, cold baths, large pools, massage; they had them all. The ruins of the magnificent Baths of Caracalla, which covered nearly thirty acres, are a popular tourist attraction today. Moderns didn't invent the health spa either. In fact, the term *spa* comes from the name of a village of the same name that was popular for its naturally occurring hot springs when the Roman Legions were on the march. Throughout history, people have used heat and cold in combination to make themselves feel better. At least as far back as the Middle Ages, Scandinavians enjoyed the invigorating experience of first sweating in a sauna and then rolling in a snowbank.

Sweating It Out: The idea of sweating out an illness has a long tradition in folk medicine everywhere. In the United States, Native Americans call their superheated healing rooms "sweat lodges." Treatment usually includes herbs and other medications as well as heat. Often the patient leaves the sweat lodge and leaps into an icy stream just as the Scandinavians do.

Modern-day deodorant manufacturers have given sweat a bad name, but it is actually the body's natural air-conditioning system. Sweat cools the body by evaporation and keeps us from becoming dangerously overheated when the temperature soars and during exercise. In general, people who are physically active sweat more—and at a lower temperature—than do sedentary people. In just a couple of hours on a hot day, an athlete can lose as much as eight pounds of water. Women don't begin to sweat as quickly as men. On average, a woman's body temperature is a full degree higher than a man's before she begins to "glow," as they used to say in the days when sweating was considered unfeminine.

In Elizabethan times, the odor of sweat was considered an aphrodisiac, and lovers exchanged peeled apples they had worn under their armpits. Today most people try to keep their sweat odorless, but profuse sweaters can be proud of the rivers running down their faces; it's a sign their bodies are in good working order.

INSTRUCTIONS

Heat therapy is one of the easiest and least expensive treatments available, and because it has such wide applications, it is ideal for self-care. Just remember a few basic principles, and you'll be able to find all sorts of applications for heat. For many conditions, heat can be combined with cold for a one-two punch against health problems.

Heat increases the heart rate and opens up the blood vessels to increase circulation, whereas cold constricts the blood vessels and slows down the heart and circulation. Therefore, heat is *not* a good treatment for inflammation because it brings more blood to an area that is already congested. A good criterion to use to decide whether to use heat or cold is the temperature of the affected body part. If it's already hot and swollen, then use cold as the treatment. If not, then heat may help.

Hot baths work wonders for a variety of problems including:

- Aches and pains following exercise
- Arthritis
- Initial symptoms of colds or flu
- Stress

For the most part, you shouldn't use heat on swelling, but experts say that a warm sitz bath can ease hemorrhoid or post-childbirth pain. Put a few inches of water in the tub and sit with your knees drawn up for about fifteen minutes.

You can use heat on one part of your body to make another part of your body feel better. For example, you may be able to unclog congested nasal passages by heating up your feet. (Use a hot foot bath, hot water bottle, or heating pad.) The way it works is that the heat dilates the blood vessels in your feet, causing more blood to flow toward that part of your body and away from your head. As blood leaves the nasal area, congestion decreases. This treatment often works for sinus headache and congestion from cold symptoms.

Contrast Therapy: When circulation increases to an area, blood brings in more vital oxygen and carries away waste products and toxins, thus promoting healing. To rev up circulation, try contrast therapy. Contrast therapy uses alternating heat and cold to dilate and then contract blood vessels. Alternate dilation and contraction forces the pumping action that carries blood swiftly throughout the body.

Contrast baths can really help reduce muscle and joint pain and stiffness from a variety of ailments, including arthritis and sports-related problems. Soak the sore area in a tub, bucket, or basin of water at about 104° F. for about five minutes. Then plunge it into cold water (about 59° F.) for a minute or two. Keep alternating between cold and hot for fifteen to twenty minutes. Some experts believe that contrast baths are twice as effective as either hot or cold therapy by themselves.

You might also try contrast treatment on a migraine headache. It doesn't work for everybody, but some people get relief by taking a hot shower followed by a cool one. (Contrast therapy gives your system quite a jolt, so don't try it without a healthcare practitioners' okay if you are pregnant or have heart-related problems or diabetes. When in doubt, check first.)

You'll find plenty of uses for heat therapy (and heat combined with cold) if you'll remember that heat increases blood flow to an area, whereas cold reduces it. The two together produce a pumping action that improves circulation.

FURTHER READING

Dail, Clarence W., and Charles S. Thomas. *Simple Remedies for the Home*. Banning Calif.: Preventive Healthcare and Education Center, 1985.

Horay, Patrick. *Hot Water Therapy*. Oakland, Calif.: New Harbinger Publications, 1991.

Licht, Sidney Herman, and Herman Kamenetz. *Therapeutic Heat and Cold*. New Haven, Conn.: E. Licht, 1965.

Michlovitz, Susan L., and Steven L. Wolf. *Thermal Agents in Rehabilitation*. Philadelphia: Davis, 1986.

HYDROTHERAPY (WATER THERAPY, SEE ALSO THALASSOTHERAPY)

DEFINITION

Hydrotherapy is the internal or external use of hot or cold, fresh or mineral water for healing.

APPLICATIONS

Physiological: Muscle aches, sprains, arthritis, rheumatism, eczema, psoriasis, blood circulation, pain, inflammation, hemorrhoids, back pain, colds, flu, headache, infections, joint stiffness, overweight, chronic pain, sinus problems, wounds
Psychological: Stress, tension, insomnia, inability to concentrate, nervousness, phobias, smoking addiction

COLLATERAL CROSS-THERAPIES

Thalassotherapy, swimming, water exercises, aromatherapy

RECOMMENDED ADJUNCT ACTIVITIES AND BEHAVIORS

During prolonged soaks, you may want to read or listen to music. Be sure to keep the source of the music away from the water and don't adjust the controls while you're wet.

CONTRAINDICATIONS

Most forms of hydrotherapy are safe for anyone, but people with heart conditions should avoid extremes in temperature.

EQUIPMENT & MATERIALS

Depending upon the form of therapy, you may need a tub, pool, spa, whirlpool, or shower. You may also need wet cloths or towels, and you might like to add aromatic oils or herbs to your bath.

ORIGIN

Water is essential to all forms of life, so it is not surprising that this wonderful refreshing fluid has been used for healing since humankind first appeared. Ruins of ancient civilizations almost all include some form of bath. Cretans, Egyptians, and Babylonians all soaked themselves for health and relaxation, and they practiced other forms of water therapy as well. So did the Hindus in long-ago India.

In the fifth century B.C. the Greek physician Hippocrates touted natural spring water for its healthful effects, and somewhat later another physician, Galen, developed a whole regimen of exercise, massage, and bathing for the sick.

Sparta, the Greek city-state that rivaled Athens, was famous for the toughness of its people. To ensure that their babies grew up strong and healthy, the Spartans dunked newborns into cold water. They also believed that this frigid introduction into the world would immunize the children against disease.

Romans Loved Their Baths: The Romans weren't the first to build baths, but they certainly carried bathing to a high art. They built huge, spacious, beautifully decorated buildings to house their baths, which were large enough for swimming and exercising in the water. Bathing was an elaborate ritual that began with scraping the dirt and sweat from the body with a special tool called a strigil. After that, it was off to the bath for a swim or a relaxing soak. Then the Roman of leisure could nip into the steam room and perhaps follow that with a quick plunge into a smaller bath with the temperature of his choice: hot, warm, or cold. To top it all off, our well-pampered Roman might finish with an invigorating massage.

There were many elaborate bathing palaces scattered throughout Rome, but the most spectacular was the Baths of Caracalla, which covered nearly thirty acres. The remnants of this bath still stand, and today operas are sometimes performed there. The famous Roman aqueducts carried water to the baths, so they could build one wherever it struck their fancy.

When the Roman Legions went on the march, they carried their bathing customs with them. In fact, the bath house was one of the first buildings they built when they conquered new territory. The city of Bath, England, is so-named because the Romans built a bath there, the remains of which can still be seen. The Romans were also fond of mineral springs and often visited the waters at Spa, a village in what is now Belgium. It is from this village that the modern name for a luxurious bathing retreat is derived.

We're all familiar with the term "Turkish Bath," and it really did originate in Turkey. The first Turkish baths were built in Istanbul, which was then called Constantinople, in the fifteenth century.

During the Middle Ages, bathing became unpopular throughout much of Europe, but the Scandinavians were ardent devotees of the sauna even then. They sat in small rooms heated by log fires until the temperature became unbearable, then dashed outside to roll in the snow or plunge into an icy pool. To make the experience even more invigorating, they slapped their skin with bunches of birch or pine twigs after the plunge. Today many people still take their saunas this way.

Water therapy was repopularized in Europe in the mid-19th century by a German priest, Father Sebastian Kneipp, who developed a cold-water treatment that apparently cured his own tuberculosis. Father Kneipp's treatment, known as the "Kneipp Cure," later featured not only cold water, but sunshine, fresh air, and regular activity. The cure also included walking barefoot in dew-moistened grass or snow, alternating hot and cold baths, and warm wraps.

The Kneipp Cure was well-known in Europe for many years before it finally came to the United States in the early 1900s. Kneipp wrote several books about his treatment, the most famous of which was *Meine Was-serkur* ("My Water Cure").

Dr. John Harvey Kellogg was an American physician, surgeon, and inventor of medical devices. He was also a proponent of many forms of natural medicine, and in his sanitorium in Battle Creek, Michigan, he treated patients with hydrotherapy, diet, and other non-drug therapies. His book *Rational Hydrotherapy* became a model text on the subject.

Kneipp and Kellogg helped to make hydrotherapy known in the United States, but it had actually been practiced here all along. Native Americans built "sweat lodges" that were similar to saunas to cure disease. Healing herbs were often added for their aromatic vapors. After inhaling the vapors in the sweat lodge, the patient would go outside for a cold plunge into a nearby river or snowbank.

Hydrotherapy is probably as popular today as it has ever been, although most people relaxing in a sauna or hot tub probably don't realize they're giving themselves a "treatment."

INSTRUCTIONS

The ways in which you can use water as therapy are nearly limitless, and you probably already know most of them. Here's a quick list to jog your memory:

- Drink six to eight glasses of pure water daily. (Mineral water is fine.)
- Soak your feet in a tub of very warm water after a long day. Then quickly run cold water over them and give them a brisk rubdown.
- To ease tension, soak your whole body in a tub filled with warm water. Add your favorite herb or scented oil for a special treat.
- For relief of arthritis, soak in a hot tub (temperature no higher than 104° F.) for no more than fifteen minutes. Put a cold washcloth on your head to prevent headache or congestion. Obviously, if you have a real "hot tub," you can use this instead, but don't exceed the time and temperature. (Hot tubs are not recommended for pregnant women or people with circulation problems, high blood pressure, nerve impairment, diabetes, or heart disease.) After the hot bath, splash with cool or lukewarm water to normalize your blood vessels.
- Fill a basin or the washbowl with very hot water, drape a towel over your head and inhale the steam. Add some herbs if you want to. This is a great skin treatment, and it can help clear your nasal passages if you have a cold or sinus congestion. Try adding some eucalyptus oil if congestion is your problem.
- Lie down and cover your eyes and forehead with a warm wet towel to banish stress and/or relieve a minor headache.

- Swim or do water exercises to keep yourself fit.
- Turn your shower on to needle-sharp or pulsating mode to massage aching muscles.
- Try alternating hot- and cold-water baths/showers or wet packs to soothe pain. Hot, then cold, baths are called contrast baths. They promote healing in a variety of conditions by causing the blood vessels to alternately dilate and contract. This sets the blood pumping and improves circulation. Start with four minutes of hot (104° F.) water, then one minute of cold (59° F.) water. Repeat the process five or six times.
- Relax (if you can) in a warm sitz bath to relieve the discomfort of hemorrhoids. (For a sitz bath, just put a few inches of water in the tub and sit with your feet flat so that your knees are raised.)
- Either a cold or warm sitz bath can help relieve the pain and swelling after childbirth.
- Have trouble falling asleep? Try a just-above-skin-temperature (about 100° F.) bath just before bed. Soak for as long as a half hour, dry off, and go to bed immediately.
- Got a migraine? A hot shower followed by a cool one might help.
- Try using your feet to alleviate a cold or cure a sinus headache. Soaking your feet in a hot tub pulls blood from the head to the feet and may unclog your nasal passages.

Here are a couple of more exotic water therapies you might try if you have access to the facilities. There's a new form of water therapy called *watsu*. Watsu is shiatsu done in warm water. Watsu was developed in the early 1980s at Harbin Hot Springs in northern California by Harold Dull, a Zen shiatsu master. Watsu practitioners are licensed by the Worldwide Aquatic Bodywork Association. If you're interested, contact them to find a practitioner in your area.

For the ultimate in relaxation, you might like to try a session in a flotation tank. A flotation tank is the updated version of what used to be known as a "sensory deprivation" tank, but don't let that name scare you. It doesn't deprive you of *your* senses, only the distractions of the outside world. The tank is a completely dark, soundproof chamber in which you float effortlessly in skin-temperature water treated with epsom salts. (It's the epsom salts that keep you afloat.) For the claustrophobic, there's an intercom to connect you with the outside. Some tanks have dim lights and Jacuzzi attachments, but you'll relax more if you tune out everything and just float. Where can you find a flotation tank? Try a stress-management or pain-control center, or an athletic camp. In some places, there are also commercial float centers.

FURTHER READING

Berson, Dvera, and Sander Roy. *Pain-Free Arthritis*. Brooklyn: S&J Books, c1982. (Hydrotherapy and exercise; book is also available in large type.)

Buchman, Dian Dincin. *The Complete Book of Water Therapy*. New Canaan, Ct.: Keats Publishing, c1994.

Horay, Patrick, and David Harp. *Hot Water Therapy*. Oakland, Calif.: New Harbinger Publications, 1991.

Lawrence, D. Baloti. *Waterworks: with Therapies for Health and Fitness*. New York: Perigee Books, c1989.

RESOURCE GROUPS

Flotation Tank Association
PO Box 1396
Grass Valley, CA 95945-1396
Phone: 916/432-3794

Membership $25; *Floating* magazine; directory of flotation centers

United States Water Fitness Association, Inc.
PO Box 3279
Boynton Beach, FL 33424
Phone: 407/732-9908

Publications, videos; information about water exercising; referrals for programs, instructors

HELIOTHERAPY/PHOTOTHERAPY (LIGHT THERAPY)

DEFINITION

Heliotherapy is treatment of disease with sunlight. Phototherapy treats disease with artificial light.

APPLICATIONS

Physiological: Hair loss, impotence, rickets, dermatitis, jet lag, leukemia, psoriasis, rheumatoid arthritis, scleroderma, vitiligo, eczema
Psychological: Depression, insomnia, irritability, seasonal affective disorder, alcohol abuse

COLLATERAL CROSS-THERAPIES

Color therapy

RECOMMENDED ADJUNCT ACTIVITIES AND BEHAVIORS

None

CONTRAINDICATIONS

Sunlight has many beneficial effects, but it can also cause serious damage as can artificial lights like suntan lamps. The incidence of skin cancer has risen dramatically over the past few years. This may be due in part to the thinning of the ozone layer, which allows greater penetration of ultraviolet rays, but it is also related to people's desire to have a "healthy tan." There is nothing "healthy" about a suntan. Exposing your skin to the sun for the purposes of tanning greatly increases your risk of skin cancer, and it also leads to premature aging (wrinkling) of the skin. Sunscreens help protect against damaging rays, but the safest way to get a tan—if you must have one—is from a bottle.

Sunlamps carry the same risk as natural sunlight. Many people have suffered severe burns and permanent scarring from having fallen asleep under a sunlamp.

When you're going to be outdoors in the daytime, always wear a sunscreen with a protection factor of 15 or better, even on a cloudy day. Use sunblock if you have the type of skin that burns easily. Wear sunglasses to protect your eyes.

EQUIPMENT & MATERIALS

Full-spectrum light bulbs, sunlight

ORIGIN

From the time the first human warily opened an eyelid and looked to the east, the rising sun has signaled a new beginning, a fresh start on this business of living. Natural phenomena were the most powerful influences on our early ancestors, so it is not surprising that they personified the sun and the moon and called them gods. Then as now, dawn was something special, and it had its own godly status. Some cultures worshipped the sun god as the all-powerful creator of everything on earth. *Sun Worship in Central America:*   In Central America, the Aztecs kept the sun god supplied with the still-beating hearts of human and animal sacrificial victims to ensure that the vital life energy continued to flow to earth. The god's appetite for hearts was so voracious that the Aztecs were forced to fight wars, not for conquest of territory, but for captives that could be sacrificed, sometimes thousands at a time.

The Mayas practiced sun worship and sacrifice as well. And in Peru, the emperors of the Incas derived their divine right to rule from the sun because they were its children.

The Egyptians, Greeks, and Romans: Most cultures had a long list of gods that they worshipped, with the sun god generally being the most powerful. Ancient Egypt was no exception, but in the fourteenth century B.C. the ruling pharaoh revolutionized society by decreeing that thereafter, the Egyptians would worship only one god: Aton, the sun god. To honor the god, the pharaoh changed his name from the royal patronym Amenhotep to Akhenaton.

The sun was a god to both the Greeks and the Romans. The Roman sun god was Sol, a name for the sun that we still use today. Both the Greeks and the Romans knew more about astronomy than they did about most other sciences. Among other achievements, the Greeks accurately predicted solar eclipses, and the Romans named all the constellations.

Solstice Celebrations: Unless we have a special interest, most of us today don't follow the changing seasons that closely, but for our ancestors, the phases of the moon, the solstices, and the equinoxes were significant (and often worrisome) events. Throughout the world, people celebrated the summer and winter solstices, which are the longest and shortest days of the year, respectively. At the summer solstice, people lit huge bonfires in the vain hope that they could rekindle the sun's waning energy and keep the days from shortening as the season moved toward winter. This never worked, of course, but they kept trying. Even today, some European towns preserve the tradition of the fire festival at the solstice.

Worry about what the sun was going to do was at the root of most religious rituals. What if people woke up one morning and it *wasn't* morning: the sun didn't rise? Worse, what if the sun went away somewhere and never came back? (And we moderns think *we* have a lot of stress!) People knew that their very lives depended upon the sun's continuing to follow the cycle of the seasons, and they spent a great deal of time fretting about the hideous possibility that the sun might capriciously decide to chuck it all and disappear. As you can imagine, a solar eclipse was a truly terrifying event that had to be countered with all sorts of rituals to induce the sun's return.

Some cultures also believed that the sun god could impregnate women. A Colombian Indian legend has it that a powerful chieftain wanted his daughter to have a child by the sun, so he ordered her to climb the east side of a mountain every morning to receive the first rays. In due time, the daughter gave birth to an emerald, which miraculously evolved into a human boy.

Other creation myths deal with the birth of the sun itself. One African legend tells that the sun was originally a human being endowed with the extraordinary ability to emit sunlight by raising his arms. This was wonderful for those nearby who could bask in its glow, but people wanted more. They wanted sunlight to shine down on the whole world, so they all got together and with a mighty heave they flung the man into the sky where he has remained ever since.

Moonstruck: For thousands of years, people also revered the moon as a god. They celebrated the new moon and the full moon, but a waning moon made them fearful. Depending upon their attitudes toward these events, various peoples honored the moon as the benefactor of the menstrual cycle and of birth or viewed it as a vengeful god who heaped its wrath upon women once a month.

Historically, people also connected the moon with rain, tides, and the growth of living things. Of course, the sun was also associated with growth cycles. Among others, the Mayans and the Indians of the U.S. Southwest determined the vernal equinox by means of precisely placed slits in specially constructed buildings through which the sun shone just at the equinox and only then. Thus they knew that planting time was near. (The vernal equinox is the midpoint between the winter and summer solstices when day and night are the same length. There is also an autumnal equinox.)

Health and Cycles of Light: Early on, people discovered that the earth's cycles of light were related to cycles within the human body and to health. At least 5,000 years ago, Chinese physicians recognized that the human body has its own rhythms that change within the course of each day, with the seasons, and, in women, with the stages of the menstrual cycle. Somewhat later, the Greek physician Hippocrates made similar observations, but many centuries passed before western scientists found proof that the body is governed by an internal twenty-four hour clock known as the *circadian system.*

Hippocrates and his colleagues used heliotherapy (from Helios, the Greek sun god) for various ailments. They prescribed sunbaths to help heal wounds and to strengthen muscles. The Romans too took sunbaths for health. Wealthy Romans built solariums atop their houses where they could bask in sunshine privately.

With the advent of Christianity, heliotherapy declined in the western world. The Christians treated anything that smacked of sun worship as pagan and banned it.

In the 1700s the writings of French philosopher Jean Jacques Rousseau brought a renewed interest in the so-called "natural life," and people once again experimented with using the sun to heal. Toward the end of the century, French physicians reported curing leg ulcers and cancer with sunlight. For the latter disease, they used optical lenses to focus the rays.

It was an eighteenth-century experiment with the heliotrope flower (named for the Greek sun god Helios) that led to the proof of the existence of circadian rhythms. The heliotrope opens at dawn, turns to follow the passage of the sun throughout the day, and closes as the sun sets. A French scientist found that the heliotrope followed this pattern even when it was kept in the dark and could not "see" the sun.

People thought this was interesting, but they didn't do any serious follow up on circadian rhythms until the twentieth century. Now we know that all living things have internal clocks that follow an approximate twenty-four-hour cycle. Our bodies change throughout the day according to our own personal rhythms. The fact that one person is a "morning" person while another can't add two and two until midday is governed by each person's internal clock. Normally our clocks are "set" by the twenty-four-hour cycle of light and darkness. If you were to spend your life in a cave, your body would still run on a daily cycle, although it might get out of whack with the cycle in the outside world.

A Light in Your Eyes: The eyes are the primary organs through which light affects the body. Sunlight enters the body through the skin too, but it doesn't penetrate very far. When light enters the eyes, it is transformed into electrical impulses that travel to the brain by several different pathways. One pathway leads to the visual cortex, which allows us to see images. Another leads to the hypothalamus, the regulator of many of our vital functions.

Located deep in the brain, the pea-sized, cone-shaped pineal gland receives light information from the eyes via the hypothalamus. Until recently, scientists weren't quite sure what the pineal gland did or even whether it did anything useful at all. Studies now reveal that the pineal gland is attuned to light changes in the environment. The pineal secretes a hormone called melatonin in rhythm with daily and seasonal light-dark cycles. The pineal secretes the most melatonin in total darkness and the least in bright light. Melatonin acts as a sort of on-off switch for the body's other functions, telling them when to work and when to rest. Melatonin travels through the bloodstream so it affects all our bodily processes and keeps them functioning according to their own rhythms.

Did you ever wonder how your cat "knows" to put on a thicker winter coat even though there isn't a snowflake in sight yet? The pineal gland notes the ever-shortening hours of daylight and signals the cat's body to get out the heavy-duty fur. The reproductive cycle is governed in the same way.

Until the invention of the electric light bulb, all the light that affected our health came from the sun. Today workers who toil all day in windowless offices illuminated by fluorescent lights may rarely see the sun. Sunlight contains the full spectrum of light necessary to maintain life, but most artificial light is deficient in some areas of the spectrum. Light bulbs come in cool-white, warm-white and a number of other configurations, including full-spectrum light that simulates natural sunlight. The latter is the only one that provides all the benefitsofsunshine.Despitetheall-pervasivenessofartificiallight,most people (and many scientists) remain unaware that the type of artificial light source can affect health, productivity, and emotional well-being.

Scientists have, however, developed artificial lights with specific spectrums for treatment of various illnesses. This type of therapy with artificial light is known as *phototherapy*. Another form, photodynamic therapy, involves the use of certain chemicals that are light-activated. Although still experimental, photodynamic therapy has shown promising results in thousands of cancer patients worldwide, and researchers are investigating its use in a number of other diseases.

INSTRUCTIONS

Many of the therapeutic uses of light are not available for self-healing, but there are licensed physicians in nearly every state who use phototherapy as part of their treatment protocol. The book *Light: Medicine of the Future* by Dr. Jacob Liberman lists physicians who use phototherapy as treatment for cancer, certain vision disorders, and seasonal affective disorder. (Also check **Resource Groups** at the end of this section.)

Most of the light-therapy techniques that you can use on your own are relatively simple and inexpensive, but they can have a dramatic effect upon your health and sense of well-being.

Strong Bones and Teeth: One of the beneficial effects of sunlight is that it produces vitamin D in skin exposed to ultraviolet rays. Vitamin D is essential for the proper metabolism of calcium, which builds strong bones and teeth. Some researchers believe that neither vitamin supplements nor the vitamin D in foods is adequate for this purpose. Fortunately, it takes very little sunshine to promote vitamin D synthesis. Except for areas near the poles, a thrice-weekly fifteen-minute walk with the face exposed to the sun will do the trick.

If you hardly ever get outdoors or work all day in artificial light, you may need to get a little more sunshine into your system. Even in midwinter, a short stroll in the daytime should rev up your vitamin D production and help your body absorb bone-strengthening calcium better. Older people especially need this protection to prevent hip fracture, which can be caused either by osteoporosis or adult rickets (osteomalacia).

Seasonal Affective Disorder: For a long time, people didn't understand why they often got the winter blahs. Now we know that seasonal affective disorder (SAD) is caused by the low levels of natural sunlight in the wintertime. Some people experience only minor blues on cold, gray February days, while others are so severely depressed that they can barely function at all. The condition is often worse and more prolonged in the more northern latitudes that have the fewest daylight hours. (In northern Alaska, SAD can get a grip on people as early as August.) Most people who are afflicted with SAD are adults, although it can occur in children too.

The treatment for SAD and milder winter depression is the same: exposure to bright full-spectrum light to trick the brain into thinking it's springtime. Most experts recommend a light box that contains at least six forty-watt full-spectrum fluorescent tubes that provide a brightness of 2,500 lux. (A lux is a measure of the brightness of light based on the light given off by a candle. One candle equals one lux.) Units are available that produce even brighter light: the equivalent of 10,000 lux. The brighter the light, the shorter the amount of time a person needs to be exposed.

Generally, morning and noon are the best times to use the light treatment. (The treatment can speed up or slow down your internal clock, so you may need to experiment with the time of day to avoid disrupting your sleep patterns too much.) Exposure time varies with the individual, the time of year, the climate, and the place where he/she lives. Some people get relief with only a half hour of exposure, while others require up to four hours daily.

An occasional person experiences positive effects after just one session, but most need two to four days of treatment before they feel better. If you skip the treatment for only a couple of days, your symptoms are likely to return, so you should continue the daily treatments for the entire period during which environmental light is insufficient for your needs. (If you want to, you can replace some of your regular bulbs with full-spectrum bulbs for everyday lighting. These bulbs do cost a little more.)

Scientists are developing new portable units to be worn on the head like visors. These will allow a person to be mobile while receiving treatment, and they will be a boon to travelers. Other features that are now available include a timer that gradually increases and decreases the light to simulate dawn and dusk. Folks with these devices often set them to turn on just as they're waking up. (See *Resource Groups* at the end of this section for a list of manufacturers of full-spectrum bulbs and fixtures.)

Skin Disorders: If you have eczema or psoriasis, you may find that a dose of sunlight is just the ticket for alleviating these problems. There are no set rules for the amount of exposure that will help, so you'll have to experiment a bit. Start with about ten minutes a day several times a week in the morning or afternoon. Don't expose your skin at midday; the risk of damage from ultraviolet rays then outweighs any beneficial effects on your skin condition.

Give the ten-minutes-a-day regime a chance to work—several weeks, at least—before increasing your exposure. Then first try increasing the number of days of exposure before increasing exposure time. If the treatment doesn't seem to be working, you can ultimately increase exposure up to a half hour, but talk to your healthcare practitioner before going beyond that.

Sunlight is a practical treatment for skin conditions in the summer, but if you live in a northern climate, you may need to turn to a full-spectrum artificial light source in the winter. You can use the same sort of set-up as that for SAD. In fact, if your mood is a bit dark, you may find that both your spirits and your skin clear up with a simulated-sunlight treatment. (Sunlamps have such a potential for harmful exposure we hesitate to even mention them, but we suspect that someone might be tempted to use one. Do not use a sunlamp for your skin condition without checking with your healthcare practitioner or a dermatologist first.)

Jet Lag: Zooming across several time zones in the course of a single day gets you where you're going in a hurry, but it also knocks your internal clock for a loop. The result is jet lag. Fortunately, you can use ordinary light and darkness to help reset your body's clock:

- Start resetting your clock by shielding your eyes from the morning sun (until about 10 A.M.) on the day of your departure, during the flight, and on the day of your arrival. To do this, wear *very* dark sunglasses (dark goggles are even better, but you'll look a little weird on the plane) and close the blinds or pull down the shade on the plane.
- On those same days, get as much exposure to afternoon sun as you can. If you're flying during the afternoon, try to sit by a window, keep the shade up and resist the inflight movie.

Experts say this method works regardless of which direction you're flying. You can adjust your body's clock by up to three hours per day. If you're a shift worker, you can use the same principles to trick your body into resetting its clock to suit your new hours.

FURTHER READING

Babbitt, Edwin D. *The Principles of Light and Color*. Secaucus, N.J.: Citadel Press, 1980.

Douglas, William Campbell. *Into the Light*. Atlanta: Second Opinion Publishing, 1993.

Huber, Frederick C. *Light, Color and Life for the World*. New York: D. McKay Co., 1978.

Hyman, Jane Wegscheider. *The Light Book*. Los Angeles: Jeremy P. Tarcher, Inc., 1990.

Liberman, Jacob, Ph.D. *Light: Medicine of the Future*. Santa Fe: Bear & Co. Publishing, 1991.

Lillyquist, Michael J. *Sunlight & Health: The Positive and Negative Effects of the Sun on You*. New York: Dodd, Mead & Co., 1985.

Moreines, Robert L. and Patricia L. McGuire. *Light Up Your Blues*. New York: Berkley Books, 1989.

Ott, John Nash. *Health and Light*. New York: Pocket Books, 1976.

Rosenthal, Norman E. *Winter Blues: Seasonal Affective Disorder*. New York: Guilford Press, 1993.

Smyth, Angela. *SAD: Seasonal Affective Disorder*. London: HarperCollins, 1991.

RESOURCE GROUPS

College of Syntonic Optometry
c/o Jacob Liberman, O.D., Ph.D
PO Box 4058
Aspen, CO 81612-4058

The college is an organization devoted to the research and clinical application of ocularly perceived light. Dr. Liberman is the president. Write him for information on lectures and seminars.

Environmental Health & Light Research Institute, Inc.
16057 Tampa Palms Blvd., Ste. 227
Tampa, FL 33647
Phone: 800/LIGHTSU

Bimonthly newsletter *Modern Wellness* ($29.95)

Light Therapy Information Service, New York Psychiatric Institute
Phone: 212/960-5714

National Organization for Seasonal Affective Disorder (NOSAD)
PO Box 40133
Washington, D.C. 20016

Organization for seasonal affective disorder. Newsletter and D.C.-area support groups; information on other support groups in U.S.

Society for Light Treatment and Biological Rhythms
PO Box 478
Wilsonville, Ore. 97070
Phone: 503/694-2404

Newsletter, information about light treatments, lists of manufacturers and suppliers of light therapy products

Dinshah Health Society
100 Dinshah Drive

Malaga, NJ 08328
Phone: 609/692-4686

Membership: $3; newsletter, *Breath Forecast* (light calculations based upon the new moon); books, pamphlets

Listed below are some manufacturers of full-spectrum light bulbs. If you can't find the product in a local store, call the 800 number for the nearest dealer.

Duro-Test Corporation (VITA-LITE), 800-289-3876
G.E. Lighting (Chroma 50), 800-626-2000
GTE Products Corporation (Design 50), 800-225-5483
North American Philips (Colortone 50), 800-752-2852
Ott Light Systems, Inc. (Ott Light; this is a complete fixture, not just a bulb), 800-234-3724

MAGNETIC THERAPY (MAGNOTHERAPY, MAGNETIC FIELD THERAPY, BIOMAGNETISM, AND BIOMAGNETIC THERAPY)

DEFINITION

Magnetic therapy is the biological use of magnetism to promote healing in human beings or animals. Magnets or magnetic fields do not themselves cure ailments. Rather, they stimulate the body's own natural processes. For example, magnetism might be used to increase blood circulation to an injured area.

APPLICATIONS

Physiological: Sprains, strains, bruises, broken bones, chronic pain, wounds, circulatory problems, burns, cancer, rheumatoid disease, headache, infections, toothache, kidney stones, edema
Psychological: Insomnia and sleep disorders, environmental stress

COLLATERAL CROSS-THERAPIES

Reflexology

CONTRAINDICATIONS

Pregnant women should not use magnetic therapy on the abdomen.

EQUIPMENT & MATERIALS

Therapeutic magnets. Standard horseshoe-shaped and bar magnets are not therapeutic magnets. Some therapeutic magnets are hard and inflexible, while others are flat and flexible. The magnetic material may be ceramic, plastiform, or neodymium (a rare earth chemical element).

Regardless of the type or composition, all therapeutic magnets have a permanent magnetic charge.

Flexible pad magnets are available in various sizes and shapes to fit different body parts. You can also buy bracelets, necklaces, pillows, mattress pads, and shoe insoles that contain therapeutic magnets. (The shoe insoles may be used in conjunction with foot reflexology.) Some biomagnets are called boji stones.

ORIGIN

Human beings first investigated the healing power of magnetism thousands of years ago. We know that the ancient Greeks, Chinese, Egyptians, and Indians all knew about magnetism and used it to heal.

No one knows who first discovered magnetism, but legend tells that a shepherd boy tending his sheep strolled near a large rock while carrying his iron staff. An unseen force pulled him irresistibly toward the rock, finally grabbing his staff and holding it fast. Some say the boy's name was Magnes and that the rock was named the Magnes Stone in his honor. Another version tells that the boy made his discovery in a country called Magnesia in Asia Minor. Either way, the attraction of the mineral for iron became known as magnetism. An early name for iron ore with magnetic properties was lodestone, which it is still called today. The iron ore itself is magnetite.

People were awed by the way lodestone attracted iron, and many thought lodestones possessed magical powers. They often wore small pieces of the mineral as amulets around their necks or wrists. About 200 years before the birth of Christ, the Greek physician Galen found that he could relieve pain from illnesses by placing pieces of these natural magnets on various parts of the body.

The ancient Chinese also knew about magnetism. About 100 B.C., Chinese healers wrote about the way that the earth's magnetic field affected the body. But there is an interesting story about another use of magnetism long before that. It is said that the Moon Gate of the imperial palace of O-Fang, built over 2,000 years ago, was made entirely of one solid piece of lodestone. Visitors to the palace approached through this gate. If a person bent on mischief attempted to enter with a knife hidden in his clothing, the gate attracted the metal, and alert guards apprehended the miscreant. If this story is true, the Moon Gate at O-Fang beat the modern-day inventors of the metal detector by more than twenty centuries.

Despite the early use of lodestone for medicinal purposes in various parts of the world, many hundreds of years passed before people discovered that a magnet hung from a string turned until one end was pointing toward the North Pole and the other end toward the South Pole. This discovery led to the invention of the compass, which has been a godsend ever since for people who don't know in which direction they're going. (At the time, the compass made it possible for sailors to navigate without having to see the stars.)

Although people trusted the compass, they didn't know why it worked until the time of Queen Elizabeth I in England. In 1600, Dr. William Gilbert showed that the earth itself was one gigantic magnet and that it attracted the ends of the magnetic needle of the compass. Gilbert is considered the father of the scientific study of magnetism, although it can be argued that many of the ancients also understood a great deal of what Gilbert later described.

Toward the end of the eighteenth century, an Austrian physician named Franz (or Friedrich) Anton Mesmer worked with magnets to cure disease. He later abandoned this technique when it was frowned upon by the Viennese medical profession. Mesmer then developed a theory he called "animal magnetism" to explain human disease. He thought that the body contained a magnetic fluid and that disease resulted from the absence or improper distribution of this fluid. Mesmer developed a hypnotic technique—mesmerism—designed to restore magnetic fluid to sick people. In Paris, Mesmer was a sensation when he demonstrated his technique in sessions he called seances. However, the French Academy of Science appointed a commission to investigate his methods, and the commission denounced him as a fraud. (As the American representative in Paris, Benjamin Franklin was on this commission as were the famous French chemist Antoine Lavoisier and Joseph Guillotin, a physician for whom the guillotine is named.)

Although Mesmer was discredited at the time, his work laid the groundwork for the development of hypnotic techniques, and his earlier studies helped develop an interest in magnetic healing.

More recently, scientists in both Russia and Japan have worked with magnets to induce healing. During World War II, Soviet army doctors used magnets to relieve pain from battlefield wounds, and after the war, they used them to relieve leg pain before and after amputation and also to speed the healing of wounds. Some Canadian physicians have also applied magnets for faster wound healing.

Russian scientists, who call the use of therapeutic magnets "magnetobiology," treat some types of heart and nerve diseases with magnets attached to the wrists. They've also worked with using magnets to help lower blood pressure.

At present, biomagnetic therapy is better known outside of the United States. In Germany, for example, magnetic devices are well known and their use for some conditions is covered by health insurance. In Japan, tiny *tai-ki* magnets are used to stimulate acupuncture points.

In the United States, biomagnetism is still not generally accepted. At least one state (California) prohibits licensed healthcare practitioners from using magnets for treating illness and disease. However, therapeutic magnets are available for self-use and practitioners not bound by licensing requirements offer biomagnetic therapy.

INSTRUCTIONS

How does magnetic therapy work? First, the magnets themselves don't heal; they simply enhance the body's own inner healing process. In part, the body's system is governed by differing patterns of ionic currents and electromagnetic fields. Static magnetic fields can be produced by natural or artificial magnets. These magnetic fields are able to penetrate the human body and affect the functioning of the nervous system, organs, and cells. A negative magnetic field can increase metabolism, which in turn stimulates the flow of blood and oxygen to damaged cells. This negative energy acts something like an antibiotic by promoting oxygenation and reducing the body's acidity. The body thrives on a well-oxygenated alkaline environment, but disease-causing bacteria don't.

Most researchers in this field believe that the negative pole has a calming effect and works toward normalizing metabolism. In contrast, the positive pole promotes stress, and with long exposure, may actually interfere with metabolism and induce illness.

All magnets have a positive pole and a negative pole. However, researchers disagree as to how to name the poles, so in order to be sure you know which is which, you'll need to use a compass. The arrow pointing to "N" or "North" is pointing toward the magnet's negative pole.

The magnets are used therapeutically by placing one or more on the body above various organs, on various points on the head, on lymph nodes, and above the sites of bruises and other injuries. Treatments can last from a few moments to overnight. Depending upon the condition, magnets can be applied at various times during the day or for days or even weeks at a time. Some people use a negatively charged mattress pad or blanket for long-term treatment.

A negative magnetic field applied to the top of the head relaxes a person and helps induce sleep. Researchers believe that the negative energy stimulates the production of the hormone melatonin, which reduces stress and retards aging.

If you want to try magnetic therapy on your own, it's best to get the advice of a practitioner before you begin. He or she can tell you how to best apply the magnets to treat your particular problem. When properly used, magnetic therapy is safe, but you should heed these guidelines:

- Because it can promote stress and induce illness when improperly used, don't use the positive magnetic pole without professional supervision.

- Limit use of a magnetic blanket/bed to no more than ten hours per day.
- Wait an hour and a half after meals to use magnetic therapy on the abdomen so as not to interfere with digestion.
- Don't use magnets on the abdomen during pregnancy.

FURTHER READING

Bansal, H.L., and R.S. Bansal. *Magnetic Cure for Common Diseases.*

Becker, Robert O., M.D. *Cross Currents: The Promise of Electromedicine.* New York: St. Martin's Press, 1990.

Burke, Abbot George. *Magnetic Therapy: Healing in Your Hands.* Oklahoma City: Saint George Press, 1980.

Davis, Albert Roy, and Walter C. Rawls. *Magnetism and its Effects on the Living System.* Kansas City, Mo.: Acres U.S.A., 1993.

———. *The Magnetic Blueprint of Life.* Hicksville, N.Y.: Exposition Press, 1979.

Hacmac, Edward A. *An Overview of Biomagnetic Therapeutics,* 1991.

Jenkins, Richard Dean. "The Healing Power of Magnets," *Men's Fitness,* February 1992.

Philpott, William, and Sharon Taplin. *Biomagnetic Handbook.* Chocktaw, Okla.: Enviro-Tech Products, 1990.

Resonance (quarterly magazine; subscription: $6), PO Box 64, Sumterville, FL 33585; phone 904/793-8748.

Schiegl, Heinz. *Healing Magnetism: The Transference of Vital Force.* York Beach, Me.: Samuel Weiser, 1983.

Verschuur, Gerrit L. *Hidden Attraction: The History and Mysticism of Magnetism.* New York: Oxford University Press, 1993.

RESOURCE GROUPS

Albert Roy Davis Research Center
PO Box 655
Green Cove Springs, FL 32043.
Phone: 904/264-8564

Books, reports, magnets, and magnetic products.

Bio-Electro-Magnetics Institute
2490 West Moana Lane
Reno, NV 89509-3936
Phone: 702/827-9099

Publishes monthly journal, *BEMI Currents.*

Enviro-Tech Products
17171 SE 29th St.
Choctaw, OK 73020

Phone: 405/390-3499 (information) or 800/445-1962 (credit card orders)

Self-help information, books, magnets, sleep energizer system

MagnetiCo, Inc.
4562 14th St. NE
Calgary, AB, Canada T1Y 6C1
Phone: 403/291-0085

Manufactures and markets magnetic products, including a Sleep-Pad™ intended to restore energy during sleep.

Nikken Products
Ste. 250, Westwood Place
10866 Wilshire Blvd.
Los Angeles, CA 90024
Phone: 310/446-4300

Manufactures magnetic products.

Prometheus Italia SrL
Centro Commerciale, VR-EST
Viale del Lavoro 45 I-36037
S. Martino B.A. (VR), Italy.

Manufactures magnetic blankets.

THALASSOTHERAPY (SEE ALSO HYDROTHERAPY)

DEFINITION

Thalassotherapy is the therapeutic use of seawater or products derived from seawater.

APPLICATIONS

Physiological: Rheumatism, arthritis, skin diseases, metabolic imbalances, circulatory problems, cellulite
Psychological: Stress, tension

COLLATERAL CROSS-THERAPIES

Hydrotherapy, swimming, massage

RECOMMENDED ADJUNCT ACTIVITIES AND BEHAVIORS

While you're waiting for a sea mud pack or seaweed wrap to work its effects, you might want to relax with a good book or listen to some favorite music.

CONTRAINDICATIONS

Women who are pregnant or people with diabetes, heart conditions, or high blood pressure should not take seawater baths that are either extremely hot or extremely cold. The elderly and young children should also avoid extremes of heat or cold.

EQUIPMENT & MATERIALS

Seawater and/or products containing marine botanicals, such as seaweed and algae.

ORIGIN

From the Greek *thalassa*, meaning "sea," thalassotherapy really dates back to the first ocean bathers, whoever they may have been. The sea has always bewitched humankind. People have idolized it, feared it, frolicked in it, and lazed on its shores, but always they have respected its awesome power. From ancient times, people have looked to the sea for restoration and health. The Greeks, Romans, Cretans, Egyptians, and Babylonians built communal baths where they bathed in water brought from the sea. The Egyptians were fond of a vegetable known as a sea onion that grew near the shore. The sea onion was also used for medicinal purposes.

In the Orient, vegetables from the sea often grace the family table. From ancient times, Orientals have eaten various forms of seaweed and kelp, and they have used them for healing purposes.

In Victorian England, people flocked to the seashore for their holidays. At that time, hot and cold seawater baths were among the amenities offered by coastal resorts.

Although products from the sea have been used for healthful purposes for a long time, the term *thalassotherapy* is a relatively recent one. In 1869, a French physician coined the name for therapy that uses seawater and sea vegetables for a variety of treatments that include baths, facials, massages, body wraps, and cosmetic products. The French are still devotees of thalassotherapy; many French spas use piped-in seawater for their baths and showers, and personal-care products containing marine botanicals abound.

Sea plants and the water itself are rich in vitamins, amino acids, metalloids, and minerals. Proponents of thalassotherapy claim that these elements can be taken into the body through the skin to stimulate the body's own natural immune system, boost circulation, and hasten the elimination of wastes and toxins. Interestingly, the salts in seawater and sea vegetables are very similar to those found in human blood serum. Some people feel that this suggests that humans had an aquatic ancestor or two. Others merely cite the resemblance as evidence for why thalassotherapy works.

INSTRUCTIONS

Some spas and holistic health centers offer thalassotherapy treatments, but you don't have to live on the coast or fork out big bucks to see what thalassotherapy can do for you. There are a variety of personal-care products on the market that you can use at home. (If you use sea salt for cooking, you've already made a tiny entry into the field.)

Most of these products contain seaweed, a vegetable rich in iodine, calcium, magnesium, potassium, sulfur, sodium, trace elements, and vitamins A, D, and E. Believers say that seaweed conditions and nourishes hair and skin and helps them retain moisture. You can buy cleansers, masks, moisturizers, shampoos, lotions, bath salts (a popular product comes from the Dead Sea), shower products, slimming gels, and creams that purport to control cellulite. If you want to emulate a spa experience, you might also want to try a seaweed body wrap. Follow that with a Sea Mud Mineral Soak (Erno Laszlo), which instantly turns your bathwater a beautiful cerulean blue, and you'll be transported to the Mediterranean without ever leaving home!

Here's a partial list of the purported benefits of seaweed:

- Softens and soothes dry skin and makes it more supple and elastic
- Plumps the skin so wrinkles are less visible
- Promotes cell division and regeneration
- Adds body, sheen, and softness to hair; controls dandruff
- Helps remove cellulite from the hips and thighs by releasing and eliminating toxins.

Oil of algae is another marine botanical that is said to have restorative powers. Massaged into the skin several times daily, it is purported to control fungal skin infections, such as athlete's foot and fingernail fungus. Mothers also use it to prevent diaper rash and cradle cap in their babies.

FURTHER READING

Hirschhorn, Howard H. *Helping Yourself to Health from the Sea*. West Nyack, N.Y.: Parker Publishing Co., 1979.
Inglis, Brian, and Ruth West. *Alternative Health Guide*. New York: Knopf, 1983.
Lord, Shirley, ed. "Holistic Treatments." *Vogue*, December 1991.
Wilson, Roberta. "Skin Care from the Sea," *Let's Live*, January 1993.

EATING FOR HEALTH

Our ideas about what constitutes a healthful diet have undergone some radical changes in the last thirty years or so. At the dawn of history, human beings ate mostly plant foods, adding a bit of meat, fish, or fowl when they got lucky. A crash course on human anatomy shows that people were probably designed to consume mostly plant foods. We don't have the teeth or the digestive systems of carnivores.

Nevertheless, over the course of centuries, people—particularly in affluent countries—began to consume more and more meat and other rich foods. However, as recently as 100 years ago, people in the United States still got two thirds of their protein from plants like beans and grains. Today about 70 percent of our protein comes from animal products.

Until fairly recently we applauded ourselves for our meat-rich, high-protein diets. Carbohydrates were foodstuffs to be careful we didn't eat too much of, but meat? Wolf it down to your heart's content! It's good for you.

Now with mounting evidence that the typical Western diet contributes to clogged arteries, hypertension, and dangerously elevated cholesterol levels, nutritionists have done an about-face. Today we are told we should cut out those animal products with their saturated fats and high cholesterol, and take it easy on the salt. It seems that the once-scorned vegetarian was on the more healthful course after all.

New findings in nutrition bode well for disease prevention too. Research shows that certain foods can actually protect you against major diseases like cancer and stroke.

In this section, we offer a variety of eating plans, some for general good health and others for specific conditions. Enjoy.

ARTHRITIS DIETS (NO-NIGHTSHADE DIET AND DONG DIET)

DEFINITION

Diets for people with osteoarthritis and rheumatoid arthritis

APPLICATIONS

Physiological: Pain and stiffness of arthritis

COLLATERAL CROSS-THERAPIES

Special exercises for arthritis; aerobic exercise, herbalism, healing diets, vegetarianism

CONTRAINDICATIONS

None, unless you have sensitivity or allergy to suggested foods

EQUIPMENT & MATERIALS

Ordinary kitchen equipment for preparing food

ORIGIN

From ancient times, people have used foods to try to cure various diseases, including arthritis. The Ebers Papyrus, a sort of medical encyclopedia compiled by the Egyptians about 2,000 years ago, lists food remedies for many diseases, including arthritis. Today we know that arthritis has no "cure" as such, but the symptoms can be relieved, and possibly diet can help.

There are dietary folk remedies that purport to help people with arthritis. One such diet that has a small but enthusiastic following endorses wheat germ, avocados, brewer's yeast, bananas, and pecans. These foods must be eaten, but beyond that, the diet's users claim, a person can eat anything else he or she likes. Some people who've tried it say they've become pain free within just a few weeks. (For general good health, no one should eat *just* these foods but have an all-round balanced diet.)

Other people claim to have gotten relief by adding tea made from alfalfa seeds to their diets. To make the tea:

> Simmer one ounce of untreated alfalfa seed in 2½ cups of water for half an hour. Strain, cool, and refrigerate. You should have a strong infusion. To use, dilute with an equal amount of water (or to taste), sweeten with honey if you like, and reheat. Drink a cup four to seven times a day for several weeks. The tea should be made fresh each day.

If, after several weeks, you find you've gotten relief, continue with the regimen for several months. After that, you may be able to cut down on your consumption, a little at a time. Some people find that they can maintain their pain-free state with just a few cups a week.

Other people swear by eating cherries, watercress, or parsley. None of these things will hurt you, even in large quantities. Just remember to eat a healthful diet in addition to the special foods you add.

One problem with evaluating nutritional changes to the diet to relieve arthritis pain is that people often make several changes at a time, so it's hard to tell which one did the trick. For example, one woman who vows that alfalfa tea works also changed her general diet radically, omitting meat, sugar, processed foods, white flour, and foods with chemical additives. She added more vegetables and fruits and more natural fiber.

Certainly the woman's diet seems to be on the right track. The Arthritis Foundation does not recommend any specific diet, but it urges arthritic people to:

- Eat a variety of foods.
- Maintain proper weight.
- Reduce intake of fat and cholesterol.
- Eat sugar sparingly.
- Eat foods with plenty of starch and fiber.
- Cut down on sodium (salt) intake.
- Drink alcohol in moderation.

Some health practitioners recommend a diet high in calcium-rich foods, and some suggest calcium supplements. Although there is little evidence that it helps, others recommend taking pantothenic acid supplements. Garlic and parsley are two foods that herbalists use to treat arthritis.

There are two other dietary prescriptions that some alternative practitioners recommend for people with arthritis. They are the No-Nightshade Diet and the Dong Diet.

INSTRUCTIONS

Dong Diet: The Dong Diet was developed by Collin H. Dong, M.D., a Stanford University–educated physician. Dr. Dong developed the diet to treat himself. While still in his thirties, Dr. Dong found himself overweight and with a progressively worsening arthritic condition. Being a physician, he tried all the traditional remedies his colleagues had to offer, but with no relief.

As a child of Chinese parents, Dr. Dong had eaten a simple diet consisting of small portions of meat or fish and lots of fresh vegetables and rice. As he grew older and more affluent, his diet changed to one that was more typically American. Dr. Dong began to experiment with a diet that more closely resembled the one of his childhood. Eventually, he settled on a regimen of seafood, vegetables, and rice.

Before long, Dr. Dong lost weight, and the stiffness and pain in his joints had been greatly relieved. He found that he was able to resume many everyday activities that he had had to give up. Dr. Dong continued to treat patients into his seventies and to lead a full, active life.

The Dong Diet includes seafood, vegetables, and rice. Some good seafood choices are mackerel, herring, sardines, anchovies, whitefish, and salmon, which are all rich in omega-3 fatty acids. (Other types of diet therapists also recommend foods rich in omega-3 fatty acids for arthritis.) The diet also *excludes* a number of foods and additives. If you want to follow the Dong Diet, omit:

- meats
- fruits (including tomatoes, which are considered fruits, not vege-tables)
- all preservatives
- pepper of all kinds
- other hot spices
- all dairy products (cheese, milk, butter, cottage cheese, etc.)
- all chemical additives and dyes (especially monosodium gluta-mate [MSG])
- alcoholic beverages (particularly wine)
- all nuts
- chocolate
- vinegar and other strongly acetic foods
- carbonated soft drinks

Dr. Dong wrote both a book and a cookbook that you can consult for more information and recipes. His cookbook is widely available at public libraries. (See **Further Reading** below.)

No-Nightshade Diet: The No-Nightshade diet was also developed by a person who suffered from arthritis himself. Norman F. Childers had a doctorate in horticulture, so he was aware of the toxic potential of plants in the nightshade family. When he began to experiment with dietary changes to help his arthritic condition, Dr. Childers thought first of tomatoes. He realized that every time he ate tomatoes, his joints soon became even more painful than usual. Dr. Childers decided to eliminate from his diet not only tomatoes but also all other foods in the nightshade family. Within months, his pain and stiffness had subsided.

Dr. Childers recruited other arthritis sufferers to test whether the No-Nightshade Diet worked for them too. His data, collected from hundreds of volunteers, led him to believe that eliminating all foods in the nightshade family helped alleviate arthritis symptoms in people sensitive to these plants. If you happen to be one of the estimated 10 percent of people who may be sensitive to edible nightshade foods, this diet may help relieve the pain and stiffness of arthritis. To follow the diet, simply eliminate:

- tomatoes
- eggplant
- white potatoes
- peppers, including hot peppers like jalapeños

Unlike the Dong Diet, the No-Nightshade Diet does allow ground white and black peppercorns for seasoning. This diet is relatively easy to follow, except that you have to be on the alert for foods that are thickened with potato starch. In the context of this diet, "white" potatoes would include new, unusual varieties with yellow and purple flesh. Sweet potatoes and yams are not included and may be eaten.

Because arthritis is so prevalent and so debilitating, many people are interested in finding a diet that will alleviate its symptoms. Some of these people are researchers, but others are just folks with the problem who experiment with various foods to see what will help. Although the Dong Diet and the No-Nightshade Diet have large followings, it's possible that neither will work for you. If you hear of some other dietary program that purports to ease pain and stiffness, there's no harm in trying it provided you use common sense. Be sure the diet is a sensible one nutritionally, that is, that it includes a balanced group of healthful foods. Beware of diets that ask you to consume large quantities of a supplement about which little is known or of those that make too-extravagant claims. As a precaution, always check with your healthcare practitioner before you start on a diet that deviates from nutritionally sound principles, no matter what the claims.

FURTHER READING

Childers, Norman Franklin. *A Diet to Stop Arthritis*. Somerville, N.J.: Horticultural Publications, 1981.
Dong, Collin H., M.D., and Jane Banks. *New Hope for the Arthritic*. New York: Ballantine Books, 1976.
———. *The Arthritic's Cookbook*. New York: Crowell, 1973.

RESOURCE GROUPS

Arthritis Foundation (Check your phonebook for the nearest local chapter.) The AF can provide you with their latest information on diet and arthritis.

FASTING

DEFINITION

Fasting is the process of avoiding solid food, but not fluids, for a period of time in order to cleanse the body and help it heal.

APPLICATIONS

Physiological: Arthritis, asthma, headache, obesity, ulcers, heart disease, hypertension, allergies, inflammatory diseases
Psychological: Schizophrenia, mental fatigue

COLLATERAL CROSS-THERAPIES

Meditation, exercise, breathing exercises, visualization, music therapy, journaling

RECOMMENDED ADJUNCT ACTIVITIES AND BEHAVIORS

Reading, napping, Swedish massage

CONTRAINDICATIONS

Persons with eating disorders, diabetes, epilepsy, kidney disease, severe bronchial asthma, tuberculosis, and ulcerative colitis should not fast, nor should pregnant women or nursing mothers. No one should undertake a long-term fast without professional supervision.

EQUIPMENT & MATERIALS

You must consume fluids during your fast. Depending upon the type of fast you've decided to try, you may want to have spring water, juices, or herbal teas on hand. For making juices at home, you will need a juice extractor or blender.

ORIGIN

Early human hunter-gatherers undoubtedly fasted from time to time, but probably not by choice. Whether they ate regularly or not depended upon the available supply of food, but the bodies of both humans and animals are marvelously adapted to do without food for a while without suffering any ill effects. In fact, nature has designed our bodies so that should there be no food available, we become more alert, we need less sleep, and we may even become more energetic. Why? Nature wants us to be ready and able to pounce on food should we find some.

During food deprivation, our metabolism alters to spare protein, our bodies release ketones and make other adjustments (not all of which are entirely understood) to conserve our energy and keep us healthy until we resume normal food intake. (Obviously, we must eat before too long; these effects don't last forever.)

Thousands of years ago, the first healthcare measure that an ill person undertook was to stop eating for a time. Today we know that during a fast, the body continues to excrete toxins, but the intake of new toxins is decreased, so there's a net loss of toxicity. Also, while a person is fasting, food digestion takes much less energy than it would normally, so blood, oxygen, and other nutrients are freed up to be used in healing and normalizing the body.

Fasting was a part of life in many of the early high civilizations too. The Egyptians, Greeks, Romans, and Chinese all believed in fasting for health. In many cultures, fasting has also had other purposes. The Greek philosophers Socrates and Plato believed that fasting clarified the mind, and they often fasted for a week or more before sitting down to write their treatises.

Historically, fasting has had an important place in religion. Moses is said to have fasted for forty days before receiving the Ten Commandments, and the Bible says that Jesus also ate no food for forty days. In addition to Christians and Jews, Muslims and Hindus have fasting traditions that date back to ancient times. In the Western world, Native Americans fasted for purification and renewal.

Down through the ages, people have fasted to demonstrate self-control and power over their bodies, to achieve spiritual atonement through self-denial, to cleanse and rejuvenate themselves in mind and body, to lose weight, and to dramatize their political beliefs. For some people, the primary reasons to fast are spiritual and psychological, while for others, the desire for better health is predominant.

INSTRUCTIONS

There are almost as many ways to fast as there are reasons to do it, but let's be clear here what we're *not* talking about. Therapeutic fasting is *not* starvation, nor should one develop erratic eating habits: binging like a glutton one day and foregoing all food the next, for example. If you are morbidly obese, a long-term fast is one method that some people have used successfully to lose weight when their excess poundage threatened their health. However, a long-term fast for weight loss should never be undertaken without medical supervision, and periodic, brief do-it-yourself fasts don't have a very good track record as a method of permanently slimming down unless you also change your diet when not fasting *and* exercise on a regular basis.

Before you begin a program of fasting, you should consult your healthcare practitioner to determine your physical condition and to find out what type of fast (water, juice, modified) and duration might be best for you. This is especially important if you take any type of medication. After only a few days of fasting, your body chemistry will change, and your medication might need to be adjusted. Also, your practitioner might recommend vitamin and mineral supplements.

Some practitioners recommend drinking only purified or spring water during a fast, while others permit juices and/or herbal teas. Some even advocate modified fasts, during which small amounts of solid food may be eaten.

Those who favor water-only fasts maintain that juices are foods and, therefore, a juice fast is simply a very restricted diet that won't achieve metabolic changes as quickly as a water fast.

Proponents of juice fasts, on the other hand, claim that water-only fasts cause unnecessary fatigue and that the process of detoxification is too severe. Also, there are those who think that juice fasts are more likely to lead to healthful eating habits after the fast is broken because, during the fast, the person has learned to enjoy the taste of raw vegetables. (Fruit juices are seldom included on a fast because of their high sugar content, although grapefruit juice is sometimes recommended.) Herbal teas are also often permitted on a juice fast.

With your healthcare practitioner's approval, a one- or two-day water or juice fast is safe to perform at home. Longer fasts should be supervised. Whether you decide to opt for a water fast or a juice fast, it is best to fast on days when you do not have a heavy physical or mental schedule. All bodily processes rely on glucose for energy. If you're not ingesting calories, your blood sugar decreases, and your body may not work as efficiently. An ideal fasting time is during a weekend, when you can rest, relax, and do some light exercise.

Some people regard the day before beginning a fast as an occasion for eating as much as possible to store up for the coming deprivation. This feast-then-famine approach is not recommended because it puts too much stress on your body to handle such metabolic extremes. You should eat sparingly the day before a fast and go lightly on fats and proteins. The bulk of your food intake should consist of complex carbohydrates. You should also drink plenty of fluids, but stay away from caffeine-containing beverages or alcohol. Both have a diuretic action, so you actually lose fluids. (Obviously, neither of these types of beverages should be drunk during a fast either.)

If you decide on a water-only fast, most experts recommend drinking at least three glasses, but otherwise drinking only when you feel thirsty. Whether you're on a water or juice fast, start the day by sipping a glass of the liquid slowly. Spend the morning relaxing, taking a walk, reading, meditating, and possibly doing some stretching and/or breathing exercises. Take a nap if you like. At midmorning and at lunchtime sip some more juice or water. (If herbal tea is included in your fast, you can also have that.) Do something relaxing in the afternoon; have another glass of liquid in the late afternoon, and then go to bed early.

For a two-day fast, the second day's routine should be similar to that of the first. You may be hungry, so try to keep yourself occupied but relaxed. (Hunger usually persists for two to three days after a person begins a fast.)

When you break the fast, eat something simple like a piece of fruit or a few steamed vegetables and a little rice. You can eat more later if you're still hungry. The next morning eat a light breakfast and then resume normal eating.

If you've had nothing but water during the fast, you may want to break the fast with a glass of fruit or vegetable juice instead of solid food. The idea is to work gradually back into normal eating habits, not jolt your system with a sudden rush of nutrients to contend with.

If you're going to do a juice fast, use fresh juices if possible. Nearly all vegetables have a high liquid content, so there are many possibilities, and you can combine several together in pleasing combinations. Carrots, celery, other green vegetables, and beets are a few of the possibilities. (Eliminate the beets if you need to avoid sugar.) If you don't have a juicer to make your own, some health-food stores sell fresh juices. Also, in some cities, juice bars are popular. There you can usually find a real variety of tasty mixtures.

You should be prepared for some slightly unpleasant (but not permanently harmful) side effects during your fast. Your tongue will probably feel coated and fuzzy. Brushing it with your toothbrush and rinsing your mouth will help alleviate this problem. Also, you may notice a bad taste in your mouth, and your breath will be something others will want to stay away from. Even your body may smell unpleasant. These odors are the result of elevated levels of ketones and of the enhanced elimination of toxins. Good personal hygiene during the fast will help some, but most experts advise against using either deodorants or cosmetics to avoid introducing impurities through the skin.

Some people feel very fatigued during a fast while others have trouble sleeping. Other effects that you might have include light-headedness, dizziness, and/or nausea. People who are normally caffeine drinkers may also have headaches. These are only temporary problems, and you may not experience any of them. (We are presuming here, of course, that you have gotten your healthcare practitioner's okay for the fast and that you have not fasted more than one or two days at the most without supervision.)

If you feel cleansed and rejuvenated after your brief fast and want to consider undertaking a longer fast, you may want to consult a naturopathic physician or other healthcare practitioner who includes fasting as part of his or her treatment protocol. Practitioner-supervised fasting is used to treat a variety of ailments as well as for general health maintenance.

FURTHER READING

Bragg, Paul Chappuis, and Patricia Bragg. *The Miracle of Fasting*. Santa Barbara, Calif.: Health Science, 1985.

Chaitow, Leon. *Body/Mind Purification Program*. New York: Simon & Schuster, 1990.

Goldstein, Jack. *Triumph Over Disease—By Fasting and Natural Diet*. New York: Arco Publishing Co., 1977.

Lutzner, Hellmut. *The Secrets of Successful Fasting*. New York: Thorsons Publishers, 1984.

Mayled, Jon. *Feasting and Fasting*. Morristown, N.J.: Silver Burdette, 1987.

Meyerowitz, Steve. *Juice Fasting and Detoxification*. Great Barrington, Ma.: The Sprout House, 1992.

Perry, Paul. *Fasting Safely*. Mountain View, Calif.: Anderson World, 1982.

Salloum, Trevor K., N.D. *Fasting Signs and Symptoms—A Clinical Guide*. East Palestine, Oh.: Buckeye Naturopathic Press, 1992.

RESOURCE GROUPS

American Association of Naturopathic Physicians
2366 Eastlake Ave. E., Ste. 322
Seattle, WA 98102
Phone: 206/323-7610

Brochure explaining naturopathy and referral list of all AANP physicians in U.S.: $5

American Health Sciences Institute
1108 Regal Row
PO Box 609
Manchaca, TX 78652-0609
Phone: 512/280-5566

Correspondence course in natural hygiene; also books and tapes

American Natural Hygiene Society
PO Box 30603
Tampa, FL 33630
Phone: 813/855-6607

Membership: $25; magazine *Health Science*; referrals

Bionomics Health Research Institute
PO Box 36107
Tucson, AZ 85740
Phone: 602/297-0798

Books on lifestyle management include fasting; ten-issue newsletter ($13.50)

International Association of Professional Natural Hygienists
2000 S. Ocean Dr.
Hallandale, FL 33009
Phone: 305/454-2220

Referrals; quarterly newsletter

National College of Naturopathic Medicine
11231 SE Market St.

Portland, OR 97216
Phone: 503/255-4860

Referrals

Natural Hygiene, Inc.
PO Box 2132
Huntington Station
Shelton, CT 06484
Phone: 203/929-1557

Membership: $15; bimonthly newsletter; books, audio- and video-tapes; research service

HEALING FOODS

DEFINITION

Foods (not supplements or herbs) that can keep you healthy and prevent or sometimes help cure some diseases.

APPLICATIONS

Physiological: Obesity, heart disease, diabetes, stroke, high blood pressure, elevated cholesterol, tooth decay
Psychological: Anxiety, depression, nervousness, stress, irritability, hyperactivity

COLLATERAL CROSS-THERAPIES

Exercise, vegetarianism, arthritis diets, gardening, herbalism

CONTRAINDICATIONS

If you have allergies of any kind, always check with your allergist or other health practitioner before introducing foods you've not eaten before. Of course, you don't want to eat a food to which you know you're allergic, even if it has other health benefits.

EQUIPMENT & MATERIALS

Ordinary food-preparation equipment is all you need, but a wok, steamer, and/or microwave oven are nice for preparing foods without using fat. You can easily improvise a steamer by placing a rack or colander in the bottom of a saucepan or kettle.

ORIGIN

The diet of prehistoric peoples consisted of what was native to their area and what they could get their hands on. If someone says, "cave man," what do you think of? If you're like most people, you picture a hairy sort of fellow with a club over his shoulder getting ready to go out and bash a beast or two for brunch. Actually, if early humans had had to depend on animals for food, they would have been *very* hungry most of the time. Most animals were too agile and fast for primitive hunters. The real staples of early humans' diets were roots, berries, tubers, fruits, nuts, plants, and seeds. And it was cave *woman*, not cave man, who gathered most of these foods.

In short, early humans ate what many nutritionists tell us we should eat today: complex carbohydrates, fresh fruits, and fresh vegetables.

The teeth tell the story. The earliest fossilized teeth from our almost human ancestors show patterns of wear not unlike those of modern folks who eat no meat. Meat-eaters show tooth markings made by bone that were absent in these first people. Our immediate ancestor, *Homo erectus*, did eat some meat, but it was still a small part of his diet. Over the millennia, meat gradually assumed a larger place in the diet, but even today, it is a supplement, rather than a mainstay in the eating patterns of many people throughout the world. In the Far East, Middle East, the Mediterranean, and Mexico, starchy foods form the bulk of the diet, with small amounts of meat sometimes added as a garnish to grain and bean dishes.

Other sources of protein, like eggs and dairy products, are relatively new on the human menu too. Early people had an occasional egg stolen from a nest, but it was not until the domestication of fowl and cattle that milk and eggs became common foods.

Egypt: As the population of the world grew, people gathered in areas where there was plenty of food. In Egypt, the flood waters of the Nile River deposited some of the richest soil in the world. The climate was warm, and farmers could grow three crops each year. Much of the food the ancient Egyptians grew was the same as that we grow today: wheat, barley, lettuce, cabbage, cucumbers, beans, and peas. They also made wine and raised melons and other fruits. Sesame seed was first grown in ancient Egypt.

The Holy Land: Hebrews living in the Holy Land subsisted simply on grains, vegetables, and rice. They baked bread made from barley, lentils, or beans. A favorite food was a thick soup of lentils or beans, called "pottage."

Greece and Rome: Early Greeks and Romans ate seafood, domestic animals, breads made of wheat or barley, olives, grapes, and figs. The spread for bread was not butter but olive oil. A typical day's fare for an early Greek farmer might have been a breakfast of bread dipped in wine, a midday meal of beans or peas and perhaps an onion or a turnip. At sundown he ate his main meal, which was often bread, cheese, olives, a fig or two, and possibly a bit of meat or fish. Early Romans dined similarly.

However, as these civilizations spread and grew more sophisticated, they added food from foreign lands to their diets. The Greeks brought cherries from Persia and spices, apricots, and peaches from the Orient.

The Romans returned from their travels with oysters, truffles, and mushrooms. The Romans were the first to set out oyster beds, and they grew fish in ponds. Snails were a delicacy that they fattened on meal soaked in new wine.

Eventually, the Roman upper classes became so rich and powerful that they carried eating to excess. It became the custom among the wealthy to stuff themselves with as much rich food and drink as they could hold, politely retire to a room called a vomitorium, regurgitate what they had just consumed, and then rejoin the banquet to start all over again.

Europe: In Europe during the Middle Ages, simple foods were common. Beans and turnips were the principal vegetables, and people also ate honey, fruits, and juices. They raised grains and livestock, which they slaughtered in the fall. Meat often spoiled before it could be eaten; people knew how to preserve meat by curing it with salt, but salt was so expensive, they often couldn't afford enough. The Crusades brought a return of interest in foods from foreign lands, and trade in food once again flourished.

United States: European explorers who came to the Americas took back many native foods, including maize or Indian corn, potatoes, sweet potatoes, pumpkins, squash, and tomatoes. Cacao, the bean from which cocoa and chocolate are made, and cassava, the source of tapioca, were first found in America.

The early colonists' diet was relatively simple, but as the country prospered, eating habits gradually began to change. Historically, as people's standard of living goes up, so does their consumption of meat, sugar, and fat. Unfortunately, what soon follows is an increase in the incidence of poor health. Obesity, heart disease, stroke, and high blood pressure are among the problems that go along with a rich diet. Ironically, people in less-developed (and often poorer) nations frequently have more healthful diets than those in wealthier countries because they can't afford the things that are bad for them.

Human Anatomy: The human body is not really very well designed for a high-meat diet. Take the teeth. They look much more like the teeth of that super vegetarian, the cow, than like the family cat's. Like the cow's, our teeth were meant for grinding, whereas the cat's are pointed and sharp, just right for ripping up a defenseless field mouse.

Our intestines, too, are wrong for meat digestion. People have very long, winding intestines, well-suited for the slow digestion of fibrous foods like plants. Carnivores have short, straight intestinal tracts that quickly process meat and eliminate the resulting toxic waste products.

The human digestive system hasn't changed much for thousands of years, but the human diet certainly has. In 1890, people in the United States got two-thirds of their protein from plants like beans and grain.

Now 100 years later, more than two-thirds—around 70 percent—comes from animal products. Most people eat far more protein than they need anyway, but when it comes from animal sources, it comes with an extra dietary hazard: fat. Fat is associated with increased risk of some big-time killers like coronary artery disease and high blood pressure.

We commonly think of meat as a major source of protein, and it is, but actually the majority of calories in meats like hamburger and steak are fat calories, not protein calories. Cheese, butter, and whole milk are also fat-rich.

What else is wrong with the modern-day diet? Generally, too much salt, sugar, and refined flour as opposed to whole grains. With the busy lifestyles that many people have, they often cut corners by buying lots of prepared foods and picking up meals on the run at fast-food restaurants. Prepared foods generally contain way too much sodium (salt), and even foods that don't taste sweet often have quite a bit of sugar. (Refined sugar isn't as dangerous to the health as fat, but it doesn't provide much nutritional benefit; it adds calories and thus promotes obesity; and it contributes to tooth decay and some other problems.)

Obesity is a more severe problem than many people realize. Although there's probably more nutritional information available today than at any time before, and fitness appears to be a national obsession, the statistics indicate that the number of overweight people in the United States is growing.

A few years ago, the American Cancer Society reported that data from nearly one million subjects clearly showed that overweight people had a higher risk of several different types of cancer. Research suggests that diet plays a significant causal role in ten different types of cancer: breast, lung, colon/rectal, prostate, pancreas, ovary, bladder, stomach, and liver. These cancers account for about 73 percent of all cancer deaths. Several studies have shown that about a third of all cancers in the United States might have dietary causes. The good news is that, while the wrong foods can kill you, other foods may actually help protect against cancer and other diseases.

INSTRUCTIONS

To maintain good health, many experts recommend that adults:

- Cut fat to less than 30 percent of their daily calorie intake (some suggest an intake as low as 15–20 percent).
- Eat five or more servings of fruit and vegetables daily.
- Eat six or more servings of grains and legumes daily.
- Reduce salt intake.
- Drink alcoholic beverages in moderation, if at all.
- Reduce calorie intake sensibly if overweight.

Fiber is an important component of a healthful diet. Fiber may protect against cancers by hastening the passage of food through the intestines and by reducing the concentration of carcinogens. Dietary fiber is found in fruits, vegetables, and whole grains.

Following the guidelines for a healthful diet can help a person normalize weight and maintain robust health. However, increasingly, research shows that we may be able to do more. Certain foods appear to help prevent specific diseases, and some may help cure them. The chart following gives a sample of what some experts think are the protective—and healing—foods. There are many foods that contain nutrients like vitamins A and C. In the chart below, we've mentioned only a few, and to avoid confusion we've generally listed the same ones each time

PROBLEM	NUTRIENTS THAT HELP	NUTRIENT-CONTAINING FOODS
Acne	Zinc; vitamin A; avoiding foods containing trans-fatty acids (milk products, hydrogenated oils) and fried foods	*Zinc:* herring, wheat germ, soybeans, sunflower seeds; *vitamin A:* liver, green leafy vegetables, carrots, yams
Alzheimer's disease	Calcium; magnesium; vitamins C and E; carotene; flavonoids	*Vitamin C:* currants, parsley, citrus fruits; *magnesium:* kelp, sunflower seeds, wheat germ; *calcium:* cheese, brewer's yeast, milk; *carotene:* green leafy vegetables, carrots, yams; *flavonoids:* berries (blueberries, cherries, blackberries)
Anemia	Iron; vitamin C (helps increase absorption of iron); B vitamins	*Iron:* calf liver (also rich in B vitamins), green leafy vegetables, lecithin, wheat germ, lentils, blackstrap molasses; *vitamin C:* rose hips, parsley, citrus fruits; *B-vitamin complex:* brewer's yeast, wheat germ
Arthritis	Omega-3 fatty acids; avoiding plants in nightshade family (tomatoes, potatoes, peppers, eggplant, tobacco)	*Omega-3 fatty acids:* mackerel, herring, sardines, anchovies, whitefish, salmon; plenty of vegetables, complex carbohydrates
Bursitis	Vitamin B$_{12}$	Sardines, other fish, cheese

Cancer	Antioxidants (beta carotene, vitamins C and E, flavonoids, selenium); high-fiber foods; vitamins A and D (colon cancer); vitamin C (bladder cancer); cruciferous vegetables; foods low in saturated fat; poach, steam or broil foods instead of frying	*Beta carotene:* green leafy vegetables, carrots, yams; *high-fiber foods:* bran, whole grains, raw fruits and vegetables, dried figs and other dried fruits, dried beans and peas; *vitamin C:* currants, parsley, citrus fruits; *cruciferous vegetables:* broccoli, cauliflower, brussel sprouts, cabbage, turnips; *flavonoids:* berries (blue-erries, cherries, blackberries)
Cholesterol, high	Avoiding saturated fats, egg yolks; cutting down on red meat; eating more fruits and vegetables, omega-3 fatty acids	*Omega-3 fatty acids:* fish, seafood; *polyunsaturated fats:* corn, safflower, olive oil; oat bran; yoghurt
Constipation	High-fiber diet, fluids	Whole grains; raw fruit and vegetables; dried beans and peas; dried fruit; seeds
Cystitis		Cranberry or cherry juice; garlic
Gallbladder disease	Vitamin E, lecithin; low fat, low refined sugar; high fiber; reduced protein from meats	Fruits, vegetables, pectin, oat bran; soybeans, other vegetable protein; *vitamin E:* wheatgerm, seeds, nuts; *lecithin:* soy beans, eggs
Gout	Eliminating alcohol and such as organ meats; neither feast nor fast; slow, sensible weight reduction: reducing fats, protein	Fruits; vegetables; breads; cereals; lots of fluids
Headache	These foods apparently cause headaches in some people: alcohol (especially beer, red wine); dried beans; caffeine; cheese; chocolate; monosodium glutamate (MSG); cured meats and fish	Eliminate possible "trigger" foods one at a time; add back those that you like if they don't seem to be part of the problem
Hypertension	Potassium, calcium, fiber; reducing sodium (salt), refined sugar; sensible weight-loss diet (if appropriate); eliminating saturated fat; reducing red-meat consumption	*Potassium:* bananas, broccoli; *calcium:* cheese, brewer's yeast, milk; *high fiber:* raw fruits and vegetables, bran, whole grains

Immune system, strengthening	Vitamins A, C, and E; zinc; lipotropics (choline, methionine, inositol)	*Zinc:* herring, wheat germ, seeds; *vitamin A:* liver, green leafy vegetables, carrots, yams; *vitamin C:* currents, parsley, citrus fruits; *vitamin E:* wheat germ, nuts,seeds; *choline:* egg yolk, wheat germ, lentils; *methionine:* eggs; *inositol:* lentils, wheat germ, brown rice
Kidney stones	Magnesium; fiber; complex carbohydrates; green leafy vegetables; decreasing oxalates (cocoa, black tea, nuts, spinach, beets, strawberries); reducing purines (organ meats), dairy products, and simple carbohydrates (white bread)	*Magnesium:* kelp, sunflower seeds, wheat germ; whole-grain bread; green leafy vegetables; fresh fruits
Osteoporosis	Calcium; lactose (unless intolerant); vitamin D; phosphorus; manganese; boron; reducing alcohol, nicotine, and caffeine intake	*Calcium:* milk, yoghurt; *lactose:* milk, cottage cheese; *vitamin D:* sardines, mackerel, salmon; *phosphorus:* meat, eggs; *manganese:* oats, whole wheat; *boron:* apples, leafy vegetables, nuts
Stress	Protein; vitamins A and C; pantothenic acid; magnesium	*Protein:* soy, meat, fish, poultry; vitamin A: liver, green leafy vegetables, carrots, yams; *vitamin C:* currants, parsley, citrus fruits; *pantothenic acid:* brewer's yeast, brown rice, soybeans; *magnesium:* kelp, wheat germ, sunflower seeds
Wound healing	Vitamin C, zinc	*Vitamin C:* currants, parsley, citrus fruits; zinc: herring, wheat germ, seeds

the specific nutrient is mentioned. Space limitations forced us to curtail the list of specific nutrient-rich foods, and our selections are somewhat arbitrary. If you're interested in using foods for healing and prevention of certain diseases, you'll want to explore a much wider variety than those listed. Your local health-food store is probably a good source for books and charts on nutrition and, of course, cookbooks to help you prepare these delicious foods. When it comes to fruits and vegetables, though, the simplest preparation is often the best. Just open the refrigerator and enjoy.

FURTHER READING

Brody, Jane E. *Jane Brody's Good Food Book*. New York: W.W. Norton & Co., Inc., 1985.

Hausman, Patricia, and Judith Benn Hurley. *The Healing Foods*. New York: Dell Publishing, 1989.

Murray, Michael, M.D. and Joseph Pizzorno. *Encyclopedia of Natural Medicine*. Rocklin, Calif.: Prima Publishing, 1991.

Natural Healing Newsletter. FC&A Publishing, 103 Clover Green, Peachtree City, GA 30269. Phone: 404/487-6307 (subscription information)

Natural Health magazine. PO Box 57320, Boulder, CO 80322-7320 (subscription address)

Nutrition Action Healthletter. Center for Science and the Public Interest, 1501 16th St. NW, Washington, DC 20036. Phone: 202/332-9110 (subscription information)

Quillin, Patrick. *Healing Nutrients*. Chicago: Contemporary Books, 1987.

Salaman, Maureen. *Nutrition: The Cancer Answer*. Menlo Park, Calif.: Statford Publishing, 1984.

Salaman, Maureen, and James F. Scheer *Foods that Heal*. Menlo Park, Calif.: Statford Publishing, 1989.

Sass, Lorna. *Recipes from an Ecological Kitchen*. New York: William Morrow, 1992.

Werbach, Melvyn R. *Nutritional Influences on Illness*. Tarzana, Calif.: Third Line Press, 1988.

RESOURCE GROUPS

American Board of Nutrition
9650 Rockville Pike
Bethesda, MD 20814
Phone: 301/530-7110

This is the professional certifying board for nutritionists; referrals to certified nutritionists.

American College of Nutrition
722 Robert E. Lee Dr.
Wilmington, NC 28412-0927
Phone: 919/452-1222

American Institute of Nutrition
9650 Rockville Pike

Bethesda, MD 20814
Phone: 301/530-7050

North American Nutrition & Preventive Medicine Foundation, Inc.
1280 W. Peachtree St., Ste. 2209
Atlanta, GA 30367
Phone: 404/876-3060

Nutrition Education Association
3647 Glen Haven
Houston, TX 77025
Phone: 713/665-2946

Price-Pottenger Nutritional Foundation
PO Box 2614
La Mesa, CA 92044-2614
Phone: 619/582-4168

(See also *Resource Groups* under VEGETARIANISM.)

MACROBIOTICS (MACROBIOTIC DIET)

DEFINITION

Macrobiotics is the practice of a more natural way of life that includes proper dietary practice. A macrobiotic diet is high in complex carbohydrates and fiber and low in protein, refined sugars, and fats. Whole grains and vegetables form the bulk of the diet.

APPLICATIONS

Physiological: Cancer, high blood pressure, stroke, heart disease, hardening of the arteries, constipation, high cholesterol, overweight, rheumatoid arthritis
Psychological: Stress, anxiety, tension, insomnia

COLLATERAL CROSS-THERAPIES

Vegetarianism, natural hygiene, healthful diets, exercise

RECOMMENDED ADJUNCT ACTIVITIES AND BEHAVIORS

Moderation in lifestyle

CONTRAINDICATIONS

A macrobiotic diet includes only healthful foods, but you should check with your healthcare practitioner before you make radical dietary changes if you are taking medication, are pregnant, or have a serious illness.

EQUIPMENT & MATERIALS

Steaming is a favorite way of preparing many foods on a macrobiotic diet, so you might like to have a pot with a steamer basket. A sieve or colander placed inside a larger kettle makes a satisfactory substitute. Oriental markets often carry stacked steamer baskets that allow you to steam several foods at once, each in its own basket. A wok is another handy cooking utensil for stir-frying foods just until they're crisp-tender. The unique shape of the wok allows you to push foods up the sides to keep them from cooking too much or too quickly, and you need very little oil to cook a whole pot of food.

ORIGIN

The term *macrobiotics* means "great (or long) life" in Greek. The Greek physician Hippocrates was one of the first to advocate proper diet as essential to good health. He postulated that food nourished the "humors" in the body and that illness was the result of the humors being out of balance.

Other early writers, such as Galen and Aristotle, also advocated a diet similar to today's macrobiotics for good health and long life, but it was much later that the term *macrobiotics* came to mean specifically a naturalistic lifestyle and a simple diet consisting chiefly of grain and vegetables.

During the Renaissance, French writer and physician Rabelais praised the macrobiotic way of living in his satirical works *Gargantua* and *Pantagruel*, which poked fun at the foibles of contemporary life at the time. In the eighteenth century, a German physician, Christoph Wilhelm Hufeland, wrote a popular book called *Macrobiotics or the Art of Prolonging Life*, which helped spread the word about the benefits of a plain diet of vegetables and grains.

The principles of modern-day macrobiotics came to the United States through the teachings of George Ohsawa, who contracted tuberculosis in his youth in Japan. Told that there was no cure for his illness, Ohsawa assumed that he would die. Then—quite by accident—he came upon a book entitled *The Curative Method by Diet* by Sagen Ishizuka, M.D. Although Dr. Ishizuka had modern medical training, he believed that most diseases could be reversed by avoiding refined foods, meat, and sugar and replacing them with a simple diet consisting principally of vegetables and brown rice. Ohsawa decided to try the diet, and within a short time, his tuberculosis was completely cured.

For the next fifty years, Ohsawa devoted his life to teaching and refining the principles of macrobiotics and other precepts of Oriental healing. He spread his message throughout the world, and in 1959, established the George Ohsawa Macrobiotic Foundation in Oroville, California. Ohsawa died in 1966, but his work has been carried on by Michio and Aveline Kushi and others.

INSTRUCTIONS

Most people in the Western world are accustomed to eating lots of fats, animal protein, salt, and refined grains. What once was the diet of kings and the wealthy classes is now available to almost everyone. Ironically, most experts today believe that people would be healthier if they ate more like peasants than like kings.

Followers of macrobiotics believe that, for optimum good health, a diet should be low in fat and protein and high in complex carbohydrates and fiber. Most people who consider macrobiotics think "brown rice" and assume their diet will be monotonous, without much variety. Actually, you can eat a huge range of foods on a macrobiotic diet, although the standard macrobiotic diet does not include either meat, refined sugars, or dairy products. (Proponents believe the human body is ill-equipped to assimilate these foods well, so people should eat them very sparingly, if at all. Most followers of a macrobiotic diet are vegetarians.)

Recommendations for a macrobiotic diet break down like this:

- Whole grains: 40–60 percent
- Vegetables: 20–25 percent
- Sea vegetables and dried beans and legumes, 5–10 percent
- Vegetable, whole grain, sea vegetable, and (occasionally) sea-food soup: 5 percent, or two cups daily
- Fruit, fish and seafood, nuts and seeds, and desserts: occasionally

Besides brown rice, other suitable grains are whole wheat, millet, wild rice, barley, rye, oats, corn, and buckwheat. You can eat these grains in the form of breads, muffins, cereals, crackers, noodles, tortillas, etc. You can cook them with vegetables, sea vegetables, other grains and beans, and you can serve them in soups. You can bake them, steam them, boil them, fry them, or cook them any other way you like. The grains can be whole, flaked, puffed, cracked, or ground. In short, you can have grains in whatever way suits your fancy as long as they're not refined.

You can eat *any* vegetables, but macrobioticists recommend eating foods that are locally grown, not imported from another climate zone. Also, although dried beans are vegetables, they are considered in a separate category in a breakdown of the macrobiotic diet. You can eat fresh vegetables raw or cook them according to your taste. Steaming (just until the vegetables are crisp-tender to retain the nutrients) or stir-frying in a bit of vegetable oil or broth are popular and delicious methods for preparing vegetables.

Seaweed may not be a staple on your table today, but macrobioticists recommend that you eat a little bit every day for its high nutrient content. Some common kinds of seaweed that you'll find in your local healthfood store include: agar-agar, arame, dulse, hiziki, irish moss, kombu, mekabu, nekabu, nori, and wakame. Seaweed usually comes in a dried form (or pickled), so you can buy it from a mail-order source if you can't find it locally. You can also use powdered kelp as a seasoning instead of salt.

In the Orient, people eat sea vegetables to strengthen the heart, blood, and circulatory system. Some Japanese studies also show that sea vegetables may have anti-cancer effects. They may help to promote longevity too: People of Oki Island in Japan eat large quantities of seaweed, and they live longer than people inhabiting any other parts of Japan. They also have fewer strokes than people living elsewhere.

Another food that seems to have a protective effect against disease is miso. Miso is a flavorful, salty-tasting paste made from fermented soybeans and a variety of grains. It is usually used as the base for making broth for soup, but it also makes a savory seasoning for other foods. A very large study conducted by the National Cancer Center Research Institute in Japan found that people who ate miso soup daily had a much lower risk of dying from heart disease, cancer, and some other major illnesses than did people who hardly ever ate it or never ate it at all. Miso soup has been a staple of cuisine in the Orient for centuries, where many people believe it promotes good health and long life.

Contrary to what you may have heard, a macrobiotic diet isn't bland (unless you want it that way). You can use salt (sea salt, please), tamari soy sauce, or miso for a salty taste. Mirin and barley malt impart a sweet flavor, and vinegar, grated fresh ginger, daikon radish or horseradish, and pepper lend tang. Load up your food with fresh garlic and onions too if you like.

Pickles also lend zest to the macrobiotic table. Users of the diet believe they stimulate appetite and encourage digestion. Besides cucumbers, many other foods lend themselves to pickling: olives, cabbage (sauerkraut), carrots, onions, turnips, etc. Fruits (apricots and plums, for example) and fish can also be pickled.

If you have a sweet tooth, don't worry. You can satisfy your cravings with occasional fruits, fruit pies, cakes, and cookies, but use whole grains and natural sweeteners (not refined sugar) for the cakes and pastries. You can even make sweet desserts with dried beans (azuki) or seaweed (agar-agar)! Natural sweeteners include barley malt, rice malt, fruit juices, and date sugar.

Macrobiotic enthusiasts don't recommend regular coffee and tea, but you can substitute herb teas and coffee made from cereal grains. Instead of hard liquor, you can imbibe an occasional glass of sake, beer, or wine, preferably naturally fermented.

Although people generally think of macrobiotics as a way of eating, it is more than that. Macrobiotic practitioners pursue a life of peace, balance, and harmony, and they include exercise and meditation in their lifestyles. To learn more about the complete macrobiotic lifestyle, check your local bookstore or library for informational books and macrobiotic cookbooks.

FURTHER READING

Aihara, Cornellia, and Herman Aihara. *Natural Healing from Head to Toe*. Garden City Park, N.Y.: Avery Publishing Group, 1994.

Albert, Rachel. *Cooking with Rachel*. Oroville, Calif.: Georges Ohsawa Macrobiotic Foundation, 1989. (macrobiotic cookbook)

Diamond, Marilyn, and Harvey Diamond. *A New Way of Eating*. New York: Warner Books, 1993.

Heidenry, Carolyn. *An Introduction to Macrobiotics*. Garden City Park, N.Y.: Avery Publishing Group, 1992.

Jack, Alex. *Let Food Be Thy Medicine*. Becket, Mass.: One Peaceful World Press, 1991.

Kushi, Michio. *Standard Macrobiotic Diet*. Becket, Mass.: One Peaceful World Press, 1992.

Kushi, Michio, and Phillip Janneta. *Macrobiotics and Oriental Medicine*. New York: Japan Publications, Inc., c1991.

Ohsawa, George, and Carl Ferre. *Essential Ohsawa*. Garden City Park, N.Y.: Avery Publishing Group, 1994.

Ohsawa, George. *Essential Macrobiotics*. Oroville, Calif.: George Ohsawa Macrobiotic Foundation.

———. *Macrobiotics: An Invitation to Health and Happiness*. Oroville, Calif.: George Ohsawa Macrobiotic Foundation, 1971.

Solstice (monthly magazine: $36), 310 East Main St., Suite 105, Charlottesville, VA 22901; phone: 804/979-4427; fax: 804/979-1602

RESOURCE GROUPS

East/West Foundation
PO Box 850
Brookline, MA 02146
Phone: 617/738-0045

George Ohsawa Macrobiotic Foundation
1151 Robinson St.
Oroville, CA 95965
Phone: 916/533-7702

  Bimonthly magazine *Macrobiotics Today* ($15)

International Macrobiotic Shiatsu Society
1122 M St.
Eureka, CA 95501
Phone: 707/445-2290

Kushi Institute
PO Box 7
Becket, MA 02146
Phone: 413/623-5741

VEGETARIANISM

DEFINITION

Vegetarians eat no meat, fowl, or fish for reasons of health, ethics, and/or religious convictions. There are several subgroups of vegetarianism. *Ovo-lacto* vegetarians do eat milk, milk products (such as butter and cheese), and eggs. *Lacto* vegetarians eat dairy products but not eggs. *Vegans* eat only foods derived from plants (grains, vegetables, fruits, and nuts), and *fruitarians* eat only fruits. *Pesca* vegetarians include fish in their diets.

APPLICATIONS

Physiological: Cancer (breast, colon, and prostate), hypertension, heart disease, overweight, constipation, elevated cholesterol, rheumatoid arthritis, atherosclerosis, kidney stones, diverticulitis, non-insulin-dependent diabetes, gallstones
Psychological: Increased energy, self-esteem through weight loss

COLLATERAL CROSS-THERAPIES

Herbalism, gardening, exercise, Ayurveda, healing diets, macrobiotic diet

RECOMMENDED ADJUNCT ACTIVITIES AND BEHAVIORS

Cooking, reading vegetarian cookbooks

CONTRAINDICATIONS

If you have allergies and plan to introduce new foods into your diet, be sure to check with your allergist first.

EQUIPMENT & MATERIALS

You need nothing but ordinary food-preparation equipment, although a steamer and/or wok allow you to prepare delicious vegetarian dishes with little or no added fat. If you don't want to buy a steamer, just use a sieve or colander inside a large pot. You may also find a blender, food processor, and/or juicer convenient.

ORIGIN

Our prehistoric human ancestors didn't have much choice in what they ate. Early people lived on what they could gather or grab on their home turf. This consisted mostly of tubers, roots, berries, fruits, nuts, plants, and seeds. An occasional bird or animal appeared on the menu, but contrary to our stereotypical picture of the macho club-wielding caveman dragging home a hairy beast for dinner, primitive hunters usually came up empty-handed because most animals were too agile and swift to be felled by their weapons. Actually, woman gathered most of the largely vegetarian diet.

We know that the early diet contained little meat through the study of fossilized teeth. Teeth from our earliest ancestors show patterns of wear similar to those of modern vegetarians. They are absent the markings made by crunching on bits of bone.

As the years rolled by, meat gradually assumed a larger place in the human diet, but even today, meat is treated as a side dish or garnish in the diets of people in many parts of the world. In the Far East, Middle East, the Mediterranean, and Mexico, people fill up on grains and vegetables, not meat, although small amounts may be included in the meal. Fish, shellfish, and poultry are the principal sources of animal protein in many cultures.

Vegetarianism is an adjunct to religion in some cultures. Historians believe the Escenes, a group of early Christian mystics, were vegetarians. Hindus have been practicing vegetarianism for thousands of years.

Vegetarianism was not widely practiced in the industrialized world until about forty years ago. During the 1960s, people became more interested in fitness and in healthful lifestyles, and vegetarianism gradually began to pick up a following. Studies that showed a high rate of heart disease among populations that consume lots of animal fat helped turn the tide as did new research that showed the importance of fiber.

The trend toward vegetarianism also gained momentum as people learned more about "factory farming" as it applied to animals. Reports of veal cattle raised in pens so small they couldn't even turn around and chickens whose flesh grew around the wires they were forced to perch on caused some to renounce meat on moral grounds; others worried about the health hazards of growth-boosting hormones and high doses of antibiotics required for animals raised under such conditions.

Studies in recent years have shown that adopting a vegetarian diet can not only reduce the risk of developing heart disease, it may even be able to help reverse the effects of atherosclerosis (blockage in the arteries leading to the heart). Furthermore, vegetarians may be at lower risk for a host of other diseases, including hypertension, kidney stones, diverticulitis, breast, prostate, and colon cancer, arthritis, gallstones, and non-insulin-dependent diabetes. Because of their high carbohydrate content, vegetarian diets can also provide a remarkable boost in endurance for athletes.

INSTRUCTIONS

Not too many years ago, "balanced" vegetarian meals invariably included portions of grains, legumes, seeds, and nuts at each meal. The thinking then was that a person had to eat all those things together in order to get the complete protein that meat provided. Today we know that we need less protein than we once thought, and it doesn't matter when you eat the various types of plant protein as long as you eat a variety of foods.

Not only do vegetarian diets provide nearly all the nutrients we need, they seem to be the foods our bodies are built to process. Meat-eating animals are equipped with sharp, pointed teeth for ripping up flesh. Human teeth are more suitable for chewing like a cow than for eating one.

Our intestines too are different than a carnivore's. When a lion gulps down a gazelle, the meat passes into a straight, short intestine and is quickly eliminated. Humans, on the other hand, have long, winding intestines that are just right for the slow digestion of fibrous plants.

The type of vegetarian diet you adopt will determine whether you can get all the nutrients you need from your food. If you avoid all animal products including dairy and eggs, you may want to take vitamin B and D supplements since most plant foods lack these vitamins. Also, although some plant foods are rich in iron (dark green leafy vegetables, for example), plant-based iron is less easily absorbed than the iron in meat, so you should include a good source of vitamin C to increase iron absorption. Peppers and orange juice are two good choices.

Today's supermarkets and health-food stores offer a huge variety of fresh vegetables and fruits from around the world. Rice and beans sit side by side on the shelf with less-familiar grains like kasha and quinoa. Traditional pasta in all sizes and shapes is flanked by Japanese soba noodles and bean threads. The array of sweet, sour, spicy, and pungent condiments is staggering. And to tell you what to do with all these foods, you can find cookbooks for every skill level and palate.

A vegetarian diet is not soggy, overcooked vegetables and a plate of beans and rice. Cooking exciting nutritious vegetarian meals isn't any more difficult than cooking the old-fashioned meat-and-potatoes way. To really have fun with vegetarian cooking, you'll want to try experimenting with some of the unfamiliar vegetables and grains available today.

The most versatile food in the vegetarian lexicon is the soybean. You can use it to "cream" your coffee (soy milk), spice up your noodles (soy sauce) and make a soup (miso). The soybean also shines at overcoming one of the problems some neophyte vegetarians experience: a desire for something 'substantial" to take the place of meat. When you become a vegetarian, you don't have to give up the taste of bacon, sausage, ham, chicken, hamburger, hot dogs, or even pepperoni. Every one of these flavors is available in a meatless version, and most are made from soybeans. Years ago these substitutes tasted horrible, but today's improved products are much more appetizing.

If you're a purist who finds eating fake meat as unacceptable as eating the real thing, there are three products (two soy and one wheat) you should become familiar with. Tofu, tempeh, and seitan are meat alternatives that are low-fat and cholesterol-free. They don't mimic any kind of meat. In fact, you probably wouldn't want to eat them plain because they don't taste like much of anything. Their virtue is that when marinated, seasoned, sauced, or cooked with other foods, they absorb and hold the other flavors.

Tofu (pronounced "toe-foo") is also known as soybean cake or bean curd. Tofu is made from fresh soybean puree, and it has a velvety texture like custard. It is available fresh in four consistencies from extra-soft to extra-firm, and you can also buy it boxed from the grocery shelf. Fresh tofu needs immediate refrigeration; boxed doesn't. Tofu is extremely versatile; you can use it for everything from stir-fries to desserts. It can be baked, fried, barbecued, marinated, blanched, and simmered. Tofu absorbs other flavors easily, and it is a source of complete protein as well as iron, potassium, phosphorus, and calcium.

Tempeh (pronounced "tem-pay") is made from whole fermented soybeans. It is a powerhouse source of vegetable protein, containing 50 percent more than hamburger. Available fresh or frozen, tempeh can be grilled, fried, steamed, or baked with a sauce. Tempeh has a chewier texture and a firmer consistency than tofu. Try it with garlic and/or ginger or experiment with other seasonings and condiments.

Seitan (pronounced "say-tan") is also called "wheat meat." Made from wheat gluten, seitan has a chewy texture somewhat reminiscent of real meat. You can buy it sliced or in large blocks (usually frozen) called "roasts." A seitan roast can be cooked like a pot roast or you can cut it up and use it in stews and other cooked dishes. Because seitan contains no fat, you need to use a cooking spray, oil, or liquid to keep it from sticking to the pan while cooking.

Tofu is widely available in most supermarkets, but you may have to go to a health-food store to find seitan and tempeh. Many vegetarian cookbooks, particularly those featuring Asian cuisine, contain recipes for cooking these versatile meat substitutes.

Vegetarianism is easy to follow, even if you eat many restaurant meals. Vegetarianism is becoming so common, many restaurants now offer meatless alternatives. If you find yourself in one that doesn't, you can always fall back on some type of salad as a main course. If the salad includes ham or chicken, don't be afraid to ask the waiter to substitute cheese (or leave out the meat ingredients). Most restaurants are happy to accommodate vegetarians. Ethnic restaurants—Italian, Japanese, Chinese, Thai, Indian, Mexican, to name a few—nearly always offer a number of dishes that don't include meat. If you eat fish, your choices are even wider.

Airlines offer vegetarian meals for the traveler. Often these are tastier than the regular meals served, and they're usually more nutritious. When you buy your ticket, ask to have a veggie meal if food is served on the flight. (If you wait till you're airborne, you may have to make do with salted nuts!)

Most vegetarians like to cook with lots of herbs, spices, and condiments, but that's a matter of choice. If you're not very adventuresome in your eating habits, you can make the transition to vegetarianism by using meat substitutes that simulate the real thing. Try the veggie hot dogs, bacon, and burgers, for example. The burgers are sold as frozen patties, but you can thaw them and then crumble them up to use in any recipe that specifies ground beef. You can make a great "meat" sauce for spaghetti this way. Just saute the crumbled veggie burgers in a little oil, then add your favorite sauce recipe (or a canned sauce without meat). Think creatively, and you'll find you can adapt many of your own recipes using the simulated meat products. However, you'll be missing some real culinary delights if you don't try some veggie recipes that don't pretend to be meat. Get a good cookbook or two and experiment.

FURTHER READING

Atlas, Nava. *Vegetariana*. Boston: Little Brown, 1993.

Bernard, Neal D. *Food for Life*. New York: Crown Trade Paperbacks, 1994.

Boyd, Billie Ray. *For the Vegetarian in You*. San Francisco: Taterhill Press, 1991.

Eydie, Mae, and Chris Loeffler. *How I Conquered Cancer Naturally*. Garden City Park, N.Y.: Avery Publishing Group, 1992.

Inglis, Les. *Diet for a Gentle World*. Garden City Park, N.Y.: Avery Publishing Group, 1993.

Katzen, Mollie. *The Moosewood Cookbook*. Berkeley, Calif.: Ten Speed Press, 1992.

Klaper, Michael. *Vegan Nutrition*. Pai, Maui, Hi.: Gentle World, 1987.

Krizmanic, Judy, and Matthew Wawiorka. *A Teen's Guide to Going Vege-*
tarian. New York: Viking, 1994.

Lappe, Frances Moore. *Diet for a Small Planet*. New York: Ballantine
Books, 1991.

Lingappa, Yamuna, and B.T. Lingappa. *Wholesome Nutrition for Mind,*
Body and Microflora. Worcester, Mass.: Ecobiology Foundation International, 1992.

North American Vegetarian Society. *Vegetarianism: Answers to the Most*
Commonly Asked Questions. Dolgeville, N.Y.

Solstice. Order information: Solstice Magazine, Inc., 310 E. Main St., Suite
105, Charlottesville, VA 22901; phone 804/979-4427.

Tracy, Lisa. *The Gradual Vegetarian*. New York: Dell, 1985.

Vegetarian Times, monthly magazine. Order information: PO Box 570,
Oak Park, IL 60303; phone 708/848-8100; fax 708/848-8175.

RESOURCE GROUPS

American Vegan Society
501 Old Harding Highway
Malaga, NJ 08328
Phone: 609/694-2887

Quarterly newsletter *Ahimsa* ($18); also audio- and videotapes, vege-
tarian cookbooks, other publications

Hippocrates Health Institute
1443 Palmdale Ct.
West Palm Beach, FL 33411
Phone: 407/471-8876

Source for wheatgrass juicers and food dehydrators; also *Hippocrates*
Newsletter and book *The Hippocrates Health Program*; book and newsletter
subscription: $25.

North American Vegetarian Society
PO Box 72
Dolgeville, NY 13329
Phone: 518/568-7970

Membership: $18; quarterly newsletter *Vegetarian Voice*; also cook-
books and books on nutrition; referrals to local vegetarian organizations

Vegetarian Resource Group
PO Box 1463
Baltimore, MD 21203
Phone: 301/366-8343

Vegetarian Journal (6 issues $20); vegetarian cookbooks (including
kosher)

EXERCISING THE BODY

The phrase "use it or lose it" isn't a meaningless platitude when it comes to exercise. Our bodies are designed to do useful work. Humans can walk (or run) long distances, lift heavy loads, and swim lakes and rivers to get from here to there. Once these skills were necessary for survival and activities of daily living. Today's labor-saving devices and modern transportation have eliminated physical exercise from most of our jobs, so we have to set aside time and develop routines to be sure our bodies stay tuned up. Our ancestors would find it incredible that we have to work to exercise; they had to exercise to work.

While our forefathers and mothers might have had exercise built right into their daily routines, we today at least have the luxury of choosing the physical activities we enjoy most. This section of the book is longer than most because aerobic exercise is probably the single most important activity we can engage in to promote good health, both physically and emotionally.

Research shows that aerobic exercise not only fights stress and reduces the risk for some major killers like hypertension and heart disease, it also improves our sense of well-being. Plus it helps to normalize body weight. In fact, most studies today show that it is almost impossible to reduce excess poundage and keep it off without including an exercise component in your program.

While aerobic exercise should be your top priority, this section also includes some exercises you can do to alleviate problems with specific conditions. And we've included two Oriental disciplines—t'ai ch'i and yoga—that combine physical exercise with mental control.

There's something in this section for everyone. If you've been a couch potato for a long time, look at this section as a real key to improving your health and extending your life. There is no Fountain of Youth, but exercise is the next best thing.

AEROBIC EXERCISE

DEFINITION

The word *aerobic* means "with air or with oxygen." An aerobic exercise is any sustained physical activity that improves the body's ability to deliver and use oxygen efficiently. Aerobic exercise strengthens the cardiovascular system (heart, blood vessels, and lungs), helps shape the body, and tones muscles. Walking, swimming, and running are examples of popular aerobic exercises, but climbing stairs and vigorous vacuuming may also qualify although they aren't as much fun.

APPLICATIONS

Physiological: Strengthens the cardiovascular system; helps prevent stroke, heart attack, flu, and colds; lowers blood pressure and "bad" cholesterol; improves athletic performance and endurance; bolsters immune system; may provide some protection against cancer; aids weight loss
Psychological: Reduces stress, tension, insomnia, depression

COLLATERAL CROSS-THERAPIES

Diaphragmatic breathing, pranayama, pursed-lip breathing, healing diets, vegetarianism, yoga

RECOMMENDED ADJUNCT ACTIVITIES AND BEHAVIORS

Weight-reduction diet (if applicable), calisthenics, weight lifting/resistance training, dancing

CONTRAINDICATIONS

Nearly everyone can perform some kind of aerobic activity, but the type, intensity, and duration depend upon your fitness level when you begin, your age, and the goals that you set for yourself. Always check with your healthcare practitioner before beginning any kind of aerobic program. He or she may want you to take a stress test to see what kind of shape you're in and whether you have any cardiac abnormalities. Taking a stress test is particularly important if you fit one or more criteria that put you at risk for coronary problems. These include:

- Family history of heart disease
- Being a smoker
- Obesity
- High blood pressure (hypertension)
- Elevated "bad" (LDL) cholesterol
- High levels of tension or stress
- Sedentary behavior

For the stress test, you will be asked to pedal a stationary bicycle or walk on a treadmill at a certain pace while wearing a heart monitor. The test usually continues until your heartbeat comes close to its predicted maximum rate. If anything abnormal shows up on the monitor before that, the test will be stopped. After you stop exercising, you continue to wear the monitor until your heartbeat gets back to its normal "resting" rate.

The results of the stress test help to determine the type, intensity, and duration of the aerobic workout you should begin with. Generally, you'll also learn what your target heart rate should be during exercise. Then when you start working out, you can monitor your own pulse so you can tell when you're in the target range. The object is to get to the target rate but not to exceed it.

EQUIPMENT

The equipment you'll need depends upon the activity you've chosen. If you want to walk, run, or dance, all you'll need are a pair of good shoes and comfortable, loose-fitting clothing. Even when the weather's bad and you can't go outside, you really don't need expensive equipment to keep up your program. You can get plenty of exercise from a real stairs instead of a stepper; you can jump rope; or you can work out to a video. Excellent aerobic activities that do involve equipment include cycling, cross-country skiing, and swimming. Most aerobic activities that can be done outdoors can be simulated indoors using a treadmill, stepper, cross-country ski machine, or exercycle.

Exercise machines are a fairly major purchase, so it pays to invest in quality. Your equipment should be sturdy enough to stand up to heavy usage, and it should be comfortable. If you buy from a store that specializes in the equipment you're considering, the staff should be able to help you choose the right style and size for your needs, but you have to be the final judge. Try it out before you buy. A bicycle seat that doesn't feel right in the store will be *really* uncomfortable after a few-mile ride. And be an informed purchaser. Read up on the various brands and learn their features. You might want to check out the brand ratings in a magazine such as *Consumers Digest* or *Consumer Reports*.

Be realistic when you consider equipment. Don't buy something you're not going to use. Attics and basements are littered with barely used exercycles and the like gathering dust because their owners had good intentions they never followed up on. Their misjudgment can be your gain, however. If you're sure you *will* use it, you can often pick up a good-as-new machine for a bargain price from the classified ads.

Most sedentary people don't get much exercise because they really don't want to. They may say, "the weather's bad," "I don't have time," or some more inventive excuse, but the truth is, it's hard for them to get motivated to exercise. If you fall into this category, you *can* change your habits, and your health will be the better for it, but before you invest in expensive equipment, why not establish a pattern of low-cost exercise first? For walking or running, all you'll need is appropriate shoes and clothing you probably already own.

Get on a regular walking/running schedule. Then when you've learned to enjoy exercise and discovered the benefits, you can think about buying a piece of equipment that you know you'll use for fitness and not for a coat rack.

Once upon a time, a person wore plain old "gym shoes" for all sports and exercise. Today there's a distinctive style of shoe for nearly every activity. Walking shoes are different from running shoes, both are different from basketball shoes, and so on. This is not entirely a manufacturer's gimmick to sell more shoes. Jogging shoes, for example, have a cushioned sole to absorb the impact of running on a hard surface. The heel is wide and slightly raised to take the stress off the Achilles tendon, which is at risk when a person is running.

Buying the right shoes for a specific activity can make your feet feel better and may possibly help avoid a sports injury. Regardless of the type, you should look for shoes that fit well, feel comfortable, and have sufficient arch support.

Your workout clothes should also be appropriate for the activity. They should be loose (or stretchy) enough to allow free range of motion. If exercising outdoors in winter, you'll need a mask, ski mask, or scarf to cover your nose and mouth so that the air will be slightly warmed before it enters your lungs.

One item of clothing that you *don't* want while jogging is a rubber suit. The claim is that a rubber suit can help you sweat off unwanted pounds, but it's water, not fat, that you lose. Furthermore, the rubber doesn't "breathe," so your body can't cool off naturally through the evaporation of perspiration. The upshot is you'll be dehydrated, possibly dangerously hot, and right back where you started from, weight-wise, as soon as your body fluids are replenished.

In addition to large items like treadmills and exercycles, there is a whole host of smaller (and usually less expensive) devices purporting to help you get fit. Most don't qualify as aerobic aids because they're designed to work specific muscle groups rather than to increase your cardiovascular capacity, but there are a few things that might come in handy for your aerobic workout. A padded floor mat provides a nice cushion for jogging in place, and you can also use it for floor exercises if you want to do them in addition to your aerobics program. To add a little variety to your routine, you can get a jump rope and/or a step-aerobics set that includes a platform and blocks in various heights. Try wearing ankle and/or wrist weights or carrying small dumbbells if you want to add more huff and puff to your jogging or walking routine.

Solo exercisers often become fitness dropouts because they don't have anybody to urge them on. One way to feel as if you're part of a group is to exercise to a video. You can find videos for walking, dancing, and step aerobics as well as for ordinary aerobic routines. There are even videos made especially to use with cross-country ski machines. These combine appropriately paced music with lovely outdoor winter scenes, so that you can ski in Austria without ever leaving your home.

There are videos for all levels of fitness and for different age groups. Not all exercise videos provide aerobic exercise; some are geared to muscle-building or body-contouring. Others offer several different types of routines on one video. Aerobics videos are of two types: high-impact and low-impact. The difference is that, in low-impact aerobics, one foot is always on the floor, whereas both feet sometimes leave the floor at the same time when you're doing a high-impact program. High-impact aerobics is much more jarring and has a higher risk of injury. If you're older or a recent couch potato, you're probably better off starting with a low-impact workout.

Don't know which video to buy? Try renting from your local video rental store until you find one you like. Many public libraries also stock exercise videos that you can take out for free, just like books.

One last word about equipment: Machines or devices that require no effort from you will provide equal benefits. That is to say, none. You can't improve the capacity of your heart and lungs without making them work, nor can you tone up your muscles without using them. No device can roll, knead, jiggle, or jolt you into shape while you do nothing, so don't waste your money on such things. Buy yourself a new sweatsuit instead. It will be a lot more useful.

ORIGIN & BACKGROUND

From the beginning, people have always exercised aerobically, although, of course, prehistoric people didn't think of it that way. Early humans lived strenuous lives, and they had to be fit to survive. Without any labor-saving devices, whatever got done was accomplished with human muscle-power. If people wanted to go anywhere, it was their two feet that took them there.

People continued to get plenty of exercise just performing their daily tasks until quite recently. Even a few generations ago, no one gave planned exercise a thought. They didn't need to think about it; it was there: pitching hay, scrubbing clothes on a washboard, beating carpets, building bridges, and so forth. Then came automobiles, washing machines, dishwashers, carpet sweepers, television, and finally that ultimate laziness gadget—the remote control. People didn't even have to leave their comfortable perches to change the channel.

As labor-saving devices proliferated, fitness levels started declining. People got flabbier and flabbier. Even many children no longer engaged in enough strenuous activity to keep themselves in good shape. Gradually people began to realize that "use it or lose it" applied to the efficient functioning of the human body.

The concept of aerobic exercise for fitness developed in the 1960s and really gathered steam during the next decade. Fitness experts prescribed a taxing regimen: at least thirty minutes of serious exercise five days a week. One might do something aerobic—running, cycling, or swimming, for example—on Monday, Wednesday, and Friday. The program on Tuesdays and Thursdays might include weight lifting, resistance training, and/or calisthenics. "No pain, no gain" was the motto and high-impact aerobics the rule. In her early videos, Jane Fonda exhorted her panting followers to "go for the burn." They did, by the thousands, as more and more people climbed on the fitness bandwagon. Nearly every community of any size boasted at least one health club, and housewives everywhere rushed off to their 9 A.M. Jazzercise classes.

Not surprisingly, such a rigorous schedule spawned a lot of dropouts. Many people loved the hard routines, but others couldn't keep up the pace. So many people developed shin splints from high-impact aerobic routines that some instructors switched to low-impact, where the exerciser kept one foot on the floor at all times. Still, for the most part during the past twenty years, experts have stuck to their guns that a person needs to do thirty minutes of strenuous exercise five days a week for real fitness.

Now these rules may be changing. In late 1993, the American College of Sports Medicine and the Centers for Disease Control jointly issued new exercise guidelines. The experts still call for thirty minutes five days a week, but what has changed is the type of activity. Virtually everything that involves moving around now qualifies as a fitness exercise. This includes walking the dog, taking the stairs instead of the elevator, trotting from the far end of the supermarket parking lot to the store, and a whole lot more. And what's more, the gurus say you don't have to do your thirty minutes all at once. "Exercise lite," as it's now called, sounds wonderful to the activity-averse, but does it really work? Evidence shows that it may, but with qualifications.

Several university studies, notably those at Stanford and Brigham Young, found that exercisers who divided up their thirty-minute workouts into several segments during the day showed an equal improvement in their bodies' ability to send oxygen to exercising muscles as their counterparts who sweated it out all at once. In fact, at

Brigham Young, the short-segment folks even got an extra jolt of HDL cholesterol (good) compared to LDL cholesterol (bad).

Evidence is mounting that even moderate exercise can strengthen your heart and help you live longer. Periods of activity throughout the day also keep your metabolism revved up, which helps to burn calories faster and may flush out toxic substances quicker, before they can damage your body with diseases like cancer. At least fifteen studies have shown that burning an average of 200 calories a day exercising can help you live longer, feel better, stay healthier, and lower your risk of cancer, heart disease, and stroke to boot.

These are powerful reasons to change from being a sedentary person to a moderately active one, and everyone ought to be able to fit several short periods of exercise into even an extremely busy schedule. What if your goals are higher, though? What if you want to use exercise to lose weight and reshape your body? Then you'll have to do more. You'll also have to do more to get the boost to your immune system that exercise can provide. In the next section, we'll describe some exercise programs that can help, whatever your goals.

INSTRUCTIONS

Basic Guidelines: Regardless of the level of difficulty of the aerobics program, there are some things that you need to do to be successful:

- Check with your healthcare practitioner before beginning a new program.
- Decide on the level of fitness you'd like to achieve, and set *realistic* goals. You can't go from channel surfer to power lifter in one fell swoop, but you can always up your goals as your fitness level increases.
- Choose activities you like to do. It's unrealistic to expect that you'll stick with a running program if you hate to run, no matter how beneficial it might be. Some people prefer to do the same things all the time, while others like to vary their programs.
- Plan a schedule. This is key. Unless exercise has a preplanned time slot in your day's activities, you probably won't get around to it. Even if you opt for several short periods of exercise during the day, plan for them, at least in the beginning. If you can do it, exercising first thing in the morning is ideal. It will get you revved up so that you can attack your daily activities with more vigor. You might even find at the end of the day that you've actually *saved* time because you've accomplished your tasks more efficiently.

Preparation (warm-up): Before you begin any exercise, you need to get the blood flowing to warm your muscles and start elevating your heart rate. Even if you're only going to go for a brisk walk, your body will benefit from a warm-up routine. A lot of strains, sprains, and cramps can be traced to skipping the warm-up and plunging right into strenuous activity before the body is ready.

Stretching and limbering up are best to get your body revved for exercise. Here's a good warm-up routine that will alert your major muscles that they're going to have to get moving:

1. While standing up, hold your arms out straight and make ten big clockwise circles. Then reverse and do ten counterclockwise circles.
2. Stand up straight and hold your arms straight over your head. Rise up on your tiptoes and stretch as far as you can as if you were reaching for the sky. Pause at the height of your stretch for a few seconds, then lower your heels and slowly bend forward from the waist. Don't lock your knees. When you've bent over as far as you can, let your arms and head hang loosely for a few seconds. (If you're very limber, your fingers may brush the floor, but don't worry if they don't.) Slowly roll your body back up to a standing position. Let your arms hang at your sides. Then raise your arms over your head and repeat the whole sequence. Do this five times. Try to move slowly and rhythmically.
3. Stand with your feet about shoulder-width apart with your hands on your hips. Keep your hips facing forward and twist your upper body first to the left as far as you can and then to the right. Repeat ten times.
4   Stand at arm's length from a wall with your palms on the wall at about eye level. Keeping your body straight and your heels flat on the floor, bend your arms and lean forward until your forehead nearly touches the wall. Hold to feel the stretch in your calf muscles. Straighten your arms to push back from the wall, then repeat the cycle. Do ten repetitions.
5. Stand with one foot resting on a chair or table. (Which you use depends upon your degree of limberness. If you're pretty much out of shape, a low chair will give you plenty of stretch.) Straighten your leg and stretch your arms forward as if to touch your toes. Bend your head toward your knee and feel the stretch in your hamstrings. Hold for twenty seconds. Then switch legs and do the same thing with the other leg.
6. Squat with your feet flat on the floor. Extend one leg behind you and put your hands on the floor as if you were in the starting blocks for a race. Hold for a moment to feel the stretch, then switch legs. Repeat for a total of five cycles.
7. Lie on your back with your legs extended. Pull one knee up to your chest and hold briefly. Release. Re-extend that leg and pull the other leg in to the chest and hold. Release and return the leg to the floor. Then do both legs at once. Repeat the cycle five times altogether.

8.   Sit up, bend your knees, and spread them apart. Hold your arms out straight and parallel to the floor. Bend forward and try to grasp your toes. Slowly lower your head as far as you can, so that your forehead approaches your knees.

Your whole warm-up routine should take at least five minutes. If you're going to run, it's most important that you stretch your calf and hamstring muscles beforehand.

When you stop vigorous exercise abruptly, blood can pool in your legs and cause discomfort. To keep this from happening, always cool down at the end of your exercise routine. The cool-down is just as important as the warm-up. If you've been running, walk for the last five minutes, gradually slowing down to a snail's pace. If you've taken a brisk walk, slow down a few blocks from home. Cross-country skiing is hard work whatever the pace. When you've finished, take off your skis and stroll around the block once or twice. Do the same after an invigorating bike ride. Whatever the exercise, the idea is to let your body slowly return to its nonexercising mode.

Program for a Longer Life: This is a program for people who are now basically inactive. All you need to do is to include approximately thirty minutes of *moderate* activity in your schedule every day. You can do it all at once or in chunks. Activities can include walking, bicycling (or riding a stationary bike), calorie-burning housework, gardening, or working out to a video at a moderate pace. The goal is to burn at least 200 extra calories per day.

What will you achieve? You'll help to protect your body against the risk of heart disease, stroke, cancer, and possibly osteoporosis. You won't feel the "high" that strenuous exercisers get, but you may be more alert. This program is pretty easy to do because you don't have to work out hard, but it won't reshape your body or take off pounds. You may eventually lose some weight, but it will be very gradual. Strictly speaking, this is not an aerobic exercise program because there's no attempt to boost your heart rate into the target zone. Still cutting your risk of some major diseases is an important achievement in itself. Just don't expect to look or feel that much different. Some people may want to use this program to get started and then add higher fitness goals as they become accustomed to exercising.

Program for Cardiovascular Fitness and Strength: This program is more challenging, but you'll also experience the benefits rather quickly. To improve cardiovascular fitness, you need to perform thirty to sixty minutes of aerobic activity three to five times per week. You can walk (fast), run, bicycle, jump rope, swim, cross-country ski, aerobic dance, work out to a fast-paced video, or any other activity that keeps you moving constantly. (Start-and-stop exercises like tennis don't qualify.)

Your goal is to drive your heart rate up to at least 60 percent of its maximum.

What will you accomplish? Everything you would with the more moderate program, plus you'll feel more optimistic and less stressed. You'll reduce the ratio of bad to good cholesterol, and if you're hypertensive, you'll lower your blood pressure. This level of exercise will boost your immune system, so you'll probably have fewer colds and/or flu episodes. Your endurance will improve, and if you're overweight, you will shed pounds, particularly if you work out five days a week. You'll also strengthen the muscles that you use in performing your aerobic activities, and since muscle burns more calories than fat, more muscle means faster calorie burning.

Program for Reshaping the Body: Practically everybody knows by now that dieting alone is not very effective for permanent weight loss. You need to eat a healthful low-calorie diet (not a fad diet) *and* exercise. To burn lots of calories, perform aerobic activity for sixty minutes five days per week. Again, you want to get your heart rate up to at least 60 percent of maximum.

To really redefine the way your body looks, you'll need to add weight lifting or other resistance training, yoga, and/or floor exercises. Do these activities three times per week, but don't work with the same muscles on two successive days. Some people like to work with the upper body one day and the lower body the next. Others do their whole body routine one day and then skip a day before repeating.

What will you accomplish? You'll get all the benefits of the cardiovascular workout, and you'll have a more svelte body. Adding resistance training will build muscle, so your body will take on sleeker, less flabby contours. Be aware, though, that muscle weighs more than fat, so don't rate your accomplishments by the scale. Use the tape measure instead.

Any program that builds cardiovascular fitness has the added advantage of increasing metabolism, not just during exercise, but for hours afterward. So your body continues to burn fat at a faster rate when you go back to your sedentary job after a lunch-time run. That's what makes aerobic exercise such an effective part of a weight loss program.

How do you know whether you're exercising hard enough to make your exercise truly aerobic? There's one very simple test. If you're breathing hard but can still talk, you're probably working at about the right pace. If you're too winded to speak, you're overdoing. A more precise method is to determine your target heart rate and then take your pulse to see if you're in the zone. To find your particular range, subtract your age from 220 and multiply that number by .6 for the bottom of your target heart range and by .85 for the top. The results are measured in heartbeats per minute. For example, if you're twenty years old, the bottom of your target heart range would be 120 beats per minute, while the top would be 170 beats per minute. Your target heart rate would be somewhere within that range. At the bottom of the range, you would be exercising at 60 percent of your maximal heart rate, while at the top, you'd have worked up to 85 percent of the maximal heart rate. (Your maximal heart rate is the fastest your heart pumps while you're exercising as hard as you can. You do *not* want to reach the maximal rate during your exercise program. That's only for testing.)

As you might expect, the numbers drop with age. For a sixty-five-year-old, the bottom of the range would be 93 beats per minute and the top 132.

Keep in mind that this method is based on an average person of a certain age. It doesn't take into account individual differences, fitness levels, or specific health problems. The very best way to learn your target heart zone is to take a stress test before you begin your exercise program. Then your healthcare practitioner can tell you what your maximal rate is and what rate you should use as your target rate for exercise.

Once you've established your target heart rate, take your pulse quickly as soon as you stop exercising. (As soon as you stop moving, your heart rate begins to drop, so the reading won't be accurate if you don't do it immediately.) Find your pulse in your wrist using your first two fingers. Count the beats for ten seconds and multiply by six to get the beats per minute.

If you like gadgets, you can buy a wristwatch-style pulse monitor that measures the pulse in your finger or earlobe while you're exercising. Some models even have alarms that ring to tell you that you're overdoing and are above the target zone or that you're dogging it and have fallen below the aerobic level. You can buy pulse monitors at sporting goods stores or through mail order catalogs.

TYPES OF EXERCISES

Bicycling: Bicycling is great aerobic exercise if you enjoy it. Biking has the advantage of also being a transportation mode so you can do errands, visit friends, or go to the library at the same time that you're getting fit.

The kind of bike that you buy depends upon where and how you're going to ride it, and what is comfortable for you. Look at the chart below to see what best suits your needs.

TYPE OF BIKE	CHARACTERISTICS	ADVANTAGES	DISADVANTAGES
Ten-speed	Dropped handlebars; light weight; thin tires; large wheels; narrow saddle	Easy to carry up and down stairs; enough gears for most terrain; can change hand positions	Bumpy ride; unstable on rough terrain or cracked city streets; saddle may be uncomfortable, as may bent-over riding position

Mountain/ All-terrain (all-terrain is also called hybrid)	Straight handlebars; somewhat heavy; fatter tires, smaller wheels (all-terrain has slightly narrower wheels than mountain); may have twenty-one gears or more	More stable; good for city streets and rough terrain; widere saddle; softer ride; upright position may be more comfortable	Heavy to lug up and down stairs; only one hand position; usually fairly expensive
Three-speed	Usually straight handlebars; wide saddle; medium-width tires	Moderately priced; no extra frills; suits smooth, flat, and slightly hilly terrain	One hand position; hard work on hilly terrain
No speed	Your basic bike	Plenty of exercise; not a candidate for theft; inexpensive	Hard to pedal on hills; usually doesn't have hand brakes
Tandem	Bicycle built for two	Fun if you have a partner to ride with	Can't be ridden alone
Recu- ment/Semi-recumbent	Pedals are out in front so rider is semi-reclining	Comfortable ride; seat gives back support	Expensive; may be hard to get used to; not built for speed
Tricycle	Three-wheeled; heavy	Good for older people and those who can't balance a two-wheeler	Large, hard to store; can't take hills

Consider where and how you'll use the bike before you buy. You probably don't need twenty-one speeds to pedal to the grocery store unless you live on a mountaintop. By the same token, an expensive, shiny mountain bike parked at a commuter train station all day is an awfully inviting target for the dishonest. If you must haul your bike up stairs between uses, you'll want to try hoisting the bike in the store to see how hard that will be.

Don't buy a bicycle you haven't ridden. If the store owner won't let you try it out, shop somewhere else. Usually you can do your own hybridizing if you don't like all the features of the bike you've chosen. Most bicycle shop owners will let you swap a narrow saddle for a wider one, for example, or even one that's gel-filled. (An alternative that adds to saddle comfort is a pair of padded biking shorts.) If you want a mountain bike, but you like the two hand positions on a drop-handlebar bike, you can buy extensions for straight handlebars that give you another position.

If you're going to ride at night, get lights (*and* wear reflective clothing). There's a myriad of gadgets you can buy to make riding more fun, but consider where you're likely to park the bike before you invest in things that can be ripped off. Two accessories you definitely do need are a helmet and a good lock.

For safety's sake, don't listen to a radio or tape player with headphones while riding. You won't be able to hear outside noises that would warn you of danger.

Cross-Country Skiing: Cross-country skiing (sometimes called Nordic skiing) is one of the best aerobic exercises. It gives you a real cardiovascular workout, and it burns calories fast (up to 900 per hour). The gliding motion is easier on your joints than high-impact activities like running, and you're working both your upper and lower body. If you live in the right part of the country, you can do the real thing, but you can get similar benefits from an indoor ski machine. Try one before you invest, though. It isn't as easy as it looks on the TV ads, and some people have trouble with balance and coordination.

Outdoor cross-country skiers have a choice between waxless and waxable skis. The pros choose waxables so that they can vary the type of wax they use for different conditions. You may not be so fussy.

Skis are also classed as "diagonal" or "skating". As you might expect, skating skis are shorter, but—and this may be a surprise—the poles are longer. Skating skis are easier to maneuver, but diagonals are better-suited to varied terrain.

Step Aerobics: Step aerobics were developed in answer to the need for low-impact routines. In step aerobics, one foot is always on the floor so there's less chance of injury. Basically, step aerobics consists of stepping up and down on an elevated platform that varies in height from less than six inches to nearly a foot. The routines are usually done to music. Most health clubs and YMCAs now have step aerobic classes. Another place to check is your local community center. If you don't want to join a class, you can buy the platform and blocks in various heights at your local sporting goods store. Rent a video, follow the routine, and you're on your way. To make your workout a little harder, you can wear ankle and/or wrist weights.

Swimming and Pool Exercises: A swimming pool is a wonderful place to work out for fitness and fun. Even if you don't know how to swim, you can take advantage of the resistance of the water to get in a real aerobic workout with water exercises. Depending upon where you live, swimming pools may be commonplace or rare. Healthclubs and YMCAs are obvious places to look for pools, but you may also be able to swim at a local hotel or motel pool without becoming a guest. Some hostelries have standardized policies for nonguest use of the pool, but you may be able to cut a deal even if the establishment hasn't thought of it before. It doesn't hurt to ask.

The only essential equipment is a bathing suit (a simple tank suit is good for women: you'll be comfortable, and the straps won't slip), a cap, and a pair of goggles to keep the chlorine from irritating your eyes.

Wearing contact lenses in the pool without protective goggles is an invitation to disaster. If a lens comes loose and washes away, you can kiss it goodbye. Even if you manage to keep your lenses intact, germs in the pool water can contaminate them and cause infection. If water somehow gets behind your goggles, get out of the pool before you take them off. That way, if the lens is floating around, you can find it. Prescription goggles are available for those who want to leave their lenses off and still see what's going on.

If you want to, you can also wear ear plugs and/or a nose clip. For running or walking in the water, you can get a pair of water shoes with rubber soles that will help keep you from slipping. A flotation vest (similar to a life jacket) can make you more relaxed if you're a nonswimmer who wants to try water exercise.

There are some other items you can use to add more oomph to your water routine. To strengthen your legs, you might want to use a kickboard or fins. To work on your arms without kicking your legs, try one of the flotation devices that supports your lower body as you swim. Some pools supply at least some of these devices while others don't allow people to use things like boards and floats in the water, so check out your facility's equipment and rules before you buy.

Warm-up and cool-down: As with any other exercise, you need to warm up before you begin your swim or water exercise routine (and cool down afterward). You can do your land-based warm-up routine if you want to, or you can warm up in the pool. Start by sitting on the side of the pool and kicking your feet in the water, then jump in and run (or walk) for a few minutes. You want to gradually increase your heart rate and warm up your muscles.

For your arms, stand in chest-deep water with your arms out in front and alternately pull one arm and then the other down through the water as if you were swimming. Do some stretching exercises too. See *Preparation (warm-up)* in the earlier part of this section for some good ones. Some can be done in or out of the water, while others you'll have to do on land.

For the after-exercise cool-down, swim less vigorously for the last five minutes or float on your back kicking slightly and paddling with your arms. You can also get out of the pool and walk around it several times.

Lap Swimming: If you're going to swim laps, start with a comfortable number and gradually add more as your fitness level increases. Swimming laps can get tedious unless you vary the routine by changing strokes from time to time. This also helps to work different muscle groups. If a kickboard is available, swim at least a lap or two holding the board extended in front of you while doing a flutter kick. For your upper body, use only the arm movements while letting your legs trail behind. This is easier if you support your lower body with a flotation device.

Try to get into a rhythm with your lap swimming. Unless you're working on improving your stroke, don't think about what you're doing, your troubles, or how many laps you've swum. (It's better to focus on your total workout than to count laps.) Let your mind float free. Before long, your swim won't seem boring at all, and you'll finish your workout feeling relaxed in both body *and* mind.

Breathing Technique: The two things that cause people to tire quickly when swimming are improper breathing and too much thrashing about. Don't hold your breath while swimming. Inhale and exhale rhythmically.

If you don't know how to exhale with your face underwater (which you must do to perform the crawl properly), practice by standing with your face turned to one side and resting on the water's surface. Take a good breath, turn your face into the water and exhale. Repeat until the maneuver feels comfortable. Then add the arm movement. If you're turning your head to the right to take a breath, your right arm should be on its downward and backward stroke when you turn your head. (A common mistake is lifting the head up instead of rolling it to the side. This throws the body out of alignment and leads to early fatigue.) Add the kick, and you're swimming the crawl!

When you swim, cup your hands to form a miniature paddle. Cut the water cleanly, and don't twist your body from side to side. Unfortunately, if you've gotten into bad habits, simply swimming more often probably won't correct them. You'll have to concentrate on relearning the stroke or take some swimming lessons so that someone else can help you get it right.

If you're older or less fit when you begin your program, you may want to swim the sidestroke. It's less rigorous, and your face is always out of the water, so breathing is easier. Change sides from time to time so that both sides of your body get the same workout. If you're right-handed, swimming on your left side will seem a little awkward at first, but you'll soon get the hang of it.

If you're working within a target heart-rate zone, there's good news. When swimming, you don't have to raise your heart rate as high as with other exercises to get a good workout. Aim for a heart rate about 10 percent lower than you'd shoot for with land-based exercise.

Water Exercises: Don't swim? Not to worry; you can still have fun and get a good workout in the pool. The simplest exercise is to walk, run, or march in the water. If the pool is crowded, you can do these exercises in place. If you're marching, work toward raising your leg high enough so that your thigh is at least parallel to the bottom of the pool. To get your arms into the act, pump them up and down or swing them as you walk or march. Chest-deep water lets both your legs and arms work against resistance.

Another simple exercise: Hold onto a flotation device or something at the edge of the pool, stretch your legs out behind you, and kick from the hips with your knees slightly bent. Don't kick from the knees.

Health clubs and YMCAs with pools usually offer water-exercise classes that offer a wider variety of exercises than we've given here.

There is a huge variety of available aerobic activities. One of the best—walking—doesn't cost a penny, and almost anyone can do it. Aerobic exercise has proven health benefits. So what's the problem? Why doesn't everybody include this kind of activity in his or her daily routine? The excuse that most people use is that they don't have time, but we all make the time to do the things we want to do. The truth is, exercise sounds unpleasant to most couch-potato types. Either they don't begin to exercise at all, or they start out doing too much, so their worst fears are realized. *It is unpleasant.* If you're now sedentary, don't defeat yourself by undertaking an ambitious program while you're still basically unfit. Unless you have a physical condition that prevents it, start by walking for five, ten, or fifteen minutes a day, depending on your age and condition. If you do it at the same time every day, it will help to establish the habit, but that isn't necessary. Just do it once a day, no matter what. Inclement weather needn't stop you. Walk around your house if necessary. Keep up this simple, short routine until you feel you want to do more. You will eventually, so don't put pressure on yourself. If you miss a day, don't worry about it, just begin again the next day. Gradually increase the speed, duration, and/or length of your walks. It will take some time to improve your fitness level with this approach, but it is more important that you establish the habit of exercising and begin to enjoy it. Daily exercise is a program for a lifetime, and slow, steady progress is the key to replacing sedentary habits. One day you'll discover that you really enjoy being active. Really.

FURTHER READING

Austin, Denise. *Denise Austin's Step Workout.* Newark, N.J.: PPI Entertainment Group/Parade Videos, 1991. (video)

Brown, Dawn. *Aquacise I: Splash into a Refreshing New Way to Workout.* Newark, N.J.: Parade Video, c1987. (video: nonswimming water aerobics)

Cooper, Kenneth H., M.D. *The New Aerobics Way.* New York: Bantam Books, 1981.

Feinstein, Alice, ed. *Training the Body to Cure Itself*. Emmaus, Pa.: Rodale Press, 1992.

Fonda, Jane. *Lean Routine*. Beverly Hills, Calif.: Warner Home Video, 1990. (video: low-impact aerobics)

Gullion, Laurie. *Nordic Skiing: Steps to Success*. Champaign, Ill.: Human Kinetics, c1993.

Harris, Trudy. *The Larger Woman's Workout*. First Run Video, c1988. (video)

Katz, Jane, Ed.D. *Swim 30 Laps in 30 Days*. New York: Putnam Publishing Group, c1991.

————. *The W.E.T. Workout*. New York: Facts On File, 1985. (water exercises)

Kelly, Bill. *Video Awarebics: Exercise Your Right to Protect Yourself*. Awarebics, Inc., 1992. (video: combines aerobic exercise with instructions on how to use aerobic moves to protect yourself)

Koch, Bill. *Cross Country Skiing Skating Techniques*. Eugene, Ore.: ESPN Home Video, 1988. (video)

Missett, Judi Sheppard. *The Jazzercise Workout Book*. New York: Charles Scribner's Sons, 1986.

Moynier, John. *The Basic Essentials of Cross Country Skiing*. Merrillville, Ind.: ICS Books, 1990.

Pregnant and Fit. New York: Maier Communications (distributor), c1987. (video)

Sansone, Leslie. *Leslie Sansone's Walking Fat Burner Workout*. Newark, N.J.: Parade Video, c1990. (video: walking program plus firming exercises)

Senior Fitness Center. *Senior Fitness Center Presents Senior Flex*. Reseda, Calif.: Increase Video, c1986. (video)

Step Reebok. Master Class I. Stoughton, Mass.: Reebok International, c1991. (video: step aerobics; all fitness levels)

Watley, Jody. *Dance to Fitness*. Newark, N.J.: Parade Video, c1990. (video: aerobic dance)

Whitten, Phillip. *The Complete Book of Swimming*. New York: Random House, 1994.

RESOURCE GROUPS

American Running & Fitness Association
9310 Old Georgetown Rd.
Bethesda, MD 20814
Phone: 301/897-0197

Membership: $25; monthly newsletter *Running & FitNews*; also catalog on fitness booklets

United States Water Fitness Association, Inc.
PO Box 3279
Boynton Beach, FL 33424
Phone: 407/732-9908

   Publications, videos; referrals to local programs, instructors

ALEXANDER TECHNIQUE

DEFINITION

The Alexander Technique is a mind/body method of movement that
teaches people to use their bodies efficiently. By making subtle shifts in
the way they sit, stand, and walk, individuals can alter the way they look
and feel.

APPLICATIONS

Physiological: Sports performance, breathing, high blood pressure,
arthritis, back pain, neck pain, pinched nerve, posture problems,
scoliosis
Psychological: Stress, anxiety, depression, insomnia, mental fatigue,
self-image

COLLATERAL CROSS-THERAPIES

Breathing exercises

RECOMMENDED ADJUNCT ACTIVITIES AND BEHAVIORS

None

CONTRAINDICATIONS

Check with your healthcare practitioner before undertaking the Alexander Technique for a physical problem. He/she can tell you whether or
not the Technique is likely to help.

EQUIPMENT & MATERIALS

No equipment is necessary.

ORIGIN

The Alexander Technique was developed by Frederick Matthias Alexander,
who was born on the island of Tasmania in 1869. From early childhood,
Alexander yearned for a career on the stage, so he developed a repertoire
of recitations, which he delivered on small-town stages after he finished his
day job in a tin mine. After the tin mine, there were other unsatisfying jobs,

and Alexander decided that, once and for all, he would give up all other work and concentrate on making good as a recitalist and actor.

Unfortunately, Alexander had a problem that sometimes occurred during his recitals. Occasionally, he would lose his voice completely when speaking. He consulted various doctors, but they could help him only temporarily. One night during an important performance, his voice failed and he had to leave the stage. Alexander considered giving up the career that he loved, but then he decided to try to solve the problem himself.

After that, he spent ten years studying every move that he made and the way that he used his body, particularly when he was reciting. He even practiced his recitations before a mirror to further observe what was going on with his body as he spoke. Eventually, he noticed a pattern of movement that accompanied his every activity, not just his recitations on stage. He pulled his head back and down before he initiated any activity, and this created tension between his back, neck, and head. Although Alexander had acquired this habit over many years, he set about to correct it by consciously freeing his head to move upward and forward. Alexander's loss-of-speech problem disappeared, and he successfully resumed his stage career, but by this time he had developed a consuming interest in the implications of his discovery; namely, that we can use the conscious mind to change subconscious muscle movements. Alexander felt that the proper use of the body could affect the physical, emotional, and mental well-being of people with many different kinds of problems.

Before long, Alexander had refined his technique, and he soon abandoned the stage to teach his method to others. He died in 1955 at the age of 86. During his career, he had taught in England and the United States, but through his students, his teachings spread to many other parts of the world.

Many celebrities have studied the Alexander Technique, including Paul Newman, George Bernard Shaw, Lillie Langtry, Aldous Huxley, and Dr. Nikolaas Tinbergen, a winner of the Nobel Prize in medicine. Dr. Tinbergen even mentioned the technique in his Nobel acceptance speech.

The technique can also help athletes improve their performance, but proponents say anyone can benefit from the method, whether or not he or she ever appears in public life. The Alexander Technique does not treat specific symptoms, but stressed-out people and those with functional problems such as muscle and joint pain have often found relief after applying Alexander's principles.

INSTRUCTIONS

Although the Alexander Technique is popularly known as a "posture" technique, teachers of the method stress that it does not place the body in static positions. It is a way of thinking and moving in order to "use" the body efficiently. People learn to change the thoughts that trigger movement to eliminate unnecessary movements and tension.

Movements in the Alexander Technique are always preceded by a brief period of self-inspection. You can do this either while sitting or standing. With your eyes open, turn your head slowly from side to side and look at your surroundings. Tilt your head upward to look and the ceiling and then downward to look at the floor. Notice your neck as you're turning your head. Are the muscles tight? Did you twist your body too when you moved your head? Did you continue breathing rhythmically when you moved your head or did you stop or slow down your breathing? Did you hear any crackling sounds in your neck or spine?

Now move your head upward and forward as you turn your head. Allow your body to stretch forward and upward as it follows your head. Now once again tilt your head upward to look at the ceiling and then downward to look at the floor. Keep your neck "lengthened" as you do these movements. (When you move your head, do it as a whole, don't lead with your chin.)

Now move your whole torso upward from your hips. Let it follow along after your head. Allow your chest to expand. Don't try to narrow your torso as you move it upward, let it expand sideways too.

In the Alexander Technique, the body always follows the movement of the head. Practice these movements until you feel comfortable with them, remembering always to take stock of yourself before you begin.

Now see how your body reacts when you lean forward while sitting. Lean forward and sit back several times. Did any parts of your body tense up when you moved? Did you push yourself forward or did your hip joints simply bend naturally?

Again lean forward but this time move your head forward and upward as you did in the first exercise. Don't push your head upward, simply let it move naturally in that direction. Let your torso follow the upward movement and then simply bend from the hips. There should be no forcing motion.

One good way to practice these movements is to do them while eating. When you eat, do you round your back and cave in your chest so that your mouth will be closer to the food to avoid spilling? Or do you sit regally straight and perform a balancing act with the spoon all the way to your mouth? The Alexander way is to bend from the hips slightly so that your mouth is closer to the food but your body is not all scrunched up.

You can use the Alexander Technique to study and modify all your movements. Whatever movement you choose, always start with a self-assessment of the way you perform the movement now. Then begin to modify it by allowing your head to move forward and upward and let the rest of the body follow.

If you'd like to learn more about the Alexander Technique, you might want to enroll in a class. Group and individual lessons are available. *The Alexander Technique: Learning to Use Your Body for Total Energy* by Sarah Barker is a do-it-yourself guide.

FURTHER READING

Barker, Sarah. *The Alexander Technique*. New York: Bantam Books, c1991.
Barlow, Wilfred. *The Alexander Technique: How to Use Your Body Without Stress*. Rochester, Vt.: Healing Arts Press, c1990.
Gray, John. *The Alexander Technique*. New York: St. Martin's Press, 1991.
Leibowitz, Judith, and Bill Connington. *The Alexander Technique*. New York: Harper & Row, c1990.
Seldane, Bernice. *The Body-Mind Book: Nine Ways to Awareness*. New York: Messner, c1979.

RESOURCE GROUPS

American Center for the Alexander Technique
129 West 67th St.
New York, NY 10023
Phone: 212/799-0458

North American Society of Teachers of the Alexander Technique
PO Box 3992
Champaign, IL 61826
Phone: 217/359-3529

Pamphlets; referrals to practitioners

CALLANETICS

DEFINITION

Callanetics is a no-impact exercise program that works the deep muscles of the body through a series of small, precise movements. Each series of exercises is designed to work a specific body part.

APPLICATIONS

Physiological: Reshape and strengthen hips, thighs, buttocks, abdomen; prevent and alleviate backache; increase flexibility
Psychological: Self-confidence, body image

RECOMMENDED ADJUNCT ACTIVITIES AND BEHAVIORS

Weight reduction if appropriate

CONTRAINDICATIONS

Check with your healthcare practitioner before undertaking this program.

EQUIPMENT & MATERIALS

Exercise mat; workout clothing, such as shorts and shirt or leotard; table, ballet barre, or other elevated surface you can hold on to

ORIGIN

The early background of Callan Pinckney, the developer of Callanetics, hardly suggested that she would grow up to devise an exercise program. Pinckney was born with back problems, and as a child, she wore leg braces for many years to correct foot deformities. Despite her physical limitations, she took up the study of classical ballet and pursued this course for a dozen years.

As a young woman, Pinckney left her Georgia home to see the world. Over the next ten years, she saw a great deal of the world, backpacking and working her way through Europe, Asia, and Africa. Her living conditions were often primitive, and her life was frequently quite physically taxing. When she finally returned to the United States in the early 1970s, her body was sorely in need of remedial work.

Pinckney went to work in an exercise salon in New York City, but she soon found that some of the exercises she was teaching didn't make *her* feel good at all. In fact, they hurt her back. Reasoning that if the exercises were painful to her, they must affect at least some of her students that way too, Pinckney left the salon to develop her own exercise techniques.

She turned to her own experience with ballet for the basis of many of her exercises, but because of her own back pain, she proceeded very cautiously and made only tiny adjustments in position as she performed a routine. Pinckney found that the small movements didn't aggravate her back at all. In fact, within a short time, her back pain had disappeared entirely. What surprised her even more was that her muscle tone improved greatly in much less time than she would have expected. Convinced that she had found a new exercise method that achieved faster results without danger of injury, Pinckney set about teaching her techniques to others. Pinckney believes that one hour of her routine is the equivalent of about twenty hours of aerobic dance and seven hours of traditional exercise insofar as toning the body is concerned.

INSTRUCTIONS

Callanetics is suitable for both women and men, and you can begin the program at any age or level of fitness. The program is no-impact; that is, there is no hopping or jumping of any sort. Nor is the program done to a musical beat, although there are pleasant background tunes on the videos.

A typical Callanetics whole-body workout takes about an hour, but there are twenty-minute programs for specific problem areas like the stomach or the hips and buttocks (which Pinckney calls the "behind"). The routines basically combine stretching and muscle contraction. Some of the movements are ballet-like, while others are reminiscent of yoga postures. These are not huff-and-puff routines; they are graceful and fluid. (Movements are often in increments of a quarter to a half inch.) Because of its ballet heritage, Callanetics can improve coordination, poise, and balance as well as tone the muscles and shape the body.

Though you can take up Callanetics in whatever shape you're in, these exercises are by no means easy. If you're very inflexible and out of shape to begin with, you'll probably not be able to do all the repetitions nor achieve the desired positions at the outset. Not to worry. The Callanetics method stresses working at your own level until your body is ready to go further.

Because each Callanetics exercise is based on very small and precise movements and proper body positioning, it is not possible to adequately describe an exercise in writing. If you're interested in trying Callanetics, you may be able to find a class in your area, but if not, there are a number of Callanetics videos available through your library or video store. The videos are very easy to follow, and at least some feature classes of real people of all ages and fitness levels, so you can see variations in their ability to perform. (See **Further Reading** below for names of videos.)

FURTHER READING

Pinckney, Callan. *Beginning Callanetics*. Universal City, Calif.: MCA Universal Home Video, 1989. (video)

———. *Quick Callanetics*. Universal City, Calif.: MCA Universal Home Video, 1991. (series of three videos: hips and behind, legs, stomach)

———. *Super Callanetics*. Universal City, Calif.: MCA Universal Home Video, 1988. (video)

Pinckney, Callan; Sallie Batson; and Gary Moody. *Callanetics: 10 Years Younger in 10 Hours*. New York: William Morrow, 1984.

Pinckney, Callan, and Judie Bazerman. *Callanetics Countdown: 30 Days to a Beautiful Body*. New York: Avon Books, 1991.

Pinckney, Callan, and Michael Huss. *Callanetics*. Universal City, Calif.: MCA Universal Home Video, 1992. (video)

Pinckney, Callan, and Barbara Friedlander Meyer. *Callanetics for your Back*. New York: Avon Books, 1991.

EXERCISES FOR SPECIFIC CONDITIONS

DEFINITION

Depending upon the condition addressed, these exercises are aerobic (strengthen the cardiovascular system to help the body use oxygen more efficiently), resistance (strengthen and tone muscles), or stretching (promote flexibility in the joints).

APPLICATIONS

Physiological: Arthritis, headache, backache, incontinence, osteoporosis, bursitis, tendinitis, stiffness, obesity, carpal tunnel syndrome, intermittent claudication
Psychological: Stress, anxiety, insomnia, body image, self-esteem

COLLATERAL CROSS-THERAPIES

Diaphragmatic breathing, pranayama, pursed-lip breathing, healing diets, yoga, herbalism, flower remedies, yoga, t'ai chi, aikido, biofeedback, creative visualization

CONTRAINDICATIONS

These exercises are generally safe, but you should check them out with your healthcare practitioner to be sure they won't aggravate your condition.

EQUIPMENT & MATERIALS

Equipment and materials needed for an exercise are listed with each exercise.

INSTRUCTIONS

Any type of exercise program should always begin with at least a five-minute warm-up and end with a five-minute cool-down. The warm-up and cool-down routines listed in AEROBIC EXERCISE can be used for any type of exercise. If a different warm-up (or cool-down) routine would be more appropriate, it will be listed with the specific exercise to which it applies.
Arthritis: In simplified terms, our body's framework, the skeleton, consists of a series of bones hooked together end to end. So that we can move, the joint where two bones meet is flexible like a hinge. Just as a hinge does, the joints need to be lubricated to keep them working smoothly.

When the joint is healthy, synovial fluid—a thick, slippery substance contained in a capsule (synovium) surrounding the bone ends—keeps it well oiled. Rheumatoid arthritis inflames the lining of the synovium, which stretches surrounding tendons and ligaments. Synovial fluid deteriorates, and the whole joint weakens and stiffens. Obviously, this joint needs a lube job, and exercise can provide it by better distributing synovial fluid and increasing blood circulation in the area. (Blood brings nutrients and oxygen to help heal the damaged joint, and it takes away waste products and reduces swelling.)

In osteoarthritis, the cartilage (smooth surface of the bone) and underlying bone begin to break down. Sometimes the cartilage gives up the ghost altogether, leaving the rough bones to rub against each other. Again, exercise helps by keeping the synovial fluid moving over the cartilage. Exercise also improves muscle tone, which lightens the load on the joints. Resistance exercises help beef up the bone itself.

So what is the exercise prescription for arthritis sufferers? It's three-part: full range-of-motion exercises to move *all* the joints to keep them well-oiled and flexible, strengthening (resistance) exercises, and aerobic activities.

Range-of-motion exercises should be done every day. Try these:

- Stand with both arms parallel to the floor. Make large clockwise circles with both arms. Then reverse and make counterclockwise circles.
- Let your head hang forward with your chin on your chest. Slowly circle your head around on your neck in a clockwise direction. Do several of these and then reverse directions. Try to stretch your neck as far as you can with the rotation.
- Sit straight in a chair with your arms hanging at your sides. Lift your shoulders upward toward your ears. Then roll your shoulders back and down. Repeat several times.
- Rest your wrist on the edge of table so that your hand extends beyond the table. Bend your wrist up as far as you can and hold for a few seconds. Then bend the wrist down as far as you can and hold. Repeat several times.
- Hold your hands out in front of you. Stretch and spread your fingers out as far as you can. Then bend your fingers at the large knuckle, and finally make fists. Clench hard when you make the fist. Repeat several times.
- Lie on your back with your legs out straight on the floor and your toes pointed upward. Move one leg out to the side as far as you can and hold briefly. Move the leg back in and turn it to the outside as if trying to rest your ankle bone on the mat. Do the same with the other leg. Repeat several times.

This is just a sample of exercises to keep your joints moving. You can do shoulder shrugs, neck rolls, and finger stretches while watching TV or sitting at your desk. They're great antidotes for stiffness, whether or not you have arthritis, if you have to sit for long periods in one place. See YOGA for other good stretching and limbering exercises.

Aerobic activities should be part of your exercise program if you have arthritis, but some are no-nos. Stay away from sports like basketball or high-impact aerobic dance classes. You want to move your body smoothly, not thump on it. Walking, biking, and swimming are good. Try to do something aerobic for a half hour or more at least three times a week.

Strengthening exercises are particularly important for people with arthritis because they tend to be weaker than their arthritis-free peers. Walking, biking, and swimming (and other aerobic activities) strengthen the muscles as well as the cardiovascular system, but you'll get more from your program if you add resistance training. Be sure to get your health practitioner's okay before you start; he or she can recommend a safe program that suits your condition.

People usually think of resistance training as working with free weights or weight-training machines, but resistance can also come from elastic bands or, in the pool, water. The advantages of resistance training are that you can build muscle fairly rapidly, and you can work on specific muscles that need strengthening. Leave the free weights to the non-arthritic, though. It's too easy to lose control and injure yourself.

A warm-water pool is an excellent place to do some resistance exercises without the grunt and groan of weightlifting. The heat soothes aching joints, and you virtually can't overdo because the water provides resistance without impact.

The exercises you can do in the water are limited only by your imagination. You can walk across the pool, swing your arms and legs in circles and lifts, pedal with your legs, and pull your arms through the water as if you were swimming. Here are a few to get you started. Stand in chest-deep water for all of these. Do only a few repetitions to begin with, gradually work up to at least ten.

- Stand with your elbows bent and your hands in front of your chest, palms facing outward.
- Keeping your hands cupped, straighten your arms out to the sides as if you were doing the breast stroke. Your arms should now be fully extended sideways, parallel to the bottom of the pool.)
- Return your arms to the starting position. Now push your arms straight out in front of you.
- Return to the starting position and repeat the sequence.

This one's good for the wrists, elbows, and shoulders. It also gives a nice stretch to the back of the legs.

- Stand facing the side of the pool at arm's length from the edge.
- Place your palms flat on the side with your arms outstretched.
- Bend your elbows and lean forward keeping your body in a straight line.
- Straighten your elbows and push back to an upright position.
- Repeat the sequence.

Here's a stylized pool walk that's good for the legs:

- Stand up straight with your arms extended to the sides at shoulder height.
- Pretend you're a walking wind-up toy and step forward raising one leg high in front of you.
- Bring that leg down and step high with the other.
- Continue this goose-step walk for as many steps as you're able. Don't stop between steps. Try to keep up a pace.

The Arthritis Foundation has developed a YMCA Aquatic Program. If you're interested, contact your local chapter or the nearest Y.

Caution is the watchword if you're going to do resistance exercises on weight-training machines. Get an okay and suggestions for a program from your doctor. Then have someone on the staff show you how to use the machines properly. In general, you'll probably want to concentrate on the big muscles around your knees, hips, and shoulders. Start slowly with a small amount of weight and don't overdo. You may want to stick with lighter weights and increase the repetitions as your muscles strengthen.

Back Pain: Back pain plagues almost everyone at one time or another. Improper exercise can *cause* back pain, but proper exercise can help prevent it, and exercise is essential to maintaining back health after you've had a problem. Many back injuries occur when people bend over to lift things using their back muscles, when they should be squatting and lifting with their thighs.

It is much easier—and more comfortable—to try to prevent back pain than to cure it. Everyone should do a little preventive maintenance to keep a strong and healthy back. People who are desk-bound at their jobs are particularly prone to back injuries. Sitting all day keeps back muscles from stretching out and moving around. They become short, tight, frail little things. No wonder that just a sudden twist or even a violent cough can bring on the familiar complaint, "Oh, my aching back!"

On the issue of back pain, mainstream and alternative practitioners are in agreement: Exercise is the number one prescription for avoiding the problem. (If you've had one miserable back experience, you're more likely to have another, so it makes sense to get your back in shape before the fact.)

To ward off back pain, your exercise program should include exercises that promote flexibility and those that strengthen the muscles of the back, abdomen, and thighs. Keeping your spine in proper alignment—good posture—is another important factor in keeping a pain-free back.

The joints in your back need to be lubricated like any other joints. To keep your back loose and free-moving, do range-of-motion exercises. To loosen up your upper back, neck, and shoulders:

- Stand with your feet shoulder-width apart.
- Bend forward from the waist, allowing your head and arms to hang loosely.
- Make big, sweeping circles with your arms. Do at least twenty-five repetitions without stopping.

To stretch thse hip joints and spine, try this:

- Kneel on the floor or mat.
- Raise your arms over your head and bend forward from the waist until your hands, forearms, and forehead touch the floor.
- Keeping your arms straight and your thighs perpendicular to the floor, press down toward the floor with your chest.
- Hold for a few seconds, release and resume the original position
- Repeat several times.

This next exercise is called "Salute to the Sun." It's a great first-thing-in-the-morning stretcher that's not hard to do even if you're not very limber. Do it very slowly and rhythmically so you can feel your body rolling from one position to another.

- Stand up straight with your stomach tucked in, your shoulders back, and your arms hanging at your sides.
- Slowly raise your arms over your head as if they were being lifted by rising water.
- At the same time and at the same pace, rise on your tiptoes.
- When your arms are straight over your head, stretch up as far as you can as if you were reaching for the sun.
- Slowly lower your heels to the floor.
- With your arms still over your head, bend from the waist and slowly roll your spine downward, as if you were going to touch your toes. Don't lock your knees.

- When you've bent forward as far as you can without forcing, let your arms and head hang loosely for a moment.
- Then slowly roll your spine back up, vertebrae by vertebrae, until you're once again in a standing position with your arms at your sides.
- Repeat several times.

Many health practitioners recommend the knee-chest stretch. It's a good preventive exercise, but it can help loosen a back already tightened by muscle spasm too. Do this exercise a few times whenever you can during the day. It feels great after a long bout of sitting at a desk.

- Lie on your back with your legs out straight.
- Keeping the other leg straight, bend one leg and pull your knee toward your chest as far as you can without discomfort. Hold briefly, and then straighten out your leg and return it to the floor.
- Repeat with the other leg.
- Now do the same thing with both legs together.
- Finally, bring the first knee back to the chest as before and then pull it toward the opposite shoulder. You don't have to touch the shoulder. Just feel the stretch.
- Repeat with the other leg.
- Do each movement several times.

One of the best exercises for loosening up is just plain walking. Walk briskly, taking long free strides, and let your arms swing with the rhythm of the gait. This not only gets your joints lubricated, but it also stimulates blood circulation and relieves tension.

Swimming stretches and strengthens back muscles more gently than land exercise. When you're feeling stiff, a plunge in the pool can take away the creaks painlessly. If you're using swimming as your principal back limbering and strengthening exercise, head for the pool at least three times a week for no less than thirty minutes.

Weakness in other muscles can contribute to back pain. Got an ache between the shoulder blades? Your trapezius muscles may be flabby. Lower back giving you fits? It's a good bet your abdominals need help. The curl is a great exercise for this problem because it gives the back a good stretch while it's tightening abdominal muscles.

- Lie on your back with your knees bent, your feet flat on the floor, and your arms folded across your chest.
- Curl your body upward, lift your shoulder blades off the floor, and twist your right shoulder toward your left knee. Hold briefly, and then curl back down slowly.
- Repeat, twisting in the opposite direction.

Try to do at least ten repetitions of the curl on each side. If your stomach muscles resemble cooked spaghetti, you may not be able to do that many at first. Do what you can and gradually add a few reps. Work up to thirty (or more) per side.

There are several variations of the curl, which is also known as a crunch. Some people lift straight up, keeping their hands at their sides or between their legs. Others clasp their hands behind their heads and twist. If you want to do that, keep your elbows out flat like spread wings when you twist.

However you do the exercise, be conscious of the fact that you're trying to lift your body using the abdominal muscles, not the back or hips. If you want to be sure it's the abdominals that are getting the workout, lie on the floor with your legs bent at a ninety-degree angle over a chair seat. Then lift your head and shoulders from the floor.

If upper-back pain is your problem, here's a quick and easy exercise to strengthen the trapezius muscles. (The trapezius muscles are the muscles that start at the back of the head, fan out across the shoulders, and then taper back down between the shoulder blades.) This exercise requires dumbbells, which you can buy inexpensively at almost any sporting goods store.

- Stand straight with your arms at your sides and a dumbbell in each hand.
- With your elbows slightly bent, raise the weights out to the sides so that your arms are perpendicular to the floor and then on up straight over your head. This should be one continuous movement.
- Lower the weights the same way that you raised them, and then repeat.
- Do eight to twelve repetitions, rest for a minute or two, and then do another set of eight to twelve reps. Rest and repeat the set one more time.

Poor posture is an insidious culprit in back pain. Slouching, slumping, or otherwise putting your spine out of kilter may not have any immediate effects, but over time, your back will pay the price. The muscles, bones, tendons, and ligaments in the back system each have a job to do, and when the body is lined up properly, each can handle its own load. Put it out of whack, though, and one muscle shortens up while another has to stretch too far, and so on. Eventually, your whole back support system weakens. Slumping like a sack of flour also squishes your vertebrae on top of one another so that the disks between them don't have enough space to do a proper cushioning job. Sooner or later one can squeeze clear out of place. And there you are with a herniated disk and a lot of pain.

Learn—and practice—good posture before you start any weightlifting or resistance-training program. Otherwise your exercise regimen can hurt instead of help you. Arching the back while lifting weights is a common cause of back injury.

Another benefit that you get from good posture is better breathing. How can your lungs expand and contract freely if your shoulders are hovering over them like a protective mother hen? When your lungs aren't working efficiently, they're not carrying as much oxygen to other parts of your body. Breathe better and you'll feel better and more alert.

To sit or stand properly, pretend you're a puppet suspended from a string. Your spine hangs straight down from that string. To accomplish this:

- Set your head square on your neck, not lolling forward.
- Square your shoulders.
- Pull in your stomach.
- Tuck in your buttocks so that your back will be straight, not curved inward.

If you've had bad posture habits for a long time, sitting and standing properly may not seem comfortable at first. That's because your body has to readjust. Keep at it, and work on strengthening your back and abdominal muscles. Strong muscles help you maintain good posture without effort.

Good posture is important to how you feel *and* how you look to other people. The words "self-confident" are rarely applied to people who walk about as if they're looking for something they've lost. On the other hand, a person who sits, stands, and walks gracefully and regally has an impressive air.

If you'd like professional help with posture, look into the Alexander Technique. Through physical retraining and simple movements, the Alexander Technique teaches people how to put their bodies in balance and achieve greater awareness and control of body movements. You can obtain a list of teachers certified in the Alexander Technique through the North American Society of Teachers of the Alexander Technique or the American Center for the Alexander Technique, Inc. (See ALEXANDER TECHNIQUE.)

Other types of exercises that may help back pain are T'AI CHI and YOGA.

Bursitis and Tendinitis: Bursitis is an inflammation of any of the approximately 150 of the body's bursae. The bursae are fluid-filled sacs that cushion the friction of moving joints. Bursitis is fairly common in the knee and elbow—housemaid's knee and tennis elbow—but it hits the shoulder most often.

Tendinitis is also an inflammation, but of the tendons. Sometimes a swollen tendon presses upon a neighboring bursa, and the unfortunate victim ends up with both problems.

If you've ever had bursitis or tendinitis, you'll realize the wisdom of doing preventive exercises to ward them off. You should do both stretching exercises to increase flexibility and strengthening exercises to improve muscle tone. To stretch the Achilles tendon:

- Stand on a stair-step, low stool, or large book with your heels hanging off the back. (It's best to have something to hold on to so you don't lose your balance.)
- Rise up on your tiptoes, then slowly lower your feet back down until your heels are lower than your toes.
- Repeat ten times and work up to twenty or more.

Another one that's good for the Achilles tendon (and the muscles in the back of your leg):

- Stand at arm's length from a wall with your palms on the wall.
- Lean forward until your chest touches the wall.
- Push yourself back and repeat. Repeat ten times.

If you have to sit for long stretches, keep your shoulders loose by rolling them forward and then circling them back. Do this several times every half hour or so. Here's a back-of-the-shoulder stretcher that you can also do at your desk:

- Hold your arms up beside your head with your elbows bent so that both hands are behind your head.
- Grab one elbow with the opposite hand and pull until you feel the stretch.
- Reverse and pull on the opposite side.

Carpal Tunnel Syndrome: Carpal tunnel syndrome is an occupational hazard of the computer age, but it can be caused by any repetitive task that involves the forearm, wrist, and hand. The carpal tunnel is the sheath in the wrist that contains the tendons and the median nerve that lead into the hand. Repetitious movements (especially with the hands bent at an angle), continuous vibration, or prolonged gripping can cause the tendons to swell and fill the tunnel. When this happens, compression on the median nerve causes numbness and tingling. As the condition worsens, real pain develops. Eventually, a person can lose the use of the hand if nothing is done to correct the problem.

To prevent CTS, make sure your hands, wrists, and forearms are in a straight line if you work at a computer. Adjust your seat or desk height if necessary. When you do any sort of repetitive task with your hands, stop every half hour or so and shake your hands and arms loosely. Exercise your fingers by making a fist and then opening your hand and stretching the fingers as far as they will go. Do wrist curls to help strengthen your wrists. You can do them with or without light weights.

- While sitting down, place your forearms on your lap with your hands extending beyond your knees palms up.
- Bend your hands back slightly and then bring them up slightly beyond a straight line.
- Repeat ten times.
- Turn your hands over so your palms are facing down.
- Perform the same motion as before.
- Repeat ten times.

A good wrist stretcher:

- Hold your palms together at about chest height.
- Lift your elbows up and out from your body until you feel the stretch.
- Hold for several seconds.
- Return to original position and repeat.

Do these exercises several times a day. (If you already have advanced CPS, check with your healthcare practitioner; the exercises may aggravate your condition.)

Constipation: If you eat plenty of fiber, drink lots of fluids, and get enough exercise, you shouldn't have much trouble with irregularity. However, if you do all these things, and constipation is still a problem, here's an exercise you can try that may help. It's called the abdominal contraction. It works best when done before breakfast.

- Stand with your feet about shoulder-width apart and your knees bent in a quarter squat.
- Put your palms on the top of your thighs with your fingers pointing toward the inside of the thighs.
- Let your upper body be supported by your arms.
- Exhale strongly through your mouth. Try to get all the air out of your lungs.

- Without breathing in, pull inward and upward with your abdomen. (This motion will create a cavity under your ribs, but unless you're slim, you may not be able to see it.)
- Hold the upward pull briefly, and then pop your abdomen out vigorously.
- Pull up and pop out four more times before taking a breath. (This sounds harder than it is. It doesn't take as much time to do it as to read it.)
- Stand up straight and inhale. Breathe normally for a minute or two, and then return to the position and repeat the set of five pull-in, pop-out movements.

Depression: Studies have shown that aerobic exercise can help overcome depression and anxiety. Walking, running, biking, and swimming are good choices. One reason that exercise seems to work is that the brain gets a healthy jolt of oxygen when the cardiovascular system is working in high gear. Speeding up the metabolism seems to lift the spirits. You can also try resistance training, T'AI CHI, QIGONG, or YOGA. Exercise can help whether you have momentary blues or a more serious and chronic problem, but in the latter case, you should also seek professional help.

Headache: It is well-known that runners sometimes experience a feeling of extreme well-being known as "runner's high." This feeling of euphoria is caused by the release of brain chemicals—endorphins and enkephalins—which are powerful pain killers. Regular exercise may help prevent the onset of at least some kinds of headaches by keeping the levels of these chemicals elevated.

Aerobic exercise is also a good prescription if you've already got a tension headache. Breathing exercises such as ALTERNATE NOSTRIL BREATHING can help reduce tension. Also try the neck roll:

- Sit with your head erect.
- Very slowly drop your head forward and let your head hang limply.
- Keep moving your head in a rolling motion, first to the right, then back, then to the left, and finally back down to the front.
- Reverse directions and perform the same movements from left to right.

Do the neck roll *slowly* three times in each direction, alternating directions each time. Keep your eyes closed for greater relaxation.

Here's an exercise to relax the face and head. You may want to do this one with your office door shut. (Or you may want to do it in front of the person who gave you the headache.)

- Open both your mouth and eyes as wide as you possibly can.
- Stick your tongue out as far as you can. (Aim for your chin.)
- Hold the position for several seconds.
- Put your tongue back in your mouth and close your mouth.
- Relax all the muscles in your face as completely as you can.
- Repeat several times.

Migraine headaches are less likely to respond to an exercise prescription. Some people find that a sedate walk at the first sign helps. Aerobic exercise keeps your cardiovascular system fit, and that may help reduce the number of future attacks. Biofeedback and relaxation training are other methods to fight all kinds of headache pain.

Incontinence: Urinary incontinence is an embarrassing problem that most people don't want to own up to but would love to be rid of. Pills or surgery help some people, but there's a much safer and easier method: Kegel exercises (also known as pelvic floor exercises). Kegel exercises are pelvic contractions that strengthen the muscles around the vagina, urethra, and anus. Properly performed, Kegels can eliminate the problem for many people (especially those who leak when they laugh, sneeze, or lift) and provide improvement for some others.

Kegels won't work for you unless you can learn to identify the pelvic floor muscles (unpronounceably called the pubococcygeus muscles; PC for short). These are the muscles that allow a person to stop the flow of urine. To locate these muscles, try to stop the flow of urine without using any of the muscles of your abdomen, legs, or buttocks. If you can do it, then you've found the muscles you need to work with. Here's what to do:

- Contract and then immediately relax the PC muscles.
- Repeat this maneuver at least ten times and then go on to the next step.
- Contract the PC muscles and hold for at least ten seconds, then relax.
- Repeat least ten times.

Gradually increase the number of repetitions and the holding time. If you can't hold for ten seconds at first, hold as long as you can. Try to work up to a fifteen-second hold. You can test to be sure you're using only the PC muscles by putting your hand on your abdomen. If it moves when you contract, you're not doing it right. Do these exercises three times a day.

Don't expect quick results. It may take two to three months before you see improvement. People also use Kegel exercises to help control fecal incontinence and to enhance sexual performance.

Insomnia: Nearly everyone has an occasional night of fitful tossing and turning, but about thirty-three percent of people consider sleeplessness a real problem. Insomnia can result from too much caffeine, alcohol, or some medications, but most often it's caused by stress and anxiety. Since exercise helps relieve stress, it stands to reason it would help you get a better night's sleep too.

Besides relieving stress, aerobic exercise raises the brain's output of endorphins, and it tires out the body so it's ready for rest. Paradoxically, though, working out right before you go to bed may keep you awake. To use exercise as a means of fighting insomnia, take your walk, run, or ride in the late afternoon or early evening.

Researchers have found that, in general, people who are in good physical shape sleep better than those who are not very fit. And they spend more time in the two stages of slow-wave sleep, which scientists believe are the most restful. (Slow-wave sleep is a bit like hibernation: Metabolism and body temperature drop; breathing is very rhythmic; and the sleeper is difficult to rouse.) So exercise often enough and long enough to improve your physical condition (and your cardiovascular system), and you may notice a dramatic improvement in your ability to drop off and sleep like a bear in winter.

Intermittent Claudication: Intermittent claudication is an extremely painful problem. If you have it, you know what happens: You start to walk to the corner grocery and suddenly you're struck by a fierce leg cramp. Resting makes it better, so you try again to make it to the store. Then, whammo, there it is again. The pain is brought on by insufficient blood circulation in the arteries of the legs, a condition known as peripheral vascular disease. When the blood can't get through, neither can vital oxygen. Cramping may be anywhere in the leg, foot, hip, or buttocks.

People with diabetes and high cholesterol levels are at greater risk for developing intermittent claudication, but smoking is the greatest threat. About eighty percent of sufferers are smokers. Nearly half the people with the problem have coronary artery disease.

Surprisingly, although walking brings on intermittent claudication, it's also the best treatment (along with giving up cigarettes). Walking is preferable to other exercises because you use your calf muscles, which are the ones most likely to cramp up. Because you may have coronary artery disease, you should check with your healthcare practitioner before beginning any walking program, though.

Once you get the okay, start slowly. Keep walking until you begin to feel cramping. Then try to walk just a little further, even though you're in pain. Rest until the pain subsides and then walk back home. Walk every day and increase your distance gradually. You can use landmarks like houses or telephone poles to gauge your progress. If you can get to the third house on the left the first day, try for the fourth house the next.

If you do it consistently, this program can work amazingly well. People who could barely walk past their own dwelling when they began have been able to increase their distance to a mile or more after several months of walking.

Osteoporosis: Nearly everyone knows someone—usually an older woman—who falls repeatedly and each time fractures a wrist, an ankle or a hip. Chances are that person has osteoporosis. In osteoporosis, the bones gradually lose some of their mineral content and grow weak and fragile. Osteoporotic bones fracture easily, sometimes even without a fall. (In fact, experts believe that some fractures occur *before* the person falls and that the fracture causes the fall rather than vice versa.)

Men as well as women can get osteoporosis, but it's much less common in men because their bones are denser to begin with. And some women are at greater risk than others. White or oriental women and those who are thin and small-boned are more likely to develop the condition. Lifestyle and diet play a role too: Smokers, drinkers, caffeine fiends, and those who take in too little calcium and too much protein are on the risk list.

By the time a woman reaches senior citizen status, she may have lost a quarter of her bone mass, and if she lives long enough, she could lose more than half. Osteoporosis also cuts a person down to size, literally. Some people lose inches in stature, and they may develop the so-called "dowager's hump" as the back bones compress.

Fortunately, most people can stave off osteoporosis in old age by developing strong bones when they're young. It's never too late to begin, though. Even people who already have osteoporosis can stop its progression and sometimes even partially reverse it.

Weight-bearing exercises are one of the keys to developing thicker, stronger bones. A weight-bearing exercise is one that forces your bones to support your weight when you move. Examples are walking, running, aerobic dance, step aerobics, climbing stairs, and weight lifting. No matter what you do, you are going to lose some bone density with aging, but if you build up nice hefty bones when you're younger, you'll be able to spare a little when you're older without developing osteoporosis.

The flip side of exercising to build bone density is that if you *don't* become active, you'll begin to lose what you have. Bone density reaches its peak at about aged thirty-five. After that, you gain some, but you lose a little more. Minimal bone loss continues until menopause, when it accelerates. During the period from the middle thirties until menopause, it's important to do vigorous weight-bearing exercises to retard loss and build up calcium reserves for the time when bone density declines more rapidly.

The hormone estrogen helps maintain calcium in the bones. At menopause the ovaries stop producing estrogen, and bone density declines much more rapidly. Estrogen replacement therapy can help retard bone loss, but it has its own risks. What about calcium supplements? If loss of calcium is the problem, can't you just increase your calcium intake? Apparently, it isn't that simple. Researchers have studied the question over and over and the verdict is that calcium supplementation alone doesn't do the trick. However, calcium supplementation *plus* exercise does help.

One study took a group of older women—some as old as seventy—and really put them through their paces. They walked, jogged, bicycled, climbed stairs, and lifted weights for nearly two years. These women were healthy before they began the study, but they were not exercisers. Another group of nonexercisers of similar ages continued their sedentary ways throughout the study. The result: The exercisers added about 6 percent to their bone mass, while the couch potatoes added nothing.

If you're older, that may seem like too tough a program. You don't need to exercise that hard to benefit. Brisk walking alone can help beef up your bones. If you're not used to exercising, start by walking a distance and a pace you can handle three to five times a week. Gradually increase your time, speed, and distance. A good target pace to aim for is to be able to cover about a mile in thirty minutes. Continue your walk for forty-five minutes or even an hour if you can. Remember to warm up and cool down before and after walking.

You might also want to do some exercises aimed specifically at strengthening the parts of the body that are prone to fracture. These include the wrist, hip, and spine.

For the wrist, try the wrist curls described under *Carpal Tunnel Syndrome*. For the hips, try this:

- Lie on a mat on your side supporting your head with one hand. Place the other hand on the floor for balance.
- Raise the top leg as high as you can.
- Hold for a moment and then lower slowly.
- Repeat ten times.
- Do ten repetitions on the other side.

You can work up to more repetitions, or you can add resistance with elastic bands or both. Elastic bands are like large rubber bands. You can buy them at a sporting goods store. Bicycle inner tubes make a good substitute if you don't want to buy the bands. For the exercise described above, put a band around both ankles so that you're pulling against the band when you raise your leg. You can also use light ankle weights to get the same effect.

To strengthen the back, try the back extension exercise.

- Lie on a mat on your stomach with your feet anchored under a low chair or couch. Keep your arms at your sides with your hands palm up.
- Slowly try to raise just your head and shoulders from the floor.
- Hold momentarily, and then slowly lower yourself back to your original position.
- Repeat two or three times.

If you already have osteoporosis, don't try these exercises. Check with your health practitioner to see if you can safely try a walking program.
Overweight: People who are overweight have a dilemma. Exercise is one of the best slimming aids, yet it's harder to be active when you're carrying unwanted pounds. However, whether we like it or not, the only sure way to get rid of fat forever is aerobic exercise. The good news is you don't have to—in fact, shouldn't—diet. Naturally, you'll make faster progress if you combine a sensible caloric intake of healthful foods with exercise, but the exercise program is key. You won't win the battle against fat without it.

Why is exercise such a powerful fat fighter? First because it increases your metabolism, the rate at which your body converts food to energy. The more food you use as energy, the less will be stored in your body as fat. And exercise not only causes your body to burn food faster while you're exercising, it keeps your metabolism elevated for hours after you've stopped exercising.

Also, when you exercise, you build muscle. Muscle works. It lifts that barge, totes that bale. Fat just sits there taking up space. So the muscle that you build while exercising uses energy that fat doesn't. Voilà! More calories burned. When your body has used up the calories you took in as food, it starts in on the stored fat.

If you simply diet, your body reacts differently. It says, "Good grief, I'm not getting enough to eat. I'd better conserve." So instead of your metabolism speeding up, it slows down. You eat less, but your body sticks right with you and banks its calorie-burning fires so you won't waste away. You can't make much progress that way.

If you want to get rid of fat, you can't just exercise now and then, but you don't have to knock yourself out with super-strenuous activities either. The first step is to pick one or more activities that you really like to do. You're in this for the long haul, so you'd better find something you enjoy or you won't stick with it. There's a long list of activities that qualify as aerobic exercise: walking, jogging, biking, skating, swimming, stair-climbing, and cross-country skiing are among the most popular. And, of course, there are all sorts of aerobic routines on video that you can follow. Most of the things you can do outdoors you can do indoors if you have the equipment. Most authorities recommend at least twenty to thirty minutes of exercise in your target heart-rate zone three to five times a week. (See AEROBIC EXERCISE, for more information.)

It's not easy to get rid of fat, especially if you've been overweight and inactive for a long time. There's no quick road to success, but your efforts will be rewarded if you stick with it. You'll have more energy, a leaner, healthier body, and a whole new attitude about yourself. Exercise gives you more self-confidence, a feeling of control, and a better body image.

FURTHER READING

Basmajian, John V., and Steven L. Wolf. *Therapeutic Exercises*. Baltimore: Williams & Wilkins, 1990.

Carr, Rachel. *Arthritis: Relief Beyond Drugs*. New York: Harper & Row, c1981.

Fardon, David F. *Free Yourself from Neck Pain and Headache*. Englewood Cliffs, N.J.: Prentice-Hall, c1983.

Feinstein, Alice. *Training the Body to Cure Itself*. Emmaus, Pa: Rodale Press, 1992.

Goldberg, Linn, and Diane L. Elliot. *Exercise for the Prevention of Illness*. Philadelphia: F.A. Davis, 1994.

Imre, David, and Colleen Dimson. *Goodbye Backache*. New York: Ballantine Books, 1984.

Johnsgard, Keith, Ph.D. *The Exercise Prescription for Depression and Anxiety*. New York: Plenum Press, 1989.

Krewer, Semyon, and Ann Edgar. *Help for your Arthritic Hand*. New York: Cornerstone Library, c1982.

Medicine in the Public Interest. *Learning to Live with Osteoarthritis*. Boston: **MIPI**, 1983.

Meyers, Casey. *Walking: A Complete Guide to the Complete Exercise*. New York: Random House, 1992.

Painter, Jack W. *Postural Integration: Transformation of the Whole Self*. Mill Valley, Calif.: International Center for Release and Integration, 1986.

Perkins-Carpenter, Betty. *How to Prevent Falls*. New York: St. Martin's Press, 1993.

Pinsky, Mary. *The Carpal Tunnel Syndrome Book*. New York: Warner, 1993.

Sansone, Leslie. *Walk Aerobics—Senior Style*. Newark, N.J.: Parade Video, 1991. *(video)*

Steinfeld, Jake. *Better Back Workout*. Los Angeles: Hemdale Home Video, Inc., c1991. (video)

Weight Watchers International. *Weight Watchers Walk*. New York: Simon & Schuster Audio, p1994. (audiotape)

RESOURCE GROUPS

American Center for the Alexander Technique
129 West 67th St.

New York, NY 10023
Phone: 212/799-0468

Arthritis Foundation. (Check your phonebook for the nearest local chapter.)
The AF offers brochures on exercise classes and at-home exercise videotapes.

Help for Incontinent People
PO Box 544
Union, SC 29397
Hotline: 800/BLADDER; Phone: 803/579-900; Fax: 803/579-7902

Audio- and videotapes; pamphlets; quarterly newsletter ($5) *HIP Report*

North American Society of Teachers of the Alexander Technique
PO BOX 3992
Champaign, IL 61826
Phone: 217/359-3529

Simon Foundation
PO Box 815
Wilmette, IL 60091
Phone: 800/23SIMON; Fax: 708/864-758

Organization for help with incontinence; membership: $15; quarterly newsletter *The Informer*; also book; videotape.

T'AI CHI (T'AI CHI CH'UAN, TI JI)

DEFINITION

T'ai chi is a Chinese martial art that emphasizes graceful, fluid movements and the development of the qi (internal spirit). It may be practiced for its health benefits alone, but in its fullest expression, it encompasses a complete way of living.

APPLICATIONS

Physiological: Muscle tension, inflexibility, back pain, weak abdominal muscles, posture, gait, coordination, stamina, hypertension
Psychological: Stress, tension, poor self-esteem, fear of attack

COLLATERAL CROSS-THERAPIES (therapies)

Meditation, qi gong, healthful diet

CONTRAINDICATIONS

T'ai chi is the gentlest and most rhythmic of the martial arts. In China, even very old people continue to practice it with grace and precision. Because it requires almost no initial strength, people of almost any age or condition of health can begin the study of t'ai chi. However, it does require a certain degree of stamina and excellent balance. If you have any doubts about whether t'ai chi is for you, check with your healthcare practitioner. You might also want to observe a class or rent a video before you make up your mind.

EQUIPMENT & MATERIALS

The ideal way to learn t'ai chi is with an accomplished instructor, but it can be a do-it-yourself project, as long as you can see the movements. For this, you will really need a videotape. Several sources provide a series of three tapes that progress from beginner, through intermediate, to advanced. A book with good illustrations can be helpful too, but since the movements are fluid and graceful, you really need to see a person in motion to get the full benefit of the instruction. T'ai chi does not use props, but you should dress in comfortable, loose clothing that doesn't inhibit movement.

ORIGIN

Say "martial arts" to most Westerners, and they'll picture a beefy man in a robe viciously slicing a brick in half with the side of his hand, bellowing ferociously all the while. Or they'll envision Bruce Lee leaping into the midst of a host of bad guys and dispatching them all in nothing flat with a series of amazing (and painful) acrobatic kicks to their vulnerable body parts. The film industry has made big business of the so-called "hard" martial arts, but martial arts have their softer disciplines, too, and t'ai chi is the softest of them all. (Popular films notwithstanding, even the hard arts—judo, taekwondo, and karate—have as their ultimate goal the avoidance of conflict, not the infliction of punishment.)

The earliest precursor of t'ai chi dates back about 2,000 years to the Chou dynasty (1122– 221 B.C.), when a form of exercise called *daoyin* was popular in China. Practitioners of daoyin combined special breathing techniques with stylized body movements. During this period, the philosopher Lao-tzu, who was the founder of Taoism, developed the philosophy that the qi (life force) could be consciously controlled by the mind. (He himself had a legendary reputation for being able to do so at will.)

Then, in the latter part of the Han dynasty, Buddhists fanned out to China from India, bringing with them their doctrine of yoga and later the sport of boxing. The Chinese combined some of the principles of yoga with their beliefs about the qi and the ancient practice of daoyin. This amalgam was the forerunner of qigong, which eventually became part of the practice of t'ai chi. Boxing as the Buddhists practiced it was not so different from the sport today. Physical strength, courage, and the ability to hit hard were the hallmarks of a good boxer then as now. However, the sport began to change when renowned boxer Chang San-feng, who was a Taoist, not a Buddhist, developed a whole new theory of exercise based on Taoist teachings.

Chang San-feng believed that the body should be supple, not just strong, and he felt that movements should naturally flow one from another, gracefully as nature intended. Fluid body movements, the belief in the ability to manipulate the qi, and the breathing techniques of qigong came together in what we know today as t'ai chi. Initially, t'ai chi was practiced as a means of self-defense, but over the centuries it evolved into an elaborate system that is part lifestyle, part spiritual development, and part physical fitness training.

As the years passed, t'ai chi practitioners kept adding more and more variations in movement until eventually there were more than 125. Today, however, the system has again been simplified through the efforts of Cheng Man-ch'ing. His pupil, T.T. Liang, who taught t'ai chi for over fifty years, was a pioneer in introducing t'ai chi to the United States.

INSTRUCTIONS

It may seem hard to believe that boxing and dancing could be part of the same form of exercise, but in fact, t'ai chi instructors sometimes speak of "choreographing" the moves, and because of the slow and rhythmic way they're performed, the movements do appear dance-like.

T'ai chi practitioners stress that t'ai chi is an "internal" art, not simply a series of external movements. The great t'ai chi master Yang Cheng-fu remarked that "T'ai chi ch'uan is meditation in action, action within meditation."

Taoists believe that people would never suffer any physical illness or even death if they knew how to properly conserve the "Three Treasures." These are the *ching*, the *ch'i* (qi), and the *shen*, our reproductive, life-force, and spiritual energies. Through the disciplines and movements of t'ai chi, practitioners aver that one can use the ching, ch'i, and shen to promote good health and extend longevity.

T'ai chi exercises focus on developing an inner calm that allows the mind to regulate the body and "mobilize the ch'i." Movement is slow, fluid, and natural. One movement flows effortlessly into another. Generally, the stance is a semicrouching posture that preserves balance.

Throughout the routine, it is important to keep the rhythm of the breathing in unison with the body.

The many movements and "gestures" have fanciful names that often provide a wonderful mental picture of the posture. The "horse" stance, for example, resembles a pantomime of a person sitting astride an invisible mount. In "repulse monkey," the pose is about what you'd expect: hand upraised and outstretched with the palm facing forward in a "hey, get back there" gesture.

Since movement in t'ai chi is natural and not forced or strenuous, it is an ideal form of exercise for older people and those who aren't particularly strong or athletic. Benefits are both emotional and physical. Devotees say that t'ai chi improves circulation, increases flexibility and balance, and clears the mind.

If you want to learn t'ai chi, you really should try to do it in accompaniment to a video. There are some excellent books that illustrate the postures and describe the philosophy, but only by seeing someone actually performing the positions can you hope to achieve the fluid motion that characterizes t'ai chi.

FURTHER READING

Chuen, Lam Kam. *Step-by-Step Tai Chi*. New York: Simon & Shuster, 1994.

Crompton, Paul. *The Art of Tai Chi*. Rockport, Mass.: Element, 1993.

Grant, Joshua. *Tai Chi for Fitness & Health*. Troy, Mich.: Video Treasures, 1993. (beginning, intermediate and advanced videotapes)

Huang, Alfred. *Complete Tai-chi*. Rutland, Vt.: Charles E. Tuttle Co., 1993.

Kersh, Ken. *Tai Chi Chuan: Yang Style*. Monterey, Calif.: Kersh & Costanza Productions, 1993. (videotape)

Liao, Way Sui. *Tai Chi Classics*. Boston: Shambhala Publications, 1990.

Man-Ch'ing Cheng. *T'ai Chi Ch'uan: A Simplified Method of Calisthenics for Health & Self Defense*. Berkeley, Calif.: North Atlantic Books, 1981.

Montague, Erle. *Learn Tai Chi*. Los Angeles: Wood Knapp Video, 1992. (video)

Olson, Stuart Alve, compiler and translator. *Cultivating the Ch'i*. St. Paul: Dragon Door Publications, 1993.

Sieh, Ron. *T'ai Chi Ch'uan: The Internal Tradition*. Berkeley, Calif.: North Atlantic Books, 1992.

T'ai Chi (magazine). Order information: Wayfarer Publications, PO Box 26156, Los Angeles, CA 90026; phone 213/665-7773.

Tai Chi Chung for Beginners. Los Angeles: Tigerlily International Productions, 1993. (videotape)

RESOURCE GROUPS

All major cities and many smaller ones have t'ai chi schools and classes where you can go to observe and talk to the instructors. You can find books and tapes at libraries, bookstore, and some health-food stores.

YOGA

DEFINITION

Yoga comprises systems of movement, breathing, and meditation designed to unify and balance mind and body. There are many systems of yoga, some of which consist principally of breathing exercises and postures; others are concerned chiefly with contemplation and meditation. In the United States, yoga is popularly considered a form of exercise—which it is—but it is much more than that.

APPLICATIONS

Physiological: Muscle tension, inflexibility, backache, headache, poor circulation, complexion problems, posture, body configuration, overweight, constipation, asthma, menstrual disorders, varicose veins, sciatica, peptic ulcer, hemorrhoids, bronchitis, emphysema, diabetes, sore throat, sinus congestion
Psychological :Stress, tension, insomnia, chemical or nicotine dependency, anxiety, fatigue, distraction, nervousness

COLLATERAL CROSS-THERAPIES

Ayurveda, meditation, aromatherapy, herbalism, vegetarianism

CONTRAINDICATIONS

None

EQUIPMENT & MATERIALS

Exercise mat or rug

ORIGIN

Like Ayurveda, to which it is a sister, yoga comes out of the ancient Hindu tradition of India, from the teachings of the Vedas. In India, it is traditional to first study Ayurveda, the science of the body, before beginning to practice yoga. This is because a person is considered ready to undertake the more spiritual practice of yoga only when his or her body is fit.

Yoga probably originated about 5,000 to 6,000 years ago, but its roots may go back even farther. The word *yoga* comes from the Sanskrit *yuj,* which means "union." On the spiritual side, yoga seeks union with the Ultimate Being.

The man who is considered the father of yoga was called Pantanjali. Little is known about Pantanjali, but he described the eight limbs of yoga and yogic practices. They are: the natural regulation of the nervous system, discipline, cleansing, postures, concentration, contemplation, the awakening of awareness, and achieving the state of perfect equilibrium.

There are many systems of yoga, but they all have the same purpose: to unify the mind and body. The system taught most often in the United States is hatha yoga. Hatha yoga includes the well-known postures, called *asanas*, and breathing exercises (see PRANAYAMA). Some yogis don't consider hatha yoga a yoga at all but rather a system of exercise that serves other yogas. Nevertheless, it is the system that people in the West most often adopt. Hatha yoga itself has several variations.

Where hatha yoga works on the body to perfect it, and then works through the body to the mind, raja yoga works upon the mind to perfect it and then works through the mind to the body. Raja yoga is the yoga of meditation.

Kundalini yoga works toward union through the arousal of latent psychic energy. This yoga is characterized by the "serpent power" that releases and channels energy as it moves from its seat at the base of the spine and through the chakras toward the crown of the head. (See CHAKRA BALANCING.)

There are several other types of yoga, but these are the ones that are most familiar to people in the West. Most of the self-help books and videotapes available in the United States describe the system of hatha yoga. You can find information on other types of yoga, but it isn't as prevalent.

INSTRUCTIONS

The asanas (postures) of hatha yoga are relatively easy to learn at home on your own if you have a well-illustrated book. Even better is a videotape that allows you to follow along with an instructor. You can practice the asanas purely to achieve a greater degree of flexibility and better body conformation—in other words, as exercise—but you should include the proper breathing techniques too. (Some of these are described under PRANAYAMA.)

There are, however, certain asanas that are suggested for physical problems. Most people have a regular routine that they perform, usually early in the morning. If they have special physical problems, they include the postures designed to alleviate them.

Yogic postures are never forced or strained. Although some asanas look almost impossible to perform to a beginner, you should only push yourself slightly beyond the comfort level toward the completion of the posture. Yoga teachers say that if you have patience, your body will suddenly yield, and you will be able to perform the posture.

Because all yoga techniques aim to produce tranquillity, one of the first postures a beginner learns is appropriately called "the corpse." To perform the corpse:

- Lie flat on your back with your legs outstretched, heels slightly apart, and your legs flopping limply outward.
- Your arms should rest on the floor, palms up, with the fingers lying limp and slightly curled.
- Breathe through your nostrils, not your mouth. Observe your breathing. Don't change it in any way, just observe it.
- Then take two successive deep abdominal breaths, exhaling fully each time. (Your abdomen should swell out as you inhale and contract as you exhale.)
- Allow your abdominal muscles to relax and return to simply observing your breathing.
- Soon your breathing will become rhythmic and smooth.
- Now focus your attention on your body part by part, starting with the feet. Visualize a beam of light striking each part. Is there any tension there? If so, let it go.
- Continue focusing on each part of your body and releasing tension until your entire body is relaxed from the soles of your feet to your scalp.

You'll find that, as your body relaxes, each part will begin to feel heavier and warmer, with its full weight resting on the floor.

As you can tell from the foregoing posture, you can't hurry yoga. Each asana takes some time to perform properly, but unlike many more strenuous exercises, yoga postures do not depend upon numerous repetitions for their effectiveness. Some postures are performed only once during a routine, others just a few times.

There are literally hundreds of possible asanas, some of which would involve mind-boggling contortions for a beginner, so if you decide you'd like to try yoga either through taking a class or by studying a book or video, be sure to find something at the appropriate level.

FURTHER READING

Crocker, Deborah. *Stretching for Energy*. Indianapolis, Ind.: Kartes Video Communication, 1986. (video)

Groves, Dawn. *Yoga for Busy People*, San Rafael, Calif.: New World Library, 1995.

Hatfield, Roger. *Foundations of Yoga*. Troy, Mich.: Video Treasures, 1994. (2 videos)

Hewitt, James. *The Complete Yoga Book*. New York: Schocken Books, 1977.

Iyengar, B.K.S. *Light on Yoga*. New York: Schocken Books, 1976.

Jaggi, O.P. *Yogic and Tantric Medicine*. New Delhi: Atma Ram, 1973.

Lad, Vasant. *Ayurveda: The Science of Self-Healing*. Wilmot, Wis.: Lotus Press, 1984. (includes asanas for specific medical conditions)

Lidell, Lucy, with Narayani Rabinovitch and Giris Rabinovitch. *The Sivananda Companion to Yoga*. New York: Simon & Schuster, 1983.

Mehta, Mira. *How to Use Yoga*. New York: Smithmark, 1994.

Stewart, Mary and Sandra Lousada. *Yoga Over 50*. New York: Simon & Schuster, 1994.

Vanda, Scaravelli. *Awakening the Spine*. San Francisco: Harper San Francisco, 1991.

Yoga Journal. Order information: 2054 University Ave., Suite 604, Berkeley, CA 94704-1082; phone 415/841-9200 (6 issues $12).

RESOURCE GROUPS

American Yoga Association
513 S. Orange Ave.
Sarasota, FL 34236
Phone: 813/953-5859

American Yoga Association
3130 Mayfield Rd. Ste. W-301
Cleveland Heights, OH 44118
Phone: 216/371-0078

YOUR HEALING HANDS

When we bump our shins or bang our elbows on the corner of the table, we generally grab the offended part and start rubbing it to ease the pain. Human beings instinctively know that touch is therapeutic.

Rubbing usually does make a bumped shin or a banged elbow feel better. If you can ease pain by simply rubbing without any special technique, imagine what you can accomplish by learning some specific methods for using your hands to heal.

Many people occasionally engage in the luxury of a professional massage, and some do it often. Somewhere perhaps there is someone who came away and said, "I hated that," but most of us find it blissfully relaxing to be pummeled and kneaded by a masseur or masseuse. Obviously, to perform massage on yourself, you have to use somewhat different techniques, but you can accomplish a great deal in the way of relaxation, treatment for sore muscles, and rejuvenation.

Most of the techniques in this section are based on the premise that applying pressure to one part of the body will influence another part of the body, so they have a much wider application than simple relaxation. Accupressure, for example, can be used to treat a wide variety of problems. Accupressure uses the same points as acupuncture, but instead of needles, you use finger pressure. As an untrained person, it would be dangerous for you to start sticking needles in yourself, but you can try the method safely with acupressure and gain many of the same benefits.

As you might expect, many, but not all, the techniques in this section have their roots in Oriental healing practices. You can do all the techniques we talk about by yourself and to yourself, but you might enjoy learning them by practicing on a friend or family member.

ACUPRESSURE
(ACUPRESSURE MASSAGE, SEE ALSO SHIATSU)

DEFINITION

Acupressure is a healing technique similar to acupuncture, but instead of using needles, acupressure uses finger and thumb pressure to stimulate certain points on the body to promote healing in another part of the body.

APPLICATIONS

Physiological: Headache, arthritis, muscular tension, chronic pain, whole-body imbalance, tendinitis, obesity
Psychological: Insomnia, tension, fatigue, stress, smoking control

COLLATERAL CROSS-THERAPIES

Herbalism, meditation, aromatherapy

RECOMMENDED ADJUNCT ACTIVITIES AND BEHAVIORS

For relaxation, perform acupressure in a quiet room without distractions. You may want to dim the lights and play soft music also.

CONTRAINDICATIONS

Acupressure is not a suitable treatment for fractures or for people who are at risk for internal bleeding.

EQUIPMENT & MATERIALS

Chair and/or floor mat; to work on a partner, you'll also need a small, hard pillow for the neck.

ORIGIN

Acupressure is based on the same theories as acupuncture, but without the needles, so it is completely noninvasive. It is also sometimes thought of as a form of massage, although the methods are quite different from those of Swedish massage.

You may not think of it as a "treatment" when you rub a body part that hurts. It just seems to feel better, so you do it, but actually rubbing the afflicted part does induce healing by increasing the blood flow to the area. When circulation is stimulated, more vital oxygen comes in and more toxic products go out. People used this form of therapy long before they knew why it helped.

As civilization advanced, people learned more about their bodies, and they developed systems of healing. We know from *The Yellow Emperor's Classic of Internal Medicine*, which was written more than 4,000 years ago, that the ancient Chinese had already formulated the underlying theories of acupuncture and acupressure.

Oriental medicine is empirical; that is, its practices are based on observation and experience. Chinese healers noticed that various illnesses affected different points on the body. The Chinese catalogued these points and noted that some points seemed related to others. When related points were connected diagrammatically, they formed twelve pathways or meridians on each half of the body. The Chinese theorized that blockage at any point along a pathway could affect other points on the same pathway. Thus, removing blockage at a defined point in the arch of the foot would improve the function of the kidneys because they were on the same pathway. It is from this premise that acupuncture, and later acupressure, evolved.

Centuries later, Western researchers developed their theories of the way the body functions through the scientific method rather than empirically, but they also found interconnections, which they called "systems" (e.g., the circulatory system, the endocrine system, etc). In many cases, the functions of the systems closely correspond to the functions of the meridians, so the gap between Eastern and Western medical theory might not be as wide as we once believed.

The Chinese introduced acupuncture to Japan more than a thousand years ago, and it has been practiced there ever since. In the eighteenth century, the Japanese introduced a new needleless technique that combined acupuncture with a form of Oriental massage. The Japanese version of acupressure later became known as shiatsu. Although some people use the terms *shiatsu* and *acupressure* interchangeably, there are distinctions between the two.

Acupressure was virtually unknown in the United States until about twenty-five years ago. With the gradual public acceptance of acupuncture as a legitimate form of treatment, interest in acupressure grew. Its increasing popularity reflects the current movement toward self-care. Unlike acupuncture, acupressure can be self-administered, and it is a useful tool for maintaining health as well as for treating illnesses. Further, because it is noninvasive, it is an extremely safe therapy compared to potentially harmful drugs or other more drastic treatments.

INSTRUCTIONS

The bulb of the thumb is the most oft-used "instrument" in acupressure. When you want to cover a wider area, use both thumbs together. Their tips should be touching, with one thumb at about a forty-five degree angle to the other. You can also cover a wider area by using the bulbs of two or three fingers held together. Whether you use fingers or thumbs, be sure you're applying pressure with the fleshy parts of the digits, not the tips.

Professional acupressure therapists also sometimes use knuckles and even elbows, but the untrained should stick to fingers and thumbs. If you're working on a partner, you can also use the flattened palms of both hands to cover broad areas of the lower back and abdomen.

Whether you're working on yourself or a partner, you'll need to experiment to find the right amount of pressure. Be especially careful when doing acupressure on someone else not to jab fiercely, even if this feels good to you; the pressure level that works for you may be too uncomfortable for your partner.

You should also vary the pressure according to the body part you're treating. For example, well-muscled areas like the back of the shoulders can take a lot more pressure than the lower abdomen or the delicate areas of the face. The sensation you're aiming for is that middle ground between pleasure and pain. Pressure should be applied for three to seven seconds, no more. Limit repeat pressure on the same spot to three or four times.

You can use acupressure to help relieve the symptoms of a cold. As with all other cold remedies, this works best if you begin using the technique at the first sniffle. Don't wait until the cold has you firmly in its grip. Be sure to do each of the procedures below on both sides of your body and do them several times a day until your symptoms subside.

To relieve sinus congestion, find the pressure point directly above the inner corner of your eye. It should be slightly below the eyebrow. Be cautious when locating this point. You don't want to gouge out your eye. Apply pressure slowly until the spot feels somewhat tender. Keep applying this amount of pressure for three to four seconds. Stop. Repeat twice more, stopping for a few seconds between each pressure.

For nasal congestion, find the pressure point between the cheekbone and the outside edge of the nostril. Again, apply pressure for three to four seconds, stop, and then repeat twice more.

For a cough, locate the biceps tendon next to the hollow of your inner elbow. (It will be on the thumb side.) The pressure point is in the hollow, right next to the biceps tendon. Follow the same pressing and releasing steps as given above.

For generalized cold symptoms, there is a pressure point at the base of the thumb on the palm side. The point is in the hollow between the thumb and index finger. You may want to use two fingers here to be sure you've got the point covered. Follow the pressing and releasing steps above.

It's 2:00 A.M. and you're flipping and flopping like a beached fish, unable to fall asleep. You could reach for a pill, but instead why not try this acupressure technique. You can do it while sitting on the side of your bed.

- Place both hands on top of your head with the fingertips of the middle three fingers touching at the crown. Your fingers should be spread apart but not stretched to the maximum.
- Press down firmly with the middle three fingers for about three seconds then release pressure.
- Repeat twice more, pausing in between.
- Now move to the base of the skull and place the index and middle fingers of both hands in the indentation at the top of the neck.
- Press firmly for three seconds; release; repeat; release; repeat.
- Still working with the area at the base of the skull, move the two fingers on each hand about two finger-widths toward your ears.
- Press and pause as above for three repetitions.
- Move another two finger-widths toward the ears and repeat the sequence.

Before you know it, you'll feel relaxed and sleepy. You should be in the land of nod within a few minutes.

Many people use acupressure as a preventive technique to relieve stress and put the whole body in harmony. An acupressure session for the whole body takes a minimum of twenty minutes. If you want to see what the experience is like, treat yourself to a professional acupressure session. This will help you to develop your own technique. You can practice whole-body acupressure on yourself, but you might find it even more rewarding to recruit a friend or your spouse and practice on each other. Acupressure; like other therapies with Oriental origins, aims to treat the whole person, so you will get the most out of it if you involve your mind and spirit as well as your body.

If you want to learn more about acupressure, there's a large selection of books, audiotapes, and videotapes from which to choose. See the *Further Reading* section here and the one under SHIATSU.

FURTHER READING

Bauer, Cathryn. *Acupressure for Everybody*. New York: H. Holt, 1991.

————. *Acupressure for Women*. Freedom, Calif.: Crossing Press, 1987.

Coseo, Marc. *The Acupressure Warmup*. Brookline, Mass.: Paradigm Publications, 1992.

Friedman, Robert and Kelly Howell. *Sound Techniques for Healing High Blood Pressure*. Santa Fe: Brain Sync, 1993. (audiotape)

Gach, Michael Reed. *Acupressure's Potent Points: A Guide to Self-Care*. New York: Bantam Books, 1990.

————. *The Bum Back Book*. Berkeley, Calif.: Celestial Arts, 1983.

Hin, Kuan and Nancy Dargel. *Chinese Massage and Acupressure*. New York: Bergh Publishing, 1991.

Houston, Francis M. *The Healing Benefits of Acupressure*. New Canaan, Conn.: Keats Publishing, 1991.

Kenyon, Julian N. *Acupressure Techniques*. Rochester, Vt.: Healing Arts Press, 1988.

Wagner, Lindsay and Robert M. Klein. *The Acupressure Facelift*. Irvine, Calif.: Karl Lorimar Home Video, 1986. (video)

RESOURCE GROUPS

The Acupressure Institute
1533 Shattuck Ave.
Berkeley, CA 94709
Phone: 415/845-1059 or 800/442-2232

Workbooks, audiotapes; also local referrals

American Oriental Bodywork Therapy Association
50 Maple Place
Manhassett, NY 11030
Phone: 516/365-5025

G-Jo Institute
PO Box 8060
Hollywood, FL 33084
Phone: 305/791-1562

Self-healing acupressure techniques; books, audio- and videotapes

CHUA KA

DEFINITION

Chua ka is a form of deep-tissue massage that is used to dispel fear and tension as well as bodily aches and pains.

APPLICATIONS

Physiological: Inflexibility, muscle tension, cellulite reduction
Psychological: Stress, tension

COLLATERAL CROSS-THERAPIES

Meditation; other massage techniques; aromatherapy

RECOMMENDED ADJUNCT ACTIVITIES AND BEHAVIORS

Lifestyle changes as necessary to eliminate stress and tension

CONTRAINDICATIONS

Chua ka is perfectly safe for most people to perform on themselves, but if you have a serious medical condition, check with your healthcare practitioner before you try it.

EQUIPMENT & MATERIALS

You will need a ka stick, and a comfortable but relatively firm place to sit or lie while doing the massage.

ORIGIN

Chua ka has its roots in the preparations that Mongolian soldiers once made before going into battle. They performed a series of body manipulations to purge themselves of fear and past traumas, so that they could fight (and possibly die) without any remnants of past problems to interfere with their abilities to confront their enemies and vanquish them.

Chua ka is not very well known in the United States, but as interest in both Oriental and self-healing have grown, it is slowly gaining attention.

INSTRUCTIONS

Chua Ka is a deep-tissue massage technique that you can perform on yourself or on other people. The principle behind chua ka is that unpleasant experiences and emotional problems cause muscle tension in the body. Practitioners of chua ka believe that various regions of the body store different emotional stresses. When you perform chua ka, you release muscle tension in that particular zone. As the muscle tension in a certain area dissipates, the corresponding emotional problem disappears as well.

Chua ka uses three different techniques. In the first, you use firm hand pressure to massage your muscles. For the second procedure, you need a flat massage tool known as a "ka" stick. (Some health-food stores carry this stick or you may purchase one by mail order.) The ka stick is used much as the fingers are in shiatsu massage. (See SHIATSU.)

The sweeping, vertical strokes of the third technique are called "skin rolling." By using a combination of the three techniques, you loosen up your whole body, enabling it to relax fully. Practitioners of chua ka say it is excellent therapy for people who are habitually tense and stressed out. If you're interested in trying chua ka, contact the Arica Institute for information about training sessions. We haven't described specific techniques because you really should learn from a professional before working on your own.

RESOURCE GROUP

Arica Institute, Inc.
150 Fifth Ave.
New York, NY 10011
Phone: 212/807-9600

DO-IN

DEFINITION

Do-In (pronounced dough-in) is a simple form of Oriental exercise and self-massage that is based on the belief that people intuitively know what their bodies need at any given moment.

APPLICATIONS

Physiological: Prevention of muscle and joint pain and stiffness
Psychological: Prevention of stress, tension, insomnia

COLLATERAL CROSS-THERAPIES

Breathing exercises, macrobiotics, vegetarianism, meditation

RECOMMENED ADJUNCT ACTIVITIES AND BEHAVIORS

Moderation in lifestyle

CONTRAINDICATIONS

Since Do-In is based on the premise that you should exercise and massage your body in a manner that feels good to you, there are no contraindications as long as you don't deviate from that idea.

EQUIPMENT & MATERIALS

Exercise mat or rug

ORIGIN

Do-In is part of the holistic tradition of Oriental medicine that traces its roots back into antiquity. It is not an isolated practice but a part of a complete philosophy that includes dietary habits, breathing, meditation, and other forms of exercIse.

Do-In first developed in Japan, where it was the custom to make important decisions in the early morning—before dawn—because peo-ple felt that the fresh air of a new day cleared the foggy mind and helped them make sound judgments. The Do-In exercises helped awaken the mind and body and put them in harmony for the coming day. In the

Western world, we reach for a cup of coffee to jump-start our daily activities; in the Orient, many people begin the morning with Do-In instead.

Do-In isn't very well-known in the West as yet, but with the growing interest in self-care and the increased acceptance of alternative techniques, it is beginning to show up both in the literature and in practice.

INSTRUCTIONS

Do-In techniques are very simple and adaptable, so they are ideal for self-care. If you're trying to wean yourself away from a morning caffeine fix, they may be just the ticket to drive away the cobwebs and energize your mind and body for the coming busy day. (It's ideal to do Do-In first thing, but you can use the techniques any time during the day when you feel you need a pick-up.)

There's nothing mysterious about Do-In. It uses massage techniques with which you're probably already familiar: tapping, kneading, pounding, and pressing. The purpose of Do-In is to keep you moving smoothly through the various phases and paces of your day. The exercises are preventive; do them so you won't get stiff and tense.

Many of the movements are almost instinctive. If it seems as if rolling your shoulders would keep your back from tensing up during a long session at your desk, do it. Do-In doesn't take a big chunk out of your day because you can do one or two exercises whenever you feel the need.

In the morning, though, you may want to do a quick whole-body massage to pep up your circulation and get your body systems functioning smoothly. Start with the face and neck and work downward toward the feet. During the massage, breathe deeply. You may want to use some of the breathing techniques described elsewhere in this book.

Start by making a loose fist and tapping all over your head lightly. Then massage your scalp with your fingertips as if you're washing your hair. Now move on to your ears. (Oriental practitioners believe that massaging the ears helps the excretory functions and improves hearing and mental processes.) With your first three fingers, press all around the rim of the ear, pushing it against your head. Then massage the whole ear with the thumb and index finger. (You can easily do both ears at once.)

Get your face tingling by placing the flats of your palms against your cheeks and rubbing briskly up and down. (Keep taking those deep breaths.) You'll soon feel a warm glow.

The idea is to loosen up the whole body and get the juices flowing. When you get to your feet, lie down on your back with your arms positioned slightly away from your body. Raise and bend your knees. Put your feet together and rub them briskly against each other till you feel them tingle. Be sure to cover the tops, soles and toes of both feet.

Here's a good morning toner for your back and buttocks. Kneel on the floor, resting back on your heels. Make loose fists with both hands and gently pound your back and buttocks, starting as high as you can reach and working down. Then work your way back up. Do this several times.

Later in the day when you've been sitting for a while, you can comfort your back and shoulders by giving them a quick massage. Start with the lower back. Press rather firmly with both thumbs on the indentation near the bottom of your spine. It shouldn't be hard to find the spot because it'll feel good when you touch it. Press several times. Then, using your fingers, knead the whole area. Now stretch up as tall as you can, rolling your shoulders up toward your ears and contracting the shoulder muscles as you do so. Drop back and let your shoulders relax. Do this several times.

Now drop one shoulder lower than the other. Contract and relax the muscles on the "high" shoulder several times. (The lower shoulder remains relaxed.) Reverse shoulder positions and repeat with the other shoulder. Pound each shoulder a few times with a loose fist. Then knead the top of each shoulder with your fingers and palm. Finish by doing a couple more tall stretches and shoulder shrugs. Your whole back should feel revitalized.

Classically, the back picker-upper is done while kneeling on the floor, but you can easily perform it while sitting in a chair. If you're desk-bound most of the day, you might want to do it every hour or so to prevent an aching back. If you don't have time to do the whole procedure, concentrate on kneading the lower back and doing the tall stretches and shoulder shrugs.

Since Do-In is based on classic oriental philosophy, some of the massage exercises involve acupressure points along the meridians. If you want to learn more about the classic technique for Do-In and how it affects the body's specific functions, consult one of the references listed in the *Further Reading* section. Some massage schools also teach the Do-In technique.

FURTHER READING

Kushi, Michio. *The Book of Dō-In. Tokyo: Japan Publications, 1979.*

Kushi, Michio, with Alex Jack. *Diet for a Strong Heart.* New York: St. Martin's Press, 1985. (This book deals chiefly with macrobiotic diet, but it includes a short section on Do-In. The exercises described are principally for strengthening the heart and circulation.)

RESOURCE GROUP

American Massage Therapy Association
800 Davis St., Ste. 100

Evanston, IL 60201-4444
Phone: 708/864-0123; Fax: 708/864-1178

This is a professional organization, but they offer referrals to therapists and information on classes, workshops, conventions, and conferences.

BONNIE PRUDDEN MYOTHERAPY
(THE BONNIE PRUDDEN TECHNIQUE)

DEFINITION

- Myotherapy (pronounced my-oh-thair-a-pee) is a technique for relieving chronic muscular pain through the application of pressure to a specific point within the muscle called a "trigger point." Trigger points can be located in any muscle anywhere in the body.

APPLICATIONS

Physiological: Birth trauma; accidents (e.g., falling down and whiplash); sports injuries (e.g., tennis elbow and shin splints); occupational trauma due to repetitive motion (e.g., carpal tunnel syndrome, lower-back pain); diseases (e.g., rheumatoid arthritis, lupus, and multiple sclerosis).

Psychological: Sense of well-being associated with pain relief

RECOMMENDED ADJUNCT ACTIVITIES AND
BEHAVIORS

Exercise to keep the body fit

CONTRAINDICATIONS

Check with your health practitioner if you have a condition that could cause internal bleeding, such as ulcers or hemophilia, or if you are taking anti-blood-clotting drugs.

EQUIPMENT & MATERIALS

None

ORIGIN & BACKGROUND

Like most other treatments, Myotherapy is based on previous discoveries. In the fourth century A.D., a Chinese man named Huang Fu wrote about treating patients by inserting needles into muscles under the skin. Subsequently, other pioneers discovered that muscles contained tender areas and that tissue at these sites appeared to be harder than in surrounding areas. In the 1930s, a German, Max Lange, measured the tender areas and found that they were up to 50 percent harder than surrounding tissue. He also noted that intense exercise *didn't* make muscles harder, just stronger and bigger.

Scientists named the hard, tender spots *myofascial trigger points*. In 1948, Dr. Janet Travell, who later became President Kennedy's White House physician, began to treat trigger points with injections to relieve pain.

A trigger point is an extremely irritable spot in the muscle that can easily be identified by its tenderness. Trigger points are found throughout the body.

Bonnie Prudden's impact on physical fitness really began in the 1940s when she proclaimed that American children were the weakest in the world and that physical education in the schools was completely inadequate to change that situation. Prudden's views attracted a lot of attention, and she became a nationally recognized fitness authority. In the next few decades, Prudden developed programs for and wrote about fitness for people of all ages.

Prudden's personal experience led her to study pain and how it should be treated. When she was twenty-two, she had a serious smash-up on a ski slope. After three months in traction, she was weak, she limped, and her muscles had atrophied. Determined to regain her former strength, she began to do all the things her doctors had told her not to: she skied and climbed mountains and before long she felt fit again. However, a series of personal stresses led to a bout of persistent back pain. Nothing helped until she discovered trigger-point injection therapy, which includes injections of pain-killing medication given at the "trigger point" (source of pain), followed by mild muscle stretches. In 1948, this treatment was pioneered by Dr. Janet Travel.

The treatment worked until the next stress attack, and then, bingo, back came the pain. Unfortunately, Prudden didn't see the connection between stress and the pain flare-ups at the time.

In 1976, through her work with physiatrist (a doctor of physical medicine) Dr. Desmond Tivy, Prudden—quite literally by accident—made the discovery that led to the development of Myotherapy. (The name was coined by Dr. Tivy.) Prudden and Dr. Tivy worked as a team: Prudden identified trigger points in a patient, and Dr. Tivy gave the trigger-point injections. One day Prudden pressed (probably harder than usual) on a point in a patient's neck. The woman screeched then suddenly said she felt fine! No injection, but no pain either. After this had happened several times, Prudden realized she was on to something. Apparently, the right kind of pressure at appropriate trigger points relieved pain without the need for pain-killing medication.

The body limits its own movements to protect itself against pain. This self-limiting process is called "armoring." For example, a boy who has a high-school football injury that causes him pain when he turns his head will unconsciously limit his extent of head-turning. Prudden discovered that similar accommodations to pain built up in layers in many of her patients. As Myotherapy removed the latest and most obvious cause of pain, it often revealed another underlying problem. As one might expect, the last trigger points to come to the surface were those activated years before in some long-forgotten accident.

Prudden realized then that it was important to learn about what had gone on before in a patient's life. She felt that emotional, as well as physical, trauma could cause armoring, and so she developed a series of tests and questionnaires that would help ferret out not just the current and obvious causes of pain and limited range of motion but also those that might have happened years before.

Prudden found that once she located the appropriate trigger points, she could alleviate muscular pain in a few sessions. Sometimes the patient was pain-free after only one session. Although there are many other methods of pain relief—heat, cold, drugs, and rest, for example—Prudden claims that the real benefit of Myotherapy is that it eliminates the underlying trigger point, not just symptomatic pain. In other words, it provides permanent relief for the original injury.

INSTRUCTIONS

The first step in learning the Myotherapy technique is to discover what a trigger point feels like:

- Lay your forearm flat on the table in front of you.
- With the knuckle of the middle finger of the other hand, slowly press straight down on your forearm one-half inch from the elbow bend. As you press, you will find a sensitive spot that becomes more painful the harder you press.
- Hold the pressure for seven seconds and then release slowly and evenly. You have just "erased"—at least temporarily—one trigger point. If you're a doubting Thomas and think that *anyplace* you pressed that hard on your arm would hurt, try it. Move further down your arm and do the same thing. Unless you have chronic pain in your wrist or hand, you will feel pressure, but not pain.

There are five major tools in Myotherapy. The first, *straight-on knuckle pressure*, you've just tried. The second tool is the *forefinger*.

- Place your forefinger against your temple.
- Press straight-on into your temple. (You may or may not feel a trigger point there.)
- Whether or not you feel pain, hold the pressure while you learn another technique, the *compass*.

- Assume the area under your finger is a compass and that your finger covers the center of the dial.
- Using steady pressure, press your skin straight north, toward the top of your head.
- Next press your skin south (toward your shoulder).
- Then try pressing the skin first east and then west.
- Somewhere in your movement through the compass dial, you will probably find a trigger point. When you do, hold the pressure for five seconds and release slowly and evenly. If you have either chronic headache or pain in the jaw (temporomandibular joint dysfunction or TMJD), all four compass points may be trigger points.

The third tool is the *fist*. The fist is used almost exclusively to work with trigger points on the skull. Try the *roller technique* to see how to use the fist:

- Place the first knuckle of your right hand on the side of your forehead at the hairline.
- Moving from knuckle to knuckle, roll your fist and press on each of the spots your knuckle touches. The last contact will be the knuckle of your little finger, which should make contact at the hairline roughly above your nose. If you feel a trigger point at any knuckle contact, hold the pressure for five seconds and then perform the compass, moving the skin north, south, east, and west. Also hold the pressure for five seconds at any compass point that appears to be a trigger point.
- When you've completed one "roll," move your fist down your forehead a half inch and repeat. It should take three rolls to cover the right side of your forehead. Then do three rolls on the left side of your forehead using the left hand.

So far we've learned three tools: the knuckle, the forefinger, and the fist, and we've practiced three techniques: straight-on pressure, the compass, and the roller. The fourth tool is the *thumb*, which we will use to locate trigger points in the *splenius capitis* muscle, one of the major culprits in headache.

- Place your thumb at the hairline on the back of your neck over the spine.
- Slide the thumb in the direction of one ear (still keeping it at the hairline) until you find a hollow just beneath the curve of your skull. Press upward against the bone to trap the trigger point and

hold for five seconds. Then, keeping the pressure on, perform the compass.
- Hold for five seconds at any trigger point you encounter.

If your thumbs are weak, you can use *two-finger* pressure instead. Put your index finger on the appropriate spot, put the third finger on top of the index finger, and then apply pressure. This alternate technique is also useful for reaching small spaces where your thumb is too large.

The *wraparound* technique uses one or more fingers to put pressure on a trigger point in a muscle underlying a bony projection. For example, if you get a pain in your side while running, try this:

- Put three fingers at the edge of the lowest rib.
- Push the skin and muscle over the rib into the chest cavity.
- Pull up under the rib to trap the pressure point against the bone.
- Hold for seven seconds.

The final tool in Myotherapy is the *elbow*. There is also another technique, the *cutback*. However, you need a partner to use either, so we won't discuss them here.

If you've been trying the techniques as you read along, you should by now have a pretty good idea of what a pressure point feels like. You may even have already gotten the benefit of pain relief in some part of your body. However, there's much more to Myotherapy than the quick overview we've given here. Bonnie Prudden has written two comprehensive books on the subject, *Pain Erasure the Bonnie Prudden Way* and *Myotherapy: Bonnie Prudden's Complete Guide to Pain-Free Living* (see **Further Reading**). These books are available at libraries, bookstores, and some health-food stores. The first book covers all parts of the body from head to toe. In it, Prudden offers methods for both short-term and long-term pain relief. The text includes a complete program of exercise and physical fitness as well as step-by-step illustrations and diagrams that show exactly which body parts and muscles are addressed. Other chapters deal with proper posture, ways that Myotherapy is used to treat specific diseases and injuries (including injuries to which people in specific occupations might be prone), and tips on preparing for aging. You can also order a videocassette that you can work along with (see **Resource Groups**). The second book offers guidelines for keeping your body pain free.

If you would like to seek professional treatment, Bonnie Prudden Inc. can provide a list of certified Bonnie Prudden Myotherapy Clinics and certified Bonnie Prudden Myotherapists in the U.S. and Canada. These therapists complete 1,300 hours of training before being certified. They accept patients only upon a physician's referral.

FURTHER READING

Prudden, Bonnie. *Myotherapy. Bonnie Prudden's Complete Guide to Pain-Free Living.* Garden City, N.Y.: The Dial Press, Doubleday & Company, Inc., 1984.
————. *Pain Erasure: The Bonnie Prudden Way.* New York: M. Evans & Co., Inc., 1980, hardcover. New York: Ballantine Books, Inc., 1982, paperback.

RESOURCE GROUPS

Bonnie Prudden, Inc.
PO Box 625
Stockbridge, MA 01262.
Phone: 413/298-3781

A one-hour do-it-yourself videocassette called *The Bonnie Prudden Approach to Pain Erasure/Myotherapy* ® is available. It is designed for people of all ages, including children (and even pets). If you would like to receive an annual brochure that indicates places and dates for Pain-Erasure Seminars and workshops, send a stamped self-addressed envelope along with your request. The brochure is free.

Institute for Physical Fitness
PO Box 58
Stockbridge, MA 01262
Phone: 800/221-4624 (referrals); 413/296-3066; or 413/296-3787

Audio- and videotapes, books, equipment; referrals to therapists

Myotherapy Institute of Utah
3018 E. 3300 South
Salt Lake City, UT 84109
Phone: 800/338-8950 or 801/484-7624; Fax: 801/467-4792

Audio- and videotapes; referrals to therapists

REFLEXOLOGY
(REFLEXOTHERAPY OR ZONE THERAPY)

DEFINITION

Reflexology is a technique of applying pressure to (or stroking) areas on the feet and/or the hands that proponents believe correspond to particular areas and organs of the body. The purpose of this form of bodywork is to relax muscles and stimulate the body's own natural ability to heal itself. Reflexology is a kissing cousin to acupuncture and acupressure in that its premise is that stimulating one part of the body can affect another.

APPLICATIONS

Physiological: Not a therapy for any specific condition, but may lead to improvement in asthma, migraine and other headaches, constipation, sinus congestion, circulatory problems, hiccups, earache, kidney problems, hypertension, chronic pain, backache
Psychological: Stress, insomnia

COLLATERAL CROSS-THERAPIES

Breathing exercises, relaxation techniques

RECOMMENDED ADJUNCT ACTIVITIES

You may want to dim the lights or use candles and play soft music to enhance relaxation.

CONTRAINDICATIONS

Stimulation to circulation could accelerate the spread of infection. Reflexology is not a treatment for emergencies or for serious illness or injury.

EQUIPMENT & MATERIALS

No equipment is used in reflexology, only the hands.

ORIGIN

From ancient times, traditional Chinese medicine and other Oriental healing systems have included techniques for massaging the feet, hands, and body to affect muscles and internal organs. Early records indicate that a form of therapy similar to reflexology may have been practiced in China 5,000 years ago. A pictograph found in an Egyptian physician's tomb from about 2300 B.C. clearly shows one person massaging another's feet.

Except for certain native tribes, reflexology wasn't known in Western countries until the twentieth century. About 1913, an American ear, nose, and throat specialist, Dr. William Fitzgerald, introduced what he called "zone therapy" into the United States. Fitzgerald's method divided the body into ten zones that began in the toes, extended through the fingers and continued to the top of the head. Fitzgerald taught that the body contained bioelectrical energy that flowed through the zones to reflex points in the hands and feet. This concept differs somewhat from the Chinese theory of energy and meridians, but both relate to the same philosophy: that an energy force within the body can be manipulated through touch.

Fitzgerald's colleague, Edwin Bowers, M.D., chose a dramatic method of demonstrating the merits of reflexology: He called for a volunteer, applied pressure to a point on the hand, and then promptly stuck the person in the face with a needle! Because the point on the hand and the needle-insertion point on the face were in the same zone, the volunteer felt no pain.

In 1938, Eunice D. Ingham, a physiotherapist, wrote a book called *Stories the Feet Can Tell*. (The book can still be found in many libraries.) In studying Fitzgerald's method, Ingham became convinced that the feet were the most important areas to work on because they were so sensitive. Accordingly, she mapped out the entire body and correlated it to zones on the feet.

Ingham established a reflexology institute, and she taught and lectured widely. Later, she was joined in her work by her nephew, Dwight C. Bowers. Over the years, thousands of reflexologists have been trained in Ingham's method, which is still popular today. Another method, the Laura Norman method, is taught in some hospitals and universities. Many practitioners also perform reflexology on the hand and other parts of the body as well as the foot.

An English naturopath Robert St. John developed an unusual variation reflexology in the 1960s. St. John was interested in his patients' psychological reaction to treatment. He formulated his own reflex-point chart of the feet, with the spine running toe to heel on the inside edge of each foot. Then he correlated each spinal point to the nine months a person spends in the womb before birth. St. John theorized that an unborn child is affected by the emotional experiences of its mother during pregnancy. When a mother is frightened or angry, her whole body reacts with a rush of hormones to cope with the crisis. The fetus experiences these reactions too and stores them up in the spinal reflexes.

St. John's method, which he called the Metamorphic Technique, aimed to alleviate stored-up prenatal traumas that contribute to ill health. In other words, where reflexology creates physiological benefits that subsequently impact on emotional health, the Metamorphic Technique puts it the other way round: improve emotional health and physical benefits will follow. Either way, the goal is better health for the whole person.

Some practitioners specialize only in reflexology, but many use it as part of an overall holistic program that includes other types of bodywork as well. They may also offer other relaxation techniques, such as breathing exercises.

Practitioners admit that there is precious little scientific proof to back up the theories of reflexologists, but there is plenty of anecdotal evidence that the technique does work. The American Podiatric Medical Association takes no official position on reflexology, and some podiatrists are proponents. "We can't explain it, but we can't discount it either," said one. "There's no proof except that people get better." Other traditional practitioners point to the benefits of relaxation and tension reduction as reasons enough to try the method.

There are several theories as to how reflexology works. All practitioners agree that stroking or applying pressure to certain points on the body removes blocks that impede the free flow of energy, but they differ as to what actually happens. One theory says that reflexology stimulates sensory receptors in the nerve fibers. The sensory receptors send impulses to the spinal cord, which then disperses energy throughout the nervous system. Another theory holds that manipulation breaks up and dissolves uric-acid-crystal deposits that have settled in the extremities and created blockage. Still others believe that the key is endorphins, pain-blocking chemicals that are released into the blood stream during the treatment. (Endorphins not only block pain but also give a person a feeling of well-being.)

Perhaps the simplest theory is that treatment is so calming that even the blood vessels relax. Circulation of blood and lymphatic fluid improves, which brings more oxygen to cells and takes away toxic waste products. (Nearly everyone can relax during foot or hand reflexology, whereas some people are uncomfortable having their whole bodies worked on.)

INSTRUCTIONS

Visiting a Therapist: When you visit a reflexologist, he or she will usually try to encourage you to relax by breathing deeply and rhythmically. You may be treated either sitting up or lying down, although lying down is typical. The session often begins with a gentle massage of both feet. Then the therapist works his or her way through the reflex points on each foot. The foot and toes may be rubbed, rotated and/or moved up and down. The therapist will sometimes use stroking motions, but sometimes he or she will apply deep pressure.

Usually you can expect no pain, but some people have an occasional, momentary, sharp stab. You may feel tingling in another part of your body; this is the area that corresponds to the foot reflex under treatment.

Reflexologists recommend a thirty-minute to one-hour session once a week for general relaxation. For a specific problem, you may need more frequent sessions. Practitioners say it may take up to six weeks to notice changes, but some people feel better after only one treatment.

Doing-It Yourself: If you want to try reflexology on yourself or a partner, it's helpful to have a book or video that illustrates both the technique and the reflex points. (See *Further Reading* at the end of the section.)

To begin your self-reflexology session, take off your shoes and socks and assume a comfortable position. You can sit in a chair with one foot in your lap, or you can lie down with both knees bent so that you can hold one foot in your hands. Experiment with both positions to see which you like best. (If you've very limber, you might find a cross-legged position comfortable.) Relax as completely as you can. To relax, use breathing techniques or another method that works for you. Then "get acquainted" with your feet. Stroke or massage them gently, starting with the top and then working your way down the sides. Finally gently rub the soles of your feet. As you go, note especially any little lumps or tender spots you find. You can come back to these later for more specific work.

Now you're ready to start the real routine. To work the bottom of your foot, hold the foot in both hands with your fingers on the top and your thumbs on the sole. Pressing firmly, slide both thumbs from the outside edge of the foot across the sole and back. Work your way down the entire sole. (This is tremendously relaxing and feels wonderful.)

Then grasp the side of your foot with both hands next to each other, again with the thumbs on the sole. Gently twist the foot first one way and then the other. Now grasp your foot with your palm on the sole and your fingers on your toes and press to flex your foot at the ankle.

Next, hold your foot with one hand and press firmly with your thumb in the middle of the ball of your foot (the solar plexus point), release, and then rotate your thumb on the point. (If you have a partner, this is even more pleasant when done to both feet at the same time.)

Now for the top of the foot. Hold one foot in both hands with your thumbs on top. Starting with the toes, use both thumbs to press, release, and rotate your way down the whole length of the foot to the ankle. While you've got both hands on your foot, wring it out like a dishcloth by grasping it with your palms on top and then gently twisting both hands in opposite directions. Finally, push it around a bit by holding one hand on each side of the foot (and perpendicular to it) and slapping it from one palm to the other. Do the entire routine on one foot at a time, then switch to the other.

The routine we've just described is used for basic relaxation. Professional practitioners use additional finger movements and techniques for specific areas of the body, but you don't need to learn them to use reflexology to help you let go of stress. As you work with your feet, you'll soon learn what feels good and relaxes you. Go with your instincts and concentrate on the reflex points that work for you.

For specific problems, you need to know more about the reflex points and the body parts to which they correspond. The reflex points in the left foot correspond to areas on the left side of the body and those in the right foot, the areas on the right. The following chart shows some major organs that are stimulated by specific areas on the foot. Except for the bone that relates to the spine, which is on the side, all other points refer to the bottom of the foot.

AREA ON THE FOOT	BODY PART STIMULATED
Toes	Head, brain, and sinuses
Joint where toes meet foot	Ears and eyes
Ball of foot	Heart and lungs
Arch	Internal organs (colon, kidneys, etc.)
Heel	Sciatic nerve and pelvic area
Bone along curving arch of foot	Spine

Of course, the complete map of the foot is much more complicated and the reflex points much more specific, but this will give you an idea of some areas you might want to work on. To do a proper job on specific problems, though, you'll need to learn some other techniques that we haven't described here. You can find them in books or videos devoted to reflexology. Check to be sure the seven basic techniques are described (and illustrated) in the book before you buy. Or better yet, take the book on loan from the library until you see whether it's useful.

Here's just one of the basic techniques to get you started. It sounds simple, but you may find it a bit tiring at first. It's called thumb-walking, and it's very important to the professional. Although you would, of course, use the technique on your feet, you can practice it to get the movement right on your hand, arm, or even a flat surface like a tabletop.) To "walk" your thumb, press it down and then move it forward gradually by bending and unbending it at the first joint. Imitate a caterpillar and you've got the idea, but you need to move in very small increments so as not to miss any reflex points. You can also walk your index finger in the same way. If your hands are very stiff, you probably won't be able to do either of these movements.

Stiffness can be a problem in self-reflexology. Because of stiffness or excess weight (or both), some people can't comfortably reach their feet to perform the technique. Obviously, if you have to huff and puff and strain just to get your foot in your hands, you won't find the experience relaxing at all. There's a silver lining to this dismal picture, though: If you can find a partner, you can practice on each other, and when it's your turn, all you'll have to do is lie there and enjoy it.

FURTHER READING

Bergson, Anika, and Vladimir Tuchak. *Zone Therapy*. Los Angeles: Pinnacle Books, 1974.

Berkson, Devaki. *The Foot Book: Healing the Body Through Foot Reflexology*. New York: HarperPerennial, 1992.

Carter, Mildred, and Tommy Weber. *Body Reflexology: Healing at Your Fingertips*. West Nyack, N.Y.: Parker Publishing Co., 1994.

Ingham, Eunice D. *Stories the Feet Can Tell*, St. Petersburg, Fla.: Ingham Publishing, 1938.

Ingham, Eunice D., and Dwight C. Byers. *The Original Works of Eunice D. Ingham*, St. Petersburg, Fla.: Ingham Publishing, 1984.

Jora, Jurgen. *Foot Reflexology: A Visual Guide for Self-Treatment*. New York: St. Martin's Press, 1991.

Kunz, Kevin, and Barbara Kunz. *Hand and Foot Reflexology: A Self-Help Guide*. Englewood Cliffs, N.J.: Prentice-Hall, 1987.

————. *The Complete Guide to Foot Reflexology*. Albuquerque: Reflexology Research Projects, 1993.

Martin, Melva. *A Complete Guide to Practical Reflexology*. Fort Lauderdale, Fla.: World Life International (distributor). (video)

Norman, Laura. *Feet First: A Guide to Foot Reflexology*. New York: Simon and Schuster, 1988.

Saint-Pierre, Gaston, and Debbie Boater. *The Metamorphic Technique*. Tisbury, Wiltshire, UK: Element Books, 1983.

RESOURCE GROUPS

American Reflexology Certification Board and Information Service
PO Box 246654
Sacramento, CA 95824
Phone: 916/455-5381

Foot Reflexology Awareness Association
PO Box 7622
Mission Hills, CA 91346
Phone: 818/361-0528

International Institute of Reflexology
PO Box 12462
St. Petersburg, FL 33733
Phone: 813/343-4811

Publications, classes, and referrals to reflexologists

International Institute of Reflexology
5650 First Ave. North
PO Box 12642

St. Petersburg, FL 33733-4811
Phone: 813/348-4811; Fax: 813/381-2807

Books, other materials for self-help; referrals to practitioners

SHIATSU, ALSO SPELLED SHIATZU
(SEE ALSO ACUPRESSURE)

DEFINITION

Shiatsu (pronounced she-ott-sue) is a form of massage based on applying pressure to key points in the body using the thumbs, fingers, knuckles, and palms. Theoretically, shiatsu opens blocked pathways within the body to allow the free flow of energy, which maintains health, increases vitality, and reduces pain.

APPLICATIONS

Physiological: Headache, back pain, tennis elbow, sexual lassitude, constipation, muscle fatigue, chronic pain, arthritis, muscular tension, tension in back, shoulder or neck, gastrointestinal disturbances, inflammation, gynecological problems, whole-body imbalance
Psychological: Stress, anxiety, insomnia, flagging energy

COLLATERAL CROSS-THERAPIES

Meditation, herbalism

CONTRAINDICATIONS

Shiatsu should not be used by people with broken bones, disorders of any internal organs, or tendencies to internal bleeding either due to physical disorders (e.g., hemophilia, duodenal or stomach ulcers) or from taking anti-blood-clotting medications.

EQUIPMENT & MATERIALS

If you're performing shiatsu on yourself, you need nothing but a straight chair, but if you're going to work with a partner, you'll need a mat, rug, or blanket and a small, hard pillow or rolled towel.

ORIGIN

The term *shiatsu* comes from the Japanese words "shi," meaning finger, and "atzu," meaning pressure. Shiatsu is a complement to other Oriental forms of healing. In the East, it is used along with—not in place of—other healing arts.

The use of touch as a form of healing is as old as humankind itself. Just as we do today, our primitive ancestors instinctively held or gently rubbed a body part that was in pain. At least 5,000 years ago, Chinese Taoist monks observed these instincts and incorporated touch as a form of self-healing into their philosophy. About 2,000 years later, at the time of the Yellow Emperor, records mention the use of acupuncture and another form of therapy based on the same principles but without needles: tien-an.

Acupuncture and Oriental Massage: Chinese acupuncture made its way to Japan over a thousand years ago, but it wasn't until the 1700s that people began to combine the principles of acupuncture with traditional Oriental massage. Practitioners of a form of massage called amma used their fingers to press and rub painful body parts. They discovered that they could apply pressure to the acupuncture points, using their fingers instead of needles, and get similar benefits. This was the beginning of shiatsu therapy, although the term *shiatsu* did not become part of the Japanese vocabulary until well into the twentieth century.

Shiatsu enjoyed a wide following in Japan until about the middle of the nineteenth century, when Western medicine was introduced. For a time, interest in shiatsu waned, but it soon regained popularity. Shiatsu became so rooted in Japanese tradition that when General Douglas MacArthur attempted to ban its practice in Japan after World War II, the Japanese people were outraged. They raised such a clamor that President Truman interceded and persuaded MacArthur to lift the ban.

Tsubos Are Key: Until fairly recently, shiatsu was virtually unknown in the West. Shiatsu came to public attention in the United States at about the same time as acupuncture, which is not surprising, since, as we've already mentioned, the two practices are based on the same principles. In acupuncture, a practitioner inserts needles into *tsubos*, key points in the body. Shiatsu uses the same body points, but instead of inserting needles, the practitioner applies pressure on the points with the thumbs, fingers, knuckles, and palms. (A professional shiatsu practitioner might also use elbows and feet on a patient, but this is pretty hard to do if you're attempting shiatsu on yourself!)

There are other differences: Acupuncture can be administered only by a trained practitioner, so it is not a do-it-yourself procedure. Lay people can easily learn shiatsu and practice it on themselves and/or their partners. Broadly speaking, acupuncture is more often used to treat problems that are already plaguing a patient, whereas shiatsu is principally a means of maintaining good health. It can be used to relieve a variety of physical problems, however.

Also, shiatsu is totally noninvasive. Because the skin isn't broken as with acupuncture, there is no danger of infection or the introduction of harmful substances into the body.

The Concept of Oneness: Shiatsu and other Eastern healing arts are based on the concept of Oneness. According to Oriental philosophers, the individual and the universe are essentially one and the same. Everything in the universe consists of the same elements and follows the same life cycle. In order to achieve Oneness, opposing forces, called yin and yang, must be kept in balance.

Yin and yang are opposites, but they also work in harmony. Yin and yang are not fixed; they are constantly changing, so that too much yin becomes yang and vice versa. Yin is the negative force and yang the positive, but these terms don't translate to "bad" and "good" as they do in western thinking. In Oriental philosophy, everything simply is what it is, neither more nor less, and the concept of good and bad doesn't apply.

The moon is yin, the sun yang; woman is yin, man yang; night is yin, day yang, and so forth. Everything in the universe is either yin or yang, but since yin and yang are in constant flux, each yin object has elements of yang and each yang object has elements of yin.

Oriental practitioners believe that health problems occur when the balance between yin and yang is disrupted. Their approach to healthcare is primarily one of prevention: Keep the body in harmony, and you will enjoy good health. However, they acknowledge that sometimes the body's balance does get out of whack, and then healing measures are needed to restore the proper equilibrium.

Experience and observation led Oriental healers to the theory of the "trigger" points (tsubos). For example, they noted that a given body point might become numb or painful. From these observations, they developed the whole theory of acupuncture, and ultimately, shiatsu.

Underlying Premises of Shiatsu: Briefly, these are the underlying premises: The body contains 657 tsubos that are connected by twenty-four pathways, which form the twelve meridians on each side of the body. Two additional meridians bisect the body. One, called the meridian of conception, begins in the genital area and runs up through the abdomen and the chest, ending at a point in the middle of the lower jaw. The meridian of conception is called that because its path includes the sexual organs.

The other bisecting meridian is called the governor meridian. It begins where the meridian of conception leaves off, starting in the upper jaw and traveling up and over the center of the face and skull and down the spine. The governor meridian ends at the tailbone. The meridian of conception is yin, while the governor meridian is yang. (The meridians are, of course, invisible to the eye.)

These two meridians control the flow of energy throughout the twelve pairs of meridians on either side of the body. In turn, the twelve-pair pathways all connect to each other to allow energy to flow throughout the body and maintain health. Illness and disease occur when a pathway becomes blocked and the energy flow is interrupted, thus throwing the body out of balance.

It is interesting to note that, although the ancient sages developed the theory of the meridians many centuries before the advent of Western medicine, their functions closely correspond to many body systems commonly recognized today: for example, the circulatory, endocrine, and nervous systems. The pathways tend to fall along the lines where blood vessels, glands, and nerves are located.

INSTRUCTIONS

Our modern world provides a machine for almost every task we need to do. Partly because of this, many people have gotten somewhat out of touch with their own bodies. Shiatsu offers you the opportunity to get back in tune with your body, soothe your aches and pains, relax, give yourself a healthier complexion, and much more.

You can easily perform shiatsu on yourself, but you might also enjoy working with a partner and practicing it on each other. Self-shiatsu is usually performed while sitting on a straight chair, though you can sit on the floor if you prefer. When you work on a partner, he or she should lie down on a mat or blanket on the floor. Use a small, hard pillow or folded towel to form a head rest when your partner is on his/her stomach. When your partner is lying face up, the head rest becomes a neck rest.

When you perform shiatsu on a partner, your arms should always be extended to their full length. You may stand up and bend over, but if this is too difficult, you can also kneel beside your partner in the appropriate position for that particular shiatsu procedure.

Although shiatsu is often called "shiatsu massage," the technique is very different from Swedish massage, which is a rather vigorous procedure. Shiatsu is accomplished through pressure on the trigger points, not through rubbing. Different shiatsu procedures require different degrees of pressure. For example, when working on the head, one generally uses moderate pressure, while the abdomen requires somewhat lighter pressure. In general, you'll want to use firm pressure on big muscles. Don't worry too much about whether you're pressing hard enough, though. If you're working on yourself, you will soon discover the amount of pressure that feels right. If you experience pain, you're using too much pressure. On the other hand, you do want to *feel* it. A little experimentation should help you get it right.

It's somewhat more difficult to tell whether the pressure is appropriate when you're working on a partner. Begin cautiously. Gradually bear down harder until your partner says "ouch." Then ease up slightly. Here is a sample shiatsu exercise that will relieve tension in the muscles of your shoulders and back. To apply pressure, you can use either your thumb, index, or middle finger, or your index and middle fingers together, whichever is most comfortable. To make it easier to follow the steps of the exercise, we've arbitrarily specified the index finger.

- Using the index finger of one hand, find the midpoint of the other shoulder (measured between the base of the neck and the outer edge of the shoulder). The point should be slightly behind the main shoulder muscle. The spot should feel tender when you press on it. Keep moving your finger until you locate this tender spot.
- When you've found the proper point, press firmly for three to four seconds with your finger. Then lift your finger without moving it from the spot. Repeat twice more.
- Find the same point on the other shoulder with the index finger of the opposite hand. Perform the same maneuver three times, pausing between pressures for several seconds.

You should feel the tension flowing out of your shoulders and back. Try to keep your finger poised above the trigger point during the pauses so that you don't have to relocate the spot. Use this technique frequently if you have to sit for long hours at a desk.

To perform this same maneuver on a partner, do this:

- Have your partner lie face down on a mat with her head turned to one side and supported by a folded towel.
- Kneel in front of your partner's head. You should be far enough away so that when your arms are extended, they reach his or her shoulders.
- Locate the trigger point in the middle of the right shoulder, using your left thumb. Your hand should be palm down, with the thumb at an approximate right angle to the fingers. (Remember that the point is a little bit behind the main shoulder muscle.) Be careful not to use too much pressure when searching for the point, because it is usually sensitive. Keep checking with your partner until you're sure you've found the right point.
- Place your right thumb atop your left thumb and press firmly for three or four seconds. Remove the pressure for a second or two and then repeat twice more, pausing between pressures.
- Do the same thing on the left shoulder. On this side, place the right thumb on your partner, with the left thumb on top. You may have to reposition yourself slightly to get the proper leverage for each side. Your arm should be aligned so that it is extended straight over the middle of the appropriate shoulder.

Here is a shiatsu maneuver you can use on a partner who has a headache:

- Have your partner lie face down as before. Only this time, his or her head should be facing straight into the towel.
- Stand with one leg on each side of your partner's body at approximately the hip line, facing the head. Bend from the waist with your knees slightly bent. Extend your arms straight down to the back of your partner's neck. Using the thumb of each hand, locate the big muscles on the back of the neck that join to the shoulder muscles. There is one of these muscles on each side of the spine. (If your fingers are more sensitive, you can use them to locate the muscles.)
- Place your left thumb on top of the left muscle at the very top, where the skull meets the neck. Your right thumb should be atop the right muscle. (If you have to cross your hands to get the right thumb on the right muscle, you're facing the wrong way!)
- Exert firm pressure for three to four seconds. Stop.
- Making sure that your thumbs stay above the muscles, move down about an inch. Again exert firm pressure for three to four seconds. Stop.
- Keep moving down in one-inch increments, pressing firmly, and then pausing for a second or two before moving on. The final pressure points are approximately at the shoulder line. You should have pressed on at least four points on each side.
- Finally, locate the midpoint just below the base of the skull where the skull meets the neck.
- Place one thumb on top of the other and press firmly for three to four seconds. Stop.
- Repeat twice more, stopping in between for a second or two.

To perform the same headache-relieving exercise on yourself, follow the steps given above. You can use one or two fingers, rather than your thumbs if you'd like.

You can also use shiatsu to help relieve the symptoms of a cold. Follow the same techniques that are described in the ACUPRESSURE section. As with all other cold remedies, this works best if you begin using the technique at the first sniffle. Don't wait until the cold has you firmly in its grip. Be sure to do each of the procedures described on both sides of your body and do them several times a day until your symptoms subside.

The procedures we've described here employ just a few of the pressure points used in shiatsu—in fact there are a lot more for headache alone—but this should give you an idea of how shiatsu works. If you find that you like it, you might like to learn to do whole-body shiatsu. There are also shiatsu techniques to relieve colds, insomnia, constipation, diarrhea, and a variety of other ailments. Check your library, bookstore, or health-food or herbal store to find a good do it-yourself shiatsu book. Videotapes are also available.

One good way to find out how the pressure ought to feel might be to treat yourself to a shiatsu massage from a professional shiatsu practitioner. Professionals have finely honed their sense of touch. By palpating various parts of the body, they can diagnose physical problems and perform the appropriate techniques to relieve them. You can also go to a practitioner just to keep your body in balance.

If you live in a moderate- to large-sized city, you shouldn't have any trouble finding a practitioner. A massage school that teaches shiatsu might be a good starting point to get a referral. There is also an organization called the Ohashi Institute that teaches shiatsu at various locations throughout the United States. (The method taught is called Ohashiatsu.®) If you just want more information about shiatsu, you can contact the American Oriental Bodywork Association, whose address is given in the *Resource Groups* section.

If you think you might be interested in a whole lifestyle system that includes shiatsu, you might like to look into macrobiotic shiatsu. Macrobiotic shiatsu combines a macrobiotic diet, breathing exercises, shiatsu, and exercise. This is a comprehensive wellness system that takes into account a person's physical, emotional, mental, and environmental condition. The system was originated by Shizuko Yamamoto, a shiatsu practitioner and macrobiotic counselor.

FURTHER READING

Goodman, Saul. *The Book of Shiatsu: A Guide to a Traditional Healing Art.* Garden City Park, N.Y.: Avery Publishing, 1990.

Irwin, Yukiko, with James Wagenvoord. *Shiatzu.* New York: J.B. Lippincott Company, 1976.

Klinger, Rebecca. *Healthy Massage.* New York: V.I.E.W., Inc., 1988. (video)

Lidell, Lucy. *The Book of Massage: The Complete Step-by-Step Guide to Eastern and Western Techniques.* New York: Simon and Schuster, c1984.

Luglio, Jerry. *Japanese Shiatsu Massage.* (videotape)

Macrobiotic Shiatsu. Eureka, Calif.: International Macrobiotic Shiatsu Soc., 1990.

Morita, Pat, and David Kawika Talisman. *Shiatsu with Pat Morita.* Honolulu: Blue Banyon Productions, 1990. (video)

Seldon, Bernice. *The Body-Mind Book: Nine Ways to Awareness.* New York: Messner, c1979.

Yamamoto, Shizuko, and Patrick McCarty. *The Shiatsu Handbook.* Eureka, Calif.: Turning Point Publications, 1989.

RESOURCE GROUPS

American Oriental Bodywork Association
50 Maple Place
Manhasset, NY 11030
Phone: 516/365-5025

International Macrobiotic Shiatsu Society
1122 M St.,
Eureka, CA 95501-2442
Phone: 707/445-2290

International School of Shiatsu
22–28 South Main St.
Doylestown, PA 18901
Phone: 215/340-9918

   Courses; referrals to practitioners

Ohashi Institute
12 West 27th St., 9th Fl.
New York, NY 10001
Phone: 212/684-4190

Ohashiatsu® Chicago
825 Chicago Ave.
Evanston, IL 60202
Phone: 708/864-1130

   This is a school, but it also has a store called Ohashiatsu® Bookstore
and Healing Arts Supply, where one can purchase books, tapes, futons,
neck rolls, and other supplies for the do-it-yourselfer.

THE BREATH OF LIFE

We've often heard the expression, "Why, that's as easy as breathing." Most of us take breathing totally for granted, and we seldom think of improving our breathing as an avenue to better health. Oh, we're well aware that *not* breathing has some pretty serious implications, but unless we're afflicted with respiratory ailments, we don't give breathing a whole lot of thought. That's too bad because virtually everyone can benefit from learning better ways to breathe. Knowing how to breathe can help you overcome anxiety (public speakers know all about proper breathing to overcome stage-fright), fight stress, and help counteract the effects of debilitating respiratory diseases such as bronchitis, emphysema, and asthma. Some oriental methods that combine breathing techniques with other mental and physical disciplines provide inner calm and an improved sense of well being. These advanced methods may even aid in the treatment of diseases of other parts of the body.

Air and the oxygen in it are vital foods for the body just as the things we eat are. We can live for quite a while without putting food into our stomachs, but deprive of us of food for our lungs, and we will die within moments. Unfortunately, most of us give our lungs a fast-food lunch instead of the healthful banquet they deserve.

Healthful breathing means deep breathing to bring in plenty of oxygen and to get rid of carbon dioxide and other waste products. Oxygen is a tonic for the whole body: A healthy dose of oxygen to the brain stimulates mental faculties; infusing the bloodstream with oxygen revitalizes cells and builds up a store of energy. The more energy we have, the better we can go about our daily tasks and the better we can fight off diseases.

Deep breathing is also a natural tranquilizer. Scientific research has shown that deep breathing produces endorphins, hormones that calm us down.

Nature intended for us to breathe deeply, but unfortunately, most of us have forgotten how. Before the industrial revolution, most everything people did required hard, physical labor. Take doing the laundry, for example. Once people scrubbed out the dirt by hand or beat their clothes on rocks in a stream. Today we simply pop our dirty things into a machine and push a button. No energy required there. Because of all of the labor-saving devices, many of us can get through our daily tasks without physically exerting ourselves *at all*. An unwanted consequence of this is that we take puny, shallow breaths from the chest only, filling the upper third of our lungs with air while the lower two thirds sit there with nothing to do. No wonder that in times of stress or unaccustomed physical exertion, we're left gasping. We're out of practice at bringing in enough good, rich oxygen to keep our bodies at peak performance.

Test the fitness of your lungs by inflating a paper bag or blowing out a candle held at arm's length. Can't do it without turning purple? Then you've got lazy lungs. Fortunately, you can learn to give your lungs the workout they deserve with a little practice. Better breathing techniques are relatively easy to master, and they're completely safe for almost anyone of any age or level of fitness and health. Best of all, they require absolutely no equipment, and they cost nothing: They're as free as the air we breathe.

PURSED-LIP BREATHING

DEFINITION

Pursed-lip breathing is a technique that helps those who are chronically short of breath breathe easier during physical activity.

APPLICATIONS

Physiological: Asthma, bronchitis, emphysema, other chronic obstructive pulmonary diseases
Psychological: Stress control incidental to better control over breathing

COLLATERAL CROSS-THERAPIES

Diaphragmatic breathing, qigong, pranayama

UNCT ACTIVITIES AND BEHAVIORS

If you are more than slightly overweight, you might want to start on a weight-loss program that includes physical activity, especially walking.

CONTRAINDICATIONS

Check with your doctor if you have a bronchial condition such as asthma or emphysema. Pursed-lip breathing can trigger bronchial spasm.

EQUIPMENT & MATERIALS

None

ORIGIN & BACKGROUND

Most people with respiratory ailments can neither inhale nor exhale deeply enough. Shallow breathing causes these people to run out of air during even light exertion like walking up a flight of stairs. Often people with breathing difficulties have airways that are constricted or filled with mucus. To help alleviate these problems, respiratory-care specialists began to teach pursed-lip breathing to their patients. Today pursed-lip breathing is taught in many respiratory-care facilities and hospitals. Use of the technique probably evolved simultaneously in various facilities rather than being developed by one individual.

INSTRUCTIONS

Pursed-lip breathing is very simple. Just inhale through your nose. Pucker your lips as if you were going to kiss someone, and then exhale slowly through your mouth. That's all there is to it. The reason this works is that this type of exhalation builds up pressure in the airways, which helps to keep them open. If you've got breathing problems, try this technique the next time you walk up a flight of stairs and see if you aren't less breathless than usual when you get to the top. Even if you don't normally have breathing problems, you probably get winded during vigorous aerobic activity. Try pursed-lip breathing to help you keep up the pace.

RESOURCE GROUPS

The respiratory services department of your local hospital may have resource and support groups for people with respiratory illnesses. Also, you might contact your local chapter of the American Lung Association.

DIAPHRAGMATIC BREATHING
(BELLY BREATHING)

DEFINITION

Diaphragmatic (pronounced dye-a-fra-mat-ic) breathing is just what it sounds like: breathing from the diaphragm rather than from the upper chest. Diaphragmatic breathing provides better air intake and strengthens the lungs; it is especially good for people with breathing problems.

APPLICATIONS

Physiological: Asthma, bronchitis, emphysema, other chronic obstructive pulmonary diseases
Psychological :Feeling of greater self-control, stress relief

COLLATERAL CROSS-THERAPIES

Pursed-lip breathing, qigong, pranayama

RECOMMENDED ADJUNCT ACTIVITIES AND BEHAVIORS

If you are more than slightly overweight, your whole body—including your lungs—is working harder than it should. Try this little experiment: Say you're sixteen pounds overweight. The next time you're in the supermarket, take a look at a sixteen-pound frozen turkey. Imagine that you have to carry that turkey around with you during all your activities. You'd soon be huffing and puffing, wouldn't you? And by the end of the day you'd be a lot more tired than if you hadn't had to haul the blasted turkey around. Well, your body is already carrying the equivalent of the turkey's weight. The body is wonderfully adaptive, so it's made adjustments, but it could function much better if you shed that excess poundage. Exercise, especially walking, goes along with any sensible weight-loss program.

CONTRAINDICATIONS

None

EQUIPMENT & MATERIALS

You will need a comfortable chair with a straight back and a mat, rug, or carpeted floor to lie on to do the strengthening exercises.

ORIGIN & BACKGROUND

People who breathe without thinking about it usually breathe from the chest only. If you have respiratory problems, chest breathing may not be deep enough to keep you from becoming short of breath upon even mild exertion. Respiratory care specialists sought a way to help people with this problem learn to pull more air into their lungs and thus to inhale and exhale more deeply. One solution—borrowed in large measure from yoga—is diaphragmatic breathing.

Today diaphragmatic breathing is often taught in the respiratory care departments of local community hospitals. Another source of information is the local chapter of the American Lung Association.

INSTRUCTIONS

Diaphragmatic breathing is just what it sounds like: breathing from the diaphragm (the muscular band that separates the cavity containing your lungs from the abdominal cavity). Diaphragmatic breathing is easy once you get the hang of it, but it may seem unnatural at first. Normally, when someone asks us to take a deep breath, we expand the chest and suck in the gut. On exhalation, we allow the gut to relax and distend. If you want to do diaphragmatic breathing, forget that. Instead *push out* the gut as you inhale, and then pull it in as you exhale slowly.

Try to develop a rhythmic motion, like a wave rising and falling. To see if you're doing it right, put your fingers under your rib cage. Your fingers should lift as the abdomen rises.

Diaphragmatic breathing takes a little practice, but it's worth learning. You can combine diaphragmatic and pursed-lip breathing by inhaling from the diaphragm and exhaling through pursed lips. It may also help to develop a rhythm that coordinates with your physical activity. While walking, for example, inhale then take three steps as you exhale. Repeat.

Exercises to Strengthen the Diaphragm: If your diaphragm is very weak, you may have to work on strengthening it before you can get the maximum benefit from diaphragmatic breathing. Doing the diaphragmatic breathing exercise itself will make your diaphragm stronger, but if you want to get results faster, try these exercises:

1.   Lie on the floor with a small pillow or folded towel under your head and shoulders. Clasp your hands behind your head. Bend your knees but keep your feet flat on the floor.

   • Inhale.
   • Exhale while bringing your elbows up toward your ears as if you were trying to touch your elbows together.
   • Inhale as you move your arms back to the floor.
   • Repeat the sequence.

2.   Lie on the floor with knees bent, feet flat. Put your hands just below your ribcage.

   • Inhale.
   • Exhale and press down with your hands.
   • Relax your hands and inhale again.
   • Repeat the sequence.

RESOURCE GROUPS

The pulmonary medicine or respiratory care departments of your local hospital may have resource or support groups for people with respiratory illnesses. You can also contact the local chapter of the American Lung Association.

QIGONG

DEFINITION

Qigong (pronounced chee-kung) is a system of spiritual, mental, and physical exercises that combine breathing techniques with stylized physical movements to balance and enhance the body's vital energy force (*qi*).

APPLICATIONS

Physiological: Asthma, digestive disorders, duodenal ulcers, stomach ulcers, immune disorders, constipation, high blood pressure, paralysis following stroke, neuromuscular conditions such as multiple sclerosis
Psychological: Stress, anxiety

COLLATERAL CROSS-THERAPIES

Meditation, visualization, yoga

RECOMMENDED ADJUNCT ACTIVITIES AND BEHAVIORS

If it is not distracting, you might find it pleasant to listen to soft music while performing qigong.

CONTRAINDICATIONS

None

EQUIPMENT

You will need a comfortable chair and a mat or carpet for the sitting and lying-down postures.

PREPARATION (WARM-UP)

Qigong uses only gentle physical motion, so you will not need a physical warm-up as you would with more strenuous exercise. But the maximum benefit will be gained from performing qigong in an environment free from outside distractions and noises. You might want to turn off your telephone or perform qigong in the early morning before you begin your busy day.

ORIGIN & BACKGROUND

The origins of qigong date back more than 2,000 years. During the Chou Dynasty (1122–221 B.C.), the Chinese practiced *daoyin*, a type of exercise that combined specific breathing techniques with body movements.

In about the sixth century B.C., the remarkable Chinese philosopher, Lao-tzu (who was the founder of Taoism), became legendary for his ability to consciously manipulate his qi (life force). Early each morning he visualized his qi as it traveled through his body. Lao-tzu became so tuned in to the rhythms of his qi that he could sense when the rhythms had gone awry and correct the balance using only the force of his mind. Apparently, this practice worked well for him; he is said to have lived more than 100 years.

Later, during the first century A.D. when Buddhism swept out of India and into China in the latter part of the Han Dynasty, the Buddhists brought with them the practice of yoga. The Chinese took yoga and combined it with their ancient practice of daoyin and the theories of Lao-tzu. This was the beginning of what we know today as qigong, literally "to work the qi."

Over the centuries, Qigong became very popular in China. People believed its conscientious practice promoted long life, robust health, and physical fitness. Martial arts aficionados added the power of the qi to physical strength in preparing for combat, but qigong was also widely used as a treatment for various diseases, both for self-healing and to treat others. Those who treated others were the qigong masters, people so adept at controlling the qi that they could manipulate it at will, even channeling its force outside the body. Supposedly, a qigong master channels qi energy through his or her hands to restore people who are ill.

Eventually qigong fell out of favor in China, and people thought it was mysticism at best and superstition at worst. During the Cultural Revolution of the 1960s, Chairman Mao banned the practice of qigong altogether, so those who still wished to practice it had to do so in secret.

Today qigong is enjoying a resurgence in China, where researchers are particularly interested in learning more about its physiological effects on the body. About sixty million Chinese now practice qigong in its many forms. There may be as many as 4,000 different styles of qigong exercises.

Qigong is not as well-known in the Western world as some of the other Oriental philosophies, but interest in it is growing. In 1988 in Beijing, a medical conference on qigong attracted hundreds of researchers from all over the world.

Because Western science is only beginning to investigate qigong, there are no published studies to substantiate that its practice can aid in the treatment of diseases. However, there are studies that show that subjects who have achieved deep relaxation have decreased heart rates, oxygen consumption, and respiration rates. Researchers have also found that the type of deep relaxation promoted by qigong seems to boost the immune system. A series of studies at Ohio State University found that students who achieved deep relaxation decreased their susceptibility to viruses by 18 percent, while at the same time, their bodies developed 38 percent more immune-system fighters to ward off disease.

INSTRUCTIONS

Qigong can be practiced either indoors or outdoors in a serene setting free of external distractions. Various practitioners may include slightly different components and exercises, but the principal techniques all include proper alignment of the body through posture, regulation of the breath, and mastery of the mind and spirit. These three elements interact synergistically with one another. Postures, movements, and breathing work together to enhance the flow of air into and out of the body and to provide a sense of deep relaxation and tranquility.

The three most common qigong exercises are the inward training exercise, the strengthening exercise, and the relaxation exercise. Movements include stretching and circular motions, performed either lying down, standing up, or sitting, depending upon the exercise. Because the movements are so gentle, nearly everyone can perform qigong, regardless of his or her level of physical fitness.

If you want to try qigong, here is a sample exercise:

- Stand up straight with your feet together.
- Look straight ahead and breathe naturally.
- As you inhale, rhythmically stretch your arms above your head as high as you can. (Let your arms pull you up on your toes as if you were reaching for the sun.)
- When you've reached as high as you can, turn your palms down, and let your arms drift slowly down to your sides as you exhale. (Pretend your arms are feathers gently floating toward the ground.)

Do this exercise as gracefully and as smoothly as you can. Qigong practitioners suggest regularly performing eight successive repetitions a day to reduce stress, but you can use it anytime you feel tense.

By themselves, the relaxation exercises can provide relief from stress and tension, but when combined with its other elements, including inner training, qigong can be an advanced form of personal development. To find out more about qigong, contact the East West Academy of Healing Arts at the address listed under *Resource Groups*.

FURTHER READING

China Sports Magazine (compilers). *The Wonders of Qi Gong*. Los Angeles: Wayfarer Publications, 1985.

Eisenberg, David, M.D., and Thomas Lee Wright. *Encounters with Qi*. New York: W.W. Norton, 1985.

Takahashi, Masaru, and Stephen Brown. *Qigong for Health*. Tokyo: Japan Publications, 1986.

RESOURCE GROUPS

East/West Academy of Healing Arts, Qigong Institute
450 Sutter St., Ste. 916
San Francisco, CA 94108.
Phone: 415/788-2227

A booklet, Qigong Update, and a teacher directory are available for $15.

Himalayan Institute of Glenview
1505 Greenwood Rd.
Glenview, IL 60025.
Phone: 708/724-0300

A brochure describing the institute's programs is available by mail.

PRANAYAMA
(YOGA BREATHING TECHNIQUES, BALANCED BREATHING)

DEFINITION

Pranayama (pronounced prah-nah-yah'-mah) is the science of correct breathing as developed by ancient Indian yogis.

APPLICATIONS

Physiological: Asthma, bronchitis, emphysema, poor complexion, colds, sinus problems, weak intestinal and abdominal muscles
Psychological: Anxiety, stress, lethargy, smoking cessation

COLLATERAL CROSS-THERAPIES

Yoga, transcendental meditation

RECOMMENDED ADJUNCT ACTIVITIES AND BEHAVIORS

If it does not detract from your concentration, you may enhance your enjoyment of pranayama by listening to soothing music during your breathing exercises. Once you've learned the techniques, you may want to do them while walking.

CONTRAINDICATIONS

None

EQUIPMENT & MATERIALS

If you choose to sit or lie down for the breathing exercises, you will need a comfortable chair with a straight back and/or a mat or carpeted floor.

ORIGIN & BACKGROUND

In Sanskrit, the ancient language of India, *prana* means "life force," and *yama* means "control." Therefore, *pranayama* is translated as "control of the life force." For thousands of years, yogis and other scholars and philosophers of the East have taught that there is a primal creative force—prana—that permeates the universe. Yogis believe that prana is the sustainer of all life, whether plant, animal, or human. When prana is present, the being is alive; when it is absent, the being is dead.

According to this philosophy, the more prana a person has, the more fully alive and healthy he or she will be. People can learn to increase their intake of prana, and they can store it in their bodies. The key to doing this is through correct breathing, which should be combined with proper living habits and use of the mind for maximum benefit.

Centuries ago, yogis observed that the animals with the shallowest, quickest breathing were more nervous than other creatures, and they had shorter life spans. The mouse is one of these animals. On the other hand, elephants and turtles breathe long and slowly. These animals are calm, and they live a very long time. It was from these observations that the yogis developed their breathing exercises. (For a further description of the origins of yoga, see YOGA.)

INSTRUCTIONS

Pranayama is an integral part of yoga, but we have included the breathing techniques separately here because you can use them on their own even if you do not wish to learn the whole discipline. Three important breathing techniques are the *cleansing breath*, the *complete breath*, and *alternate nostril breathing*.

Sitting cross-legged is the traditional way to perform yoga breathing exercises, but you may sit in a chair, stand, or even lie down for some exercises if that is more comfortable.

The Cleansing Breath: To perform the cleansing breath; which is sometimes known as bellows breath or runner's breath:

- Sit erectly in a comfortable position.
- Inhale through your nose, but not deeply—about a third of a lungful of air is about right—while at the same time expanding your abdomen outward as far as you can.
- Quickly and vigorously contract your abdomen while forcefully expelling all the air from your lungs through your nostrils. This quick exhalation should be very vigorous. (It's similar to the effect of being unexpectedly punched in the stomach.)
- Expand your abdomen outward again and inhale through your nostrils.

- Repeat the vigorous exhalation through your nostrils.

Remember, all the breathing is done through your nose. Each cleansing breath is one relaxed inhalation and one forceful exhalation. Each should be completed in one or two seconds.

Because the exhalation is so forceful, the cleansing breath removes some of the pollution and other impurities that we breathe into our lungs. It is an excellent early morning wake-up technique as well as a quick refresher any time during the day when the mind is fatigued. It's also good for clearing congested nasal passages and sinuses, and it helps to strengthen the diaphragm.

Along with the other yogic breathing techniques, the cleansing breath may help you to overcome the smoking habit, but you will probably have to practice it patiently for some time in order to have this effect. People who have used the cleansing breath to help them stop smoking say that once they've become accustomed to flushing out pollution and other impurities with the cleansing breath, they have no desire to inhale them again by smoking.

The Complete Breath: To perform the complete breath:

- Sit in a comfortable position breathing normally.
- Pull in your abdomen and exhale through your nose until you've expelled all the air from your lungs.
- Push your abdomen outward while at the same time inhaling slowly and rhythmically through the nose.
- Still inhaling smoothly, pull your abdomen in slowly and expand your chest by pushing your breastbone forward and expanding your rib cage.
- Begin exhaling, and relax your shoulders and chest.
- When all the air has been expelled, you have finished one complete breath.

The entire procedure should be rhythmic and wavelike.

You will probably have to practice the complete breath a number of times before you develop the proper rhythm. The complete breath can be performed while standing, sitting cross-legged, lying down, or sitting in an ordinary chair.

The complete breath has a wonderfully calming and relaxing effect, and it helps strengthen the abdominal and diaphragmatic muscles. The increased oxygen available during the exercise may induce the release of endorphins, which could account for its remarkable effect on stress.

The complete breath can be used in combination with the cleansing breath as well as by itself. A good practice is to perform ten cleansing breaths followed by one complete breath. The more you practice these techniques, the more you'll gain from them. They're particularly effective if you do them while walking.

Alternate Nostril Breathing: Alternate nostril breathing is a technique used to relax both body and mind. To perform it:

- Hold your hand with your right thumb next to your right nostril and one finger next to your left nostril.
- Close the right nostril with your thumb.
- Inhale through the left nostril to a count of five. (Each count should be about one second.)
- Close the left nostril with the finger and release the right nostril.
- Exhale to a count of ten through the right nostril.
- Immediately inhale through the right nostril to a count of five.
- Close the right nostril with your thumb and release the left nostril.
- Exhale to a count of ten through the left nostril.
- Then: inhale left; exhale right; inhale right; exhale left; inhale left, etc.

Describing the instructions is more complicated than the exercise. Just remember to exhale through one nostril, inhale through the same nostril and then exhale and inhale through the opposite nostril. If you have learned it, use the complete breath for inhalation and try to exhale fully.

When you have inhaled and exhaled through both nostrils, you have completed one round of alternate nostril breathing. You should do at least three rounds (without stopping) in each session; more is even better. Breathe rhythmically, allowing your breath to flow easily from one nostril to another. Concentrate on keeping a cadence as you open and close each nostril.

Some practitioners add another step: after inhaling, close both nostrils and hold your breath for a five count. Then open the appropriate nostril for exhalation.

If inhaling for five seconds and exhaling for ten doesn't feel comfortable for you, try a different count, but do try to exhale for double the time that you inhale when you first practice this exercise. The reason for this is that most people don't fully exhale when they breathe. A longer count allows you to expel all the air—and the impurities—before you take the next breath. As your lungs become stronger and you become more proficient at the technique, you may choose to keep the same rhythm for inhaling and exhaling.

Don't get hung up on counting; it's not really important. In fact, some yoga practitioners disapprove of counting at all when practicing any of the breathing techniques. They believe that the rhythm of your natural breathing is the one that's right for you and you shouldn't artificially alter it. Some people also feel that counting interferes with maintaining a tranquil state of mind. Choose the method that you like best.

Alternate nostril breathing can be performed anywhere at any time, whether you are sitting, standing, or lying down. Just remember to use correct posture to allow room for your lungs to expand properly.

Many people swear that this technique rapidly relieves headaches and sinus problems, and it has a marvelously calming effect on the emotions. Because it is so relaxing, it is often used as a cure for insomnia.

You will gain maximum benefit by using the complete breath technique during alternate nostril breathing; it is well worth learning for the extra effects it gives. We've probably all benefited from the time-honored advice to "take ten deep breaths" when we're nervous or upset. If that helps even though we breathe improperly, imagine the improved results with deep and controlled breathing.

FURTHER READING

Carter, Dixie. *Dixie Carter's Unworkout*. University City, Calif.: MCA Home Video, 1992 (video)

Chopra, Deepak, M.D. *Perfect Health. The Complete Mind/Body Guide*. New York: Harmony Books, 1991.

Folan, Lilias M., and Taylor Feltner. *Lilias! Yoga for Better Health*. Thousand Oaks, Calif.: Goldhil Video, 1995. (video)

Gordon, Neil F. *Breathing Disorders: Your Complete Exercise Guide*. Champaign, Ill.: Human Kinetics, 1993.

Hendricks, Gay. *The Art of Breathing and Centering*. Los Angeles: Audio Renaissance Tapes, 1989, (audiotape)

Conscious Breathing: Breathwork for Health, Stress Release, and Personal Mastery. New York: Bantam Books, 1995.

Jackson, Ian. *The Breathing Approach to Whole Life Fitness*. Garden City, N.Y.: Doubleday, 1986.

Loehr, James E., and Jeffrey A. Migdow, M.D. *Take a Deep Breath*. New York: Villard Books, 1986.

Mills, Gary K. *Quiet Moments Relaxation*. St. Helena, Calif.: MediaHealth Publications, 1986.

Rawls, Eugene, and Eve Diskin. *Yoga for Beauty and Health*. New York: Paperback Library, Inc., 1967.

Rosen, Marion, and Sue Brenner. *The Rosen Method of Movement*. Berkeley, Calif.: North Atlantic Books, 1991.

Zi, Nancy, Greg Dinatale and Patricia Sill. *The Art of Breathing*. Glendale, Calif.: ViVi Co., 1993. (video)

RESOURCE GROUPS

American Yoga Association
513 South Orange Ave.

Sarasota, FL 34236
Phone: 813/9535859

American Yoga Association
3130 Mayfield Rd., Ste. W-301
Cleveland Heights, OH 44118
Phone: 216/371-0078

THE MIND AS HEALER

Western medicine leads the world in the technological aspects of medicine. Scientists have developed wonder drugs and sophisticated machinery to cure the physical body, but they often ignore the tremendous powers we have within ourselves to influence our own healing. This neglect stems from the entrenched Western attitude that the mind is one thing, the body another. Other cultures take a different approach. In the Orient, for example, the healer considers the totality of the human being, including the mental and emotional (spiritual) aspects, before making a diagnosis or suggesting a treatment.

Healthcare practices in other cultures differ in another important aspect: They place much more emphasis on actively staying well, preventing illness, than do we in the West.

Western scientists are quintessential "show-me" folks. Without scientific evidence of the mind/body connection in the form of case-control studies, they were reluctant to adopt nontraditional approaches. Now that evidence is mounting, and attitudes are beginning to change, toward prevention as well as cure.

Today healthcare practitioners of all persuasions recognize that each of us has within himself or herself the ability to strongly influence the course of both our physical and emotional well-being. We know now that people can even use their minds to influence the body's autonomic processes—blood flow, heart rate, and respiration, for example—that we once thought were completely beyond our control.

This is an exciting section because it outlines some powerful techniques. Not surprisingly, some have their roots in the ancient practices of the Orient. The methods herein are listed separately, but several of them can—and should—be used together for maximum effectiveness.

AFFIRMATIONS

DEFINITION

Affirmations are positive statements used to promote physical healing and emotional and psychological well-being.

APPLICATIONS

Physiological: May be used to encourage healing of any disease or physical problem
Psychological: Stress, tension, fears, phobias, daily problems, negative behaviors

COLLATERAL CROSS-THERAPIES

Meditation, visualization, biofeedback, humor, journaling, autogenics

RECOMMENDED ADJUNCT ACTIVITIES AND BEHAVIORS

Behavior modification, reading literature with a positive message

CONTRAINDICATIONS

None

EQUIPMENT & MATERIALS

None

ORIGIN

Affirmations date back to the time when the first human said, "I can do it" when faced with a difficult problem. In other words, it's part of our nature as humans to offer ourselves and others words of encouragement in tough times. The granddaddy of all affirmations is probably "I'm fine," the almost automatic response we usually make to the equally automatic greeting, "How are you?" I'm fine says more about the way we'd like to be perceived by the other person than about the actual condition of our health.

Using positive statements to buck up one's ability to face challenges is nothing new, but it's only been in recent years that people have learned that they can "reprogram" their lives and even affect the way their bodies work through positive affirmations.

INSTRUCTIONS

Exactly what is an affirmation? An affirmation is a short positive statement that you repeat to yourself to replace negative habits with positive ones, increase self-confidence, and help yourself heal. People often use affirmations in conjunction with autogenics (self-hypnosis), meditation, and/or visualization.

As we grow up, we develop automatic responses to certain situations that are often self-defeating. "I'm hopeless at organizing my life," "I'm too shy to make friends," or "I just can't stop eating." The purpose of affirmations is to replace these negative thoughts with positive ones, such as "I have enough time and energy to organize my life exactly as I want it to be."

Keep your affirmations short and specific. "I am very wealthy" is too vague; "I am the wealthiest person in the world" is specific enough, but it's too unrealistic. "I take advantage of career opportunities, and my work brings me all the money I need" is better.

Be sure to phrase your affirmations in the present tense—not "I will," but "I am" or "I can"—as if your goal were already realized. That's not cheating. You already know you *want* to change your habits; affirmations confirm that you *are* that different person.

Avoid expressing positive thoughts in a negative manner. For example, don't say "I'll never eat too much again." Instead try "I am perfectly satisfied with one helping of food at each meal." Replace words like "never" and "won't" with the flip side of your problem: "I am" and "I can."

Start with one or two affirmations that are important to you. Write them down and keep them handy to remind yourself not to slip back into negativism. One woman found herself repeatedly saying "I don't have time" whenever anyone asked her to do anything outside her usual routine. She realized that she was in a rut and that her life lacked spontaneity. Furthermore, she sensed that making time for a change of activities would probably help her work more efficiently. She taped "How delightful. Of course I can . . " next to each of her telephones, and many times during the day she repeated this affirmation: "I have all the time I want to do everything I want to do."

Be sure that your behavior mirrors your affirmations. If you tell yourself that you are an attractive, confident person, treat yourself that way. Pay attention to your appearance; walk tall, and smile at the world. Affirmations work best (and quickest) if you help them along with positive behavior.

Expect that it will take some time to see tangible improvement. It probably took years for you to develop the patterns you want to overcome, so be patient and keep working toward your goal.

Studies show that people who have positive attitudes enjoy better health. If it's a physical problem you're trying to relieve, affirmations can help you heal, but you should seek other appropriate treatment as well. A suitable affirmation for this situation might be "My treatment is working perfectly. Every day I am getting better and better" or "I feel wonderful. I am in perfect health."

The more you repeat your affirmations the sooner they'll become part of the way you really do feel about yourself, but it's particularly important to say them when you're most in touch with your unconscious. You might try combining affirmations with meditation and / or visualization. When you first wake up and just before you go to sleep are also good times to practice.

If you're skeptical that affirmations can really work, consider this: Do you really doubt that constantly telling a child he's bad or stupid will cause him to grow up feeling that he is? We all know people who feel negative about themselves because of such childhood experiences. If negative programming is so effective, why wouldn't positive programming be equally effective?

Most people want to develop their own affirmations to suit their individual situations, but if you need some samples to get you started, there are many books available. You can even buy musical tapes that have hidden (subliminal) positive affirmations that are masked by the music. Experts disagree as to whether or not these work, but the theory is that you can play the tapes while sleeping or going about your daily tasks and receive positive reinforcement without any conscious effort. If you want to try this kind of tape, pick one that includes a description of the affirmations.

FURTHER READING

Brice, Carleen. *Walk Tall: Affirmations for People of Color*. San Diego: RPI Publishing, 1994.

Clifton, Donald O., and Paula Nelson. *Soar With Your Strengths*. New York: Delacorte Press, 1992.

Daniels, Aubrey C. *Bringing Out the Best in People*. New York: McGraw Hill, 1994.

Farmer, Steven, and Juliette Anthony. *Affirmations for Adult Children of Abusive Parents*. Los Angeles: Lowell House, 1992.

Halpern, Steven. *Effortless Relaxation*. San Anselmo, Calif.: Sound Rx, 1988. (audiotape; music with subliminal affirmations)

———. *Weight Loss*. Manhasset, N.Y.: Vital Body Marketing Co. Inc., 1987. (audiotape; music with subliminal affirmations)

Jampolsky, Gerald G., and Diane V. Cirincione. *Wake-Up Calls*. Carson, Calif.: Hay House, 1994. (2 audiotapes)

Pitzele, Sefra Kobrin. *Affirmations for When You Love Again*. Deerfield Beach, Fla.: Health Communications, Inc., 1992.

Prevention Magazine. *Be a Positive Person*. Emmaus, Pa.: Rodale Press, 1988. (audiotape)

Prudden, Suzy, and Joan Meijer-Hirschland. *Change Your Mind, Change Your Body*. San Francisco: Harper San Francisco, 1992.

Subliminal Creativity. Ojai, Calif.: Gateways Research Institute, 1986. (audiotape; music with subliminal affirmations)

Sutphen, Richard. *Sleep Programming*. Malibu, Calif.: Valley of the Sun Audio, 1992. (audiotape)

Take Control of Your Life. Ojai, Calif.: Jonathan Parker's Institute, 1988. (audiotape; music with subliminal affirmations)

AUTOGENICS (AUTOGENIC TRAINING)

DEFINITION

Autogenics uses a combination of self-hypnosis, autosuggestion, and directed meditation to focus the mind (through a series of simple mental exercises) for healing and relaxation.

APPLICATIONS

Physiological: Headaches, muscular aches, diabetes, hypertension, back pain, sexual dysfunction, overweight, ulcers, burns
Psychological: Stress, tension, substance addiction, regulation of excessive habits

COLLATERAL CROSS-THERAPIES

Meditation, affirmations, visualization, yoga, biofeedback

RECOMMENDED ADJUNCT ACTIVITIES AND BEHAVIORS

Lifestyle changes as appropriate

CONTRAINDICATIONS

People with abnormal blood pressure, diabetes, hypoglycemia, or heart conditions should check with their healthcare practitioners before undertaking autogenics. Autogenics is not appropriate for folks with serious emotional or mental problems.

EQUIPMENT & MATERIALS

Autogenics requires no equipment other than a quiet comfortable place to practice.

ORIGIN

Unlike many other self-help therapies that have ancient roots, autogenic training is not even 100 years old. In the latter part of the nineteenth century, physiologist Oscar Vogt worked at the Berlin Neurological Institute. Vogt noticed that some patients seemed to recuperate more quickly than others. To find out why, he observed these patients and discovered that they used self-hypnosis to aid in their recovery.

Intrigued by his findings, Vogt experimented with various self-hypnosis techniques, working with patients who had problems like migraine headaches and muscular tension. Patients who used the techniques several times every day soon reported that their symptoms had abated.

Vogt's methods became well known throughout the medical community. In the 1930s, they attracted the attention of Dr. Johannes Schultz, a German psychiatrist, who was already doing research in hypnosis but also in yoga. Schultz liked Vogt's approach, but he thought he could improve upon it. Vogt employed a hypnotherapist to teach patients how to use self-hypnosis for healing; Schultz believed that people could learn to do it themselves.

Together with his colleague Dr. Wolfgang Luthe, Schultz developed a series of autogenic training exercises. (Autogenic means "self-generating.") The exercises combined elements of self-hypnosis, meditation, and deep relaxation techniques.

The method proved very successful, and over the next thirty years, autogenic training became a widely-recognized self-help technique. Several important books in the field helped to spread its popularity.

INSTRUCTIONS

Autogenics doesn't "cure" anything. It simply puts your mind in touch with your body so that you can use your body's own ability to repair itself and fight off disease. Nevertheless, you can use autogenic training in a wide variety of circumstances. For example, people with burns have used it to help speed the healing process and to block out pain. Athletes sometimes use autogenics to improve their performance, and some students find that it helps them with the learning process.

However, the most popular—and successful—uses for autogenics are for stress reduction (and its associated risks of hypertension, stroke, and heart disease) and for elimination of bad habits such as smoking and overeating. Many people also swear by it as a control for migraine headaches.

To practice autogenics, you need to find a quiet room where you won't be disturbed or a secluded spot outdoors. It doesn't matter whether you sit or lie down as long as you're completely comfortable. Loosen any restrictive clothing. Turn the lights down low. Close your eyes and relax. Sit or lie in this position for a few minutes breathing quietly and rhythmically through your nostrils (not your mouth). Then repeat the following phrases five to ten times each.

- My body is quiet. My body is totally relaxed.
- My right hand and arm feel very heavy and warm (same for left side).
- My right foot and leg feel very heavy and warm (same for left side).
- My abdomen is relaxed and warm.
- My breathing is rhythmic and deep.
- My heartbeat is steady and calm.
- When I open my eyes, I will be refreshed and relaxed and I will remain that way.

Return gradually to your normal state of wakefulness by first stretching your arms and then your legs. Then open your eyes and look around you for a minute or two before getting up.

Normally our bodies regulate and rejuvenate themselves only during periods of deep sleep. Autogenic training, when properly done, replicates the same conditions and activates the body's natural healing mechanisms.

Don't try to force yourself to relax. A key element to autogenics is that your remain passive. Just let the relaxation flow; observe what's happening to your body, but don't be judgmental if it doesn't seem to respond properly. Relaxation may not come easily at first, but don't worry about it. Just keep practicing. It can take a long time to master autogenics—maybe as long as six months—but nearly everybody can do it eventually.

You should practice twice a day, morning and evening, for about twenty minutes each time. You can also use autogenics for just a few minutes during the day whenever you feel you need to slow down and get a grip on yourself After you've got the hang of it, you may find that repeating just the first few phrases will induce the relaxing effect.

During your autogenic sessions, you may experience some odd effects like tingling or involuntary movement. Experts call this "autogenic discharge," and it's simply the result of releasing tension.

If you're interested in autogenics but prefer to start with professional guidance, you might check with a biofeedback clinic. Many biofeedback practitioners are familiar with autogenics.

Autogenics is not geared toward healing any specific disease or solving a particular problem. It works by promoting general physical and emotional wellness. If you want to influence the healing process toward a specific condition, you can use self-hypnosis and directed autosuggestion to achieve this end. In the **Further Reading** section following, we have listed some books and audiotapes that you can use for guidance. The technique is very similar to that of autogenics except that your statements include positive affirmations about the specific condition you want to work on. (See also AFFIRMATIONS.)

FURTHER READING

Alman, Brian M., and Peter T. Lambrou *Self-Hypnosis: The Complete Manual for Health and Self-Change*. New York: Brunner/Mazel, 1992.

Copeland, Rachel. How to Hypnotize Yourself and Others. Hollywood, Fla.: Lifetime Books, 1994.

Fannin, Patrick, and Matthew McKay. *Time Out from Stress*. Oakland, Calif.: New Harbinger Publications, 1994. (audiocassette)

Hook, Lynne O'Neill. *Hypnotizing Yourself for Success*. Saratoga, Calif.: R&E Publications, 1988.

LeCron, Leslie M. *Magic Mind Power: Make It Work for You*. Marina del Rey, Calif.: DeVorss and Co., 1982.

Oyle, Irving, and Susan Jean. *The Wizdom Within*. Tiburon, Calif.: H.J. Kramer, 1992.

Petrie, Sidney. *Helping Yourself with Autogenics*, West Nyack, N.Y.: Parker Publishing Co., 1983.

Stone, Robert B. *Mind/Body Communication*. Niles, Ill.: Nightingale-Conant Corp., 1993. (audio)

Subliminal Affirmations for Recovering Codependents. Plymouth, Minn.: Metacom, 1990. (audio)

Sutphen, Richard. *Peace of Mind Hypnosis*. Malibu, Calif.: Valley of the Sun Publishing, 1985.

Taylor, Eldon. *Subliminal Communication: with How to Create Your Own Program*. Las Vegas, N.V.: Just Another Reality, 1990.

(There are a great many self-hypnosis audiotapes available for specific problems, such as weight loss, smoking cessation, self-confidence, etc. Harold H. Bloomfield and Sirah Vettese have done a series for Harper Audio. David Illig has done another series for Metacom. Many such tapes are also available from Nightingale-Conant.)

RESOURCE GROUPS

Autogenics is practiced more widely in Europe than in the United States. As far as we know, there are no resource groups for autogenics in the U.S., but if you want more information, you can contact:

International Committee for Autogenic Training
101 Harley St.
London W1N 1DF, United Kingdom

BIOFEEDBACK (BIOFEEDBACK TRAINING)

DEFINITION

Biofeedback is the technique of making the body's unconscious processes—heartbeat or respiration, for example—known to the senses so that these processes can be controlled consciously. To understand what this means, think of the thermostat on your furnace. Through continuous temperature monitoring and feedback to the furnace, the thermostat keeps your home at a relatively constant temperature and allows the furnace to function at peak efficiency, regardless of external influences like sudden cold spells. Biofeedback works on similar principals. A person learns to regulate the way his or her body performs in order to make it function more efficiently. Often biofeedback training involves the use of a device to help the person learn to monitor and control responses, but the device may not be necessary after the training period.

APPLICATIONS

Physiological: High and low blood pressure, chronic pain, headache, Raynaud's disease, stroke, ulcers, heart arrhythmia, paralysis, stomach disorders, arthritis, backache, muscle spasm
Psychological: Insomnia, panic attack, stress, tension, fear, depression, sexual dysfunction

COLLATERAL CROSS-THERAPIES

Exercise, healthful diet, yoga, breathing techniques, imagery, meditation

RECOMMENDED ADJUNCT ACTIVITIES AND BEHAVIORS

If appropriate, lifestyle changes to reduce stress, eliminate alcohol and/or substance abuse.

CONTRAINDICATIONS

Biofeedback involves no drugs or invasive techniques, so it is not likely to cause you any harm, but talk it over with your healthcare practitioner if you have a serious, chronic, or life-threatening condition. Many people with chronic, severe pain find that biofeedback can reduce their discomfort to a level that they can tolerate without resorting to mind-numbing drugs. However, if you have a disabling condition, you should consult a professional biofeedback therapist recommended by your healthcare practitioner.

EQUIPMENT & MATERIALS

Biofeedback training devices for home use range from simple red-bulbed thermometers costing only a few dollars to relatively sophisticated electronic equipment that can cost a thousand dollars or more. Some people successfully learn biofeedback techniques without any monitoring devices at all. Unless you've been advised to do so by your healthcare practitioner, it doesn't make much sense to invest in expensive monitoring machines without first trying low-cost options. Another inexpensive device is something called a Bio-Q fingerband. This is a small "bandage" that wraps around your finger. The band contains crystals that respond to warmth, so you can tell when you've successfully raised your temperature.

ORIGIN

Although the word *biofeedback* is a Western term, the concept of controlling the body's functions through self-discipline and self-awareness has been well-known to Eastern cultures for centuries. We've all heard stories about zen masters, yogis, and Indian fakirs who can walk barefoot on hot coals without getting burned, control their own heartbeats, lie on a bed of nails without feeling pain, and otherwise exert seemingly amazing control over their bodies' internal functions. These masters have generally devoted their lives to disciplining their minds and cultivating spiritual awareness.

The concept of using the mind to control the body doesn't involve a great leap of faith in the Orient as it often does in the Western world because Eastern philosophy has always regarded the mind and body as integrated elements of the whole person. With some notable exceptions, scientists and medical practitioners in the West have generally placed a greater degree of separation between mind and body, but that philosophy is changing.

In the West, studies of biofeedback grew out of the interest in conditioned learning. In the early part of this century, Russian physiologist Ivan Pavlov conducted a famous experiment in which he rang a bell every time he fed a dog. After a while, he simply rang the bell without giving the dog any food. Despite the fact that his bowl was empty and the bell had nothing to do with food, the dog salivated just as he would have if he'd had a tasty meal before him. The dog associated food with the bell, so his body reacted to food even when only the bell was present. The idea that the body can be conditioned to react to certain associations was revolutionary at the time, and it changed thinking about how people and animals learn.

Later, behavioral scientist B.F. Skinner set up a conditioning experiment a bit differently: the animal would have to discover for itself what stimulus produced food. Skinner put a hungry rat in a cage fitted with a lever that released food into a cup. In its search for food, the rat at first pushed the lever accidentally, but gradually, it learned to push the lever to get food.

These experiments paved the way for research into human responses to conditioning stimuli. The first experiments were crude: hook a person up to some electrodes to monitor heart rate; flash a light, and then follow the light within a few seconds with a mild electric shock. The electric shock produced an accelerated heart rate, but the idea was to produce the heart speed-up *before* delivering the shock by conditioning the subject to respond to the light because he associated the light with the shock.

Since these early years, biofeedback research has come a long way. Today, using modern methods, people can learn to control peripheral blood flow, for example, in a matter of a few weeks and without expensive electronic equipment. However, control for some bodily functions does require electronic devices.

INSTRUCTIONS

Many people think that biofeedback is either a miracle cure or a complicated and mysterious procedure that the average person couldn't understand, let alone implement. It is neither. On their own, our bodies already
change our heartbeat, respiration, and other functions in response to
outside stimuli. For example, if you were about to speak in public before
a large group, you might begin to sweat, feel your heart pounding
rapidly, and show other signs of panic. If someone were to take your
blood pressure at that moment, it might be much higher than usual.
These are normal reactions to stressful situations, but if someone were
to teach you techniques to help you control these bodily changes, you
could step out on stage relatively calmly.

Essentially, that's all that biofeedback is, a method of controlling your
body's reactions to outside stimuli when these reactions cause you
problems. The devices that are used for biofeedback training help because they give you concrete evidence of the way your body reacts under
certain conditions, and they also show you when you've achieved control over the appropriate function. However, an ordinary, inexpensive
glass-bulbed thermometer will serve quite nicely for the beginning
do-it-yourselfer to monitor temperature.

Problems related to stress and pain are two big areas where biofeedback can help a person. If you have a chronic or life-threatening
condition that causes you terribly intense pain, you will probably want
to consult a professional biofeedback practitioner to help you get started,
but if you experience less serious problems like occasional stress-related
headaches, you can probably learn to control them without outside help.
Try one of the books listed in the *Further Reading* section of this listing.

Learning biofeedback techniques is not hard, but it does require lots
of practice. As a start, you should master DIAPHRAGMATIC BREATHING.
Learning to breathe properly is the first step toward being in control of
your body and helping it to relax on cue. Once you have learned to
breathe from your diaphragm, you can begin to focus your attention on
controlling other parts of your body, such as your peripheral blood flow.
That may seem a daunting task, but it isn't as difficult as it sounds.

We all have stress in our lives; there's no escaping it. If your house
were on fire, your body would immediately go into its red-alert mode:
the fight or flight response. Your heart would begin to beat faster, your
blood pressure would go up, and your body would signal for more blood
to be sent to the skeletal system and internal organs. This response would
take away blood from the extremities, so your hands and feet would feel
cold. Such a strong response is appropriate for coping immediately with
a serious threat.

But what about less serious situations? Let's say you have an extremely busy day ahead. Too much to do and not enough time to do it. Then the phone begins ringing constantly; your cat eats the chicken you've just brought from the grocery; the dog wants to take a walk *now*; and so on. As these interruptions pile up, your body overreacts and kicks in with its red-alert response each time something new interferes with your schedule. This response is not appropriate for the level of the problem. Before long, you have a raging headache, and your nerves are really frayed. Through biofeedback training, you can learn to tone down your body's responses to a level appropriate for the situation.

As we've said, biofeedback training usually begins with learning to breathe properly. Next you may learn to control muscle tension. To do this, alternately contract and relax various muscles. Begin with your hands. Make a fist and clench it tight. Note how this feels. Then completely relax your hand and note how that feels. Do this with other muscles, each time noting the feeling when the muscles are tensed and then relaxed. As you progress, you'll learn the *feeling* that relaxing the muscles produces. Soon you'll be able to relax tense muscles at your command.

We associate relaxation with a warm and comfortable feeling. Cold hands and feet often mean your body is pumping too much blood to your skeleton and internal organs because tension has raised the fight or flight response. To normalize the blood flow and reduce tension, try imagery. Imagine that you're lying on a warm and sunny beach or that you're sitting before a roaring fire. Your hands and feet feel toasty and comfortable. Use whatever imagery works for you, in order to will your hands and feet to feel hot and heavy. To test whether your imagery is working, you can wear a Bio-Q fingerband or tape an ordinary red-bulbed thermometer to your finger. Note the temperature before and after you've practiced your imagery to warm your hands. It may take some time to get the hang of this technique, but don't get discouraged or try too hard. Just keep practicing. Eventually you'll see results. (If the temperature *drops* instead of rises, you're probably trying too hard to relax and creating tension instead.)

These techniques give you an idea of what biofeedback is all about. To learn the full range of biofeedback methods, get a book or consult a professional for a few sessions to get you started. You can also get biofeedback tapes to work with. Some books come with companion tapes and/or biofeedback monitoring devices.

FURTHER READING

Barbara B., Ph.D. *Infinite Well-Being*. New York: New Horizon Press, 1984.

Corrick, James A. *The Human Brain: Mind and Matter.* New York: Arco, 1983.

Danskin, David G. *Biofeedback an Introduction and Guide.* Palo Alto, Calif.: Mayfield Publishing Co., 1981.

Kohlenberg, Robert J. *Migraine Relief.* New York: Harper & Row, 1983.

Miller, Lyle H., Alma Dell Smith, and Larry Rothstein. *The Stress Solution: Multimedia Support Package.* Brookline, Mass.: Biobehavioral Institute of Boston, 1993. (2 videocassettes, 1 audiocassette, biofeedback device, and information sheet)

Mills, Gary K. *Quiet Moments Relaxation.* St. Helena, Calif.: MediaHealth Publications, 1986.

Norris, Patricia F., and Garrett Porter. *I Choose Life.* Walpole, N.H.: Stillpoint Publications, 1987.

Reiner, Robert H. *How to Manage Stress.* New York: Warner Audio, 1985. (audiotape)

Rosenbaum, Lilian. *Biofeedback Frontiers: Self-Regulation of Stress Reactivity.* New York: AMS Press, 1989.

Sedlacek, Keith. *The Sedlacek Technique.* New York: New American Library, 1990.

Whitbread, Jane. *Stop Hurting! Start Living!* New York: Delacorte Press, 1981.

RESOURCE GROUPS

Association for Applied Psychophysiology and Biofeedback
10200 W. 44th Ave., Ste. 304
Wheat Ridge, CO 80033 .
Phone: 303/422-8436; Fax: 303/422-8894

This is a professional association, but they offer tapes and books for sale, and they can recommend a licensed, professional practitioner in your area.

DREAM THERAPY (DREAM WORK, DREAM INTERPRETATION)

DEFINITION

Dream therapy is a technique for using dreams and the dreaming state for problem solving, self-discovery, and physical and emotional healing.

APPLICATIONS

Physiological: You can try to use dream therapy to improve any health problem, but you should not use it in lieu of other healthcare treatment.

Psychological: Stress, tension, self-actualization, problem-solving, mental acuity, fears and phobias

COLLATERAL CROSS-THERAPIES

Journaling, art therapy, meditation

RECOMMENDED ADJUNCT ACTIVITIES AND BEHAVIORS

Not to make a joke of it, the obvious concomitant activity to dream therapy is sleeping.

CONTRAINDICATIONS

Dream therapy can do you no physical harm, but if you have psychiatric problems and your dreams are disturbing, you may want to talk to your therapist before self-analyzing your dreams.

EQUIPMENT & MATERIALS

You will need to keep paper and pencil or a tape recorder at your bedside to "catch" your dreams as soon as you're aware of them.

ORIGIN

Human beings have been fascinated by what goes on in the mind since antiquity. What is the relationship between our inner selves and the outside environment? Dreams seem to provide a link between our conscious and unconscious selves, and throughout history people have attempted to interpret dreams as a means of unlocking the secrets of behavior and the mind.

The ancient Greeks were strongly influenced by signs and omens. One method of foretelling the future was studying the entrails of animals, but the Greeks also looked to dreams to predict future events. They believed that dreams could bring about cures for illness, too. Dotting the countryside were "dream temples" where people could go to be healed. People flocked to these sacred temples in the hopes of going to bed sick and waking up well through the powers of a curative dream. Failing that, their dreams might at least tell them what their fate would be.

Rituals in the temple were elaborate, for one had to prepare ahead for the curative experience. Fasting, prayer, bathing, and the use of special herbs and oils were all part of the preparation, which might take weeks. Finally, the person seeking a cure would sleep before the altar of the god or goddess to whom the temple was dedicated. It was then that the curative or prophetic dream would occur. Hippocrates was an advocate of the therapeutic power of dreams as were other influential early Greek physicians.

Belief in dreams as omens persisted throughout Europe in the Middle Ages. Shakespeare often refers to the foretelling of events (usually ominous) through dreams. Later, educated people sometimes scoffed at finding meaning in dreams as mere superstition, but there has never been a time in history when some people did not take it seriously.

Dream analysis gained scientific respectability with the teachings of Freud. Freud believed that dream interpretation was a potent tool for cure in the hands of a trained psychoanalyst. Jungian therapy relies on dream interpretation too. In fact, the patient may begin the course of treatment by describing his or her dreams to the analyst.

Dream analysis is only one part of psychotherapy. There are practitioners who specialize in dreamwork alone, but most people who want to undertake dream therapy do so on their own, often with the aid of dream dictionaries and other self-help books.

INSTRUCTIONS

There are two schools of thought on do-it-yourself dream therapy. One group of experts holds that dreams should be strictly interpreted according to a set of criteria developed by professionals in the field. If you lean toward this approach, consult a professionally written text on dream therapy. Another theory is that dreams are so personal and so intimately related to the dreamer's own life that they can only be interpreted by the person who experienced the dream.

Regardless of which theory you're more inclined to credit, you must first capture your dreams. We all dream, but few of us ordinarily recall more than bits and pieces of the dream the next morning. Surprisingly, though, it's not so difficult to develop the skill of recalling your dreams more or less in detail. With a few days of practice, you should be able to recreate a good portion of your dreams on cue.

When you go to bed, relax and try to put the thoughts of the day out of your mind. You may find it helpful to use some sort of relaxation technique. Then tell yourself several times that you *will* remember your dreams when you awaken. Don't be tentative about this. Assume that it's going to happen.

Be sure to have paper and pen on a bedside table that you can reach. Since you may awaken from a dream while it's still dark outside, don't forget to have a light handy too. Everything should be close at hand; even the few moments that it takes to get up and turn on a light or find a pen can wipe the dream right out of your mind. Some people prefer to use a voice-activated tape recorder instead of writing down their dreams.

When you awake, lie still and try to focus on your dream. At first you may remember only fragments, but if you really concentrate, one recollection will lead to another and you may be able to recapture your entire dream. If you're using a tape recorder, you can recall the dream out loud as the various scenes enter your consciousness, but if you're going to write the dream down, repeat what you've remembered several times so you don't forget any details when you begin to write.

Once you've got your dream on paper or tape, ask yourself a series of questions to try to find the kernel of meaning. As you analyze each "scene" in your dream, ask yourself what it reminds you of that you can relate to your own life. Does the storyline of the dream have anything to do with your recent or past experiences? A dream in which something didn't happen that was supposed to happen—you forgot to take an important test, for example—might mean that you're anxious about some impending deadline.

The mood of the dream can give you clues too. Was the dream frightening? If you yourself were part of the dream, how did you feel? Happy? Sad? Tense? Bewildered and lost?

Try to piece together the clues that you get from the various aspects of the dream. You can use a "dream dictionary" to give you guidance in interpreting your dreams, but don't take these explanations totally literally. They can suggest what your dream might mean, but you should look at their interpretations in light of your own experience. Many people do seem to dream the same dreams as others: falling and the aforementioned forgot-to-take-the-test themes are common, but they don't necessarily mean the same things to one person as another. It's not even a given that your own similar dreams should be interpreted the same way on different occasions.

Start by looking for the obvious dream interpretation. That means reviewing recent events and emotional experiences. If that doesn't supply the answer, then go for the more abstract. For example, one woman dreamed repeatedly about her house. It was the same house she'd lived in for twenty years, but suddenly she found a door she'd never seen before. Beyond it, there was an amazingly beautiful room, and beyond that another, and another, and so on. As she went from room to room, she was delighted to find these unexpected treasures. The dream always began the same way, with finding the door, but the hidden rooms were never the same twice. After puzzling over this nighttime bonanza for some time, the woman finally concluded that the dream was all about expanded opportunity. She owned her own small business, and things were sometimes touch-and-go. She had often thought of chucking it for more secure employment, but once she determined what the dream meant (to her satisfaction, at least), she realized why she had opted for self-employment in the first place.

Totally stumped by the meaning of a particular dream? Talk it over with a few friends that know you well. They may be able to provide you with a slant you hadn't thought of. Another technique that is sometimes helpful is to try to illustrate the dream. Draw the scenes as you saw them unfolding. Seeing a real—rather than a mental—picture of the dream can sometimes unlock hidden meaning.

Be honest when grappling with what your dreams might mean. Don't shrink from an unpleasant interpretation if it seems to be the obvious one. The whole point of dream therapy is to help you deal with the issues in your life, so confront them. If your dream interpretations are particularly threatening and/or you can't sort out your problems on your own, seek professional advice.

One interesting way to turn a distressing dream interpretation into a positive experience is to try to replay the dream with a different outcome. Before you go to sleep, tell yourself that you're going to have the offending dream again, only this time instead of throwing the stapler at your boss and making a big scene, you'll have a rational discussion about your differences.

Dream therapy is about recognizing issues and conflicts that you may be unaware of during your waking hours, but you can also use sleeptime to help solve problems you already know you have. Before you go to sleep, review the problem in your mind. Try to think of all the possible solutions and obstacles. Then tell yourself that during the night, you will have a dream that will clarify the issue. This technique is known as *dream incubation*.

If you can master problem-solving through dreams, you may be ready for the ultimate in dream-therapy techniques: knowing you're dreaming *while* you're dreaming. This technique, called *lucid dreaming*, is the most productive and the one most-often used to deal with illness and/or emotional problems. In lucid dreaming, the dreamer projects his or her conscious mind into the dream state to influence the unconscious mind.

The way lucid dreaming works is that, before you fall asleep, you rehearse a script that includes the words or a visualization that you want to use to influence your dream. For example, you might say "relieve my arthritis pain" or visualize your hands feeling flexible and pain-free. You must also tell yourself that you will be aware of your dream state when it occurs. Then, during your dream your conscious mind can interact with the unconscious to give it this message.

Lucid dreaming isn't easy, and you may have to practice over and over, but if you can achieve a state where your conscious and unconscious states interact, you can use the technique to work on a variety of personal problems and health issues.

FURTHER READING

Delaney, Gayle M.V. *New Directions in Dream Interpretation*. Albany, N.Y.: SUNY Press, 1993.

Garfield, Patricia. *The Healing Power of Dreams*. New York: Simon & Schuster, 1991.

Morrison, Sarah Lyddon. *The Modern Witch's Dreambook*. Secaucus, N.J.: Carol Publishing Group, 1990.

Robinson, Stearn, and Tom Gorbett. *Dreamer's Dictionary: from A to Z*. New York: Warner Books, 1994.

Smith, Howard Everett. *Dreams in Your Life*. Garden City, N.Y.: Doubleday, 1975.

Thomson, Sandra A. *Cloud Nine: A Dreamer's Dictionary*. New York: Avon Books, 1994.

Ullman, Montague, and Claire Limmer. *The Variety of Dream Experience*. New York: Continuum, 1987.

Ullman, Montague, and Nan Zimmerman. *Working with Dreams*, New York: Delacorte Press, 1979.

Woodman, Marion. *Dreams: Language of the Soul*. Boulder, Colo.: Sounds True, 1991. (two audiotapes)

RESOURCE GROUPS

Association for the Study of Dreams
PO Box 1600
Vienna, VA 22183
Phone: 703/242-8888

Lucidity Association
PO Box 170667
San Francisco, CA 94117

Night Visions
PO Box 402
Questana, NM 87556
Phone: 505/586-0863

HUMOR

DEFINITION

Humor and laughter can be used to help heal both mind and body.

APPLICATIONS

Physiological: Surgery, stroke, cancer, other serious medical conditions; digestion; circulation; respiration; hypertension
Psychological: Stress, tension, anxiety

COLLATERAL CROSS-THERAPIES

Meditation, visualization, journaling

RECOMMENDED ADJUNCT ACTIVITIES AND BEHAVIORS

Whatever makes you smile

CONTRAINDICATIONS

None

EQUIPMENT & MATERIALS

Your own imagination; comic books and comic strips; humorous literature, videotapes, and movies; comedy routines on records or tape

ORIGIN

The ancients knew the healing power of maintaining a positive attitude during illness. In the second century, Greek physician Galen remarked, "Confidence and hope do more good than physic." We all know the proverb, "Laughter is the best medicine." History gives us many examples of how people have used humor and laughter during times of stress and pain. In olden days, the king had his court jester to lighten the cares of his day, as a witticism or a silly antic made the king smile.

People often see the humorous side of even the most desperate situations. As he lay on his deathbed in a dingy Paris bedroom, the famed British dramatist Oscar Wilde is reported to have said, "Either that wallpaper goes or I do." A friend visiting poet Walter De La Mare during a serious illness asked him whether he would like fruit or flowers. "Too late for fruit, too soon for flowers," replied De La Mare.

Gallows humor aside, research shows that humor and laughter actually can improve people's health, both physically and mentally. That humor is a potent force for healing was proved dramatically by author Norman Cousins, who was diagnosed with a potentially fatal illness in 1964. Determined to beat the odds, Cousins began experimenting with alternative forms of therapy. He decided to adopt a positive approach to his situation and to give himself a chuckle whenever he could. He began watching comic movies, reading humorous books, and otherwise doing everything he could to keep up his spirits. To the amazement of his doctors, it worked. Although Cousins died in 1990, he had many happy, productive years during which he traveled the country promoting his philosophy of humor and confidence as a healing force.

Partly due to the publicity generated by Cousins' case, many physicians today recognize the therapeutic power of laughter. In at least one hospital, stroke patients are treated to Disney cartoons and Marx Brothers comedies. Others bring in clowns to visit hospitalized children. Patients are encouraged to read books by humorists that tickle their fancy.

INSTRUCTIONS

What can humor do for us in trying times? A belly laugh causes us to breathe faster and also works some of our muscles, so it's a bit like doing mild aerobic exercise. A good laugh also speeds up the heart rate, temporarily raises blood pressure, and increases oxygen consumption. When we stop laughing, our heart rate and breathing slow, our blood pressure drops, and our muscles relax. This makes us feel relaxed and tension-free.

Not only that, researchers have found that positive emotions give a boost to the immune system. In one study by a psychologist at a New England college, students who coped with their problems humorously had higher levels of immunoglobulin A—a substance that fights viruses—than did students who couldn't see anything funny in their predicaments.

Another study found that viewing funny movies increased immune-cell activity, and helped people cope with their everyday stresses more easily. And that's important for everybody.

Laughter can improve your life whether or not you're actually ill. To some people, laughing at life's foibles comes naturally; to others it does not. Start improving your humor quotient by opening yourself up to the humorous possibilities in otherwise irritating situations.

One technique that can help in a stressful circumstance: make it totally absurd. For example, let's say you're a salesperson and you have to get to another city to close a big deal. There you are at the airport, waiting to hop on a plane for your big moment when suddenly all flights are grounded by bad weather. If the weather doesn't clear up soon, you're going to miss your appointment. Frustrating? You bet, and there doesn't seem to be much humor in the situation. But suppose you carry the bad news to a ridiculous extreme. You'll be at the airport forever. Your children will grow up without ever knowing they had a mother. You'll become part of the furniture in the airport lounge. The cleanup crew will dust you every morning when they come through. "Who's that," people will say. "Oh, she's been waiting for a flight to Des Moines for nigh onto fifty years." If you make the situation far-fetched enough, you'll soon be able to smile and relax.

Try picturing someone who's giving you a bad time in a ludicrous costume. Imagine that the checkout clerk who's berating you for bringing in expired coupons is wearing rabbit ears and whiskers. Every time she shakes her head in irritation, her ears bob up and down and her whiskers twitch. This technique may sound silly, but it works, and it can defuse a situation before your blood pressure hits red alert.

Cultivate people who make you laugh; read the funny papers and humorous books; rent comedy videos. Be alert to what you think is funny. (Not everyone has the same sense of humor.) The idea is to tune in to the things that you get a chuckle from, so that you can increase your exposure to them. Before long, you may find you feel better physically as well as emotionally.

FURTHER READING

Cousins, Norman. *The Biology of Hope*. Chicago: Nightingale-Conant Audio, 1990. (audiotape)
———. *Head First*. New York: Penguin Books, 1990.
———. *The Healing Force*. Los Angeles: Fox Hills Video, 1987. (video)
———. *Mind Over Illness*. Chicago: Nightingale-Conant Audio, 1991. (2 audiotapes)
Cousins, Norman and M.A. Jackson. *The Celebration of Life*. Beverly Hills, Calif.: Dove Books on Tape, 1986.
Siegel, Bernie S., M.D. *Humor and Healing*. Boulder, Colo.: Sounds True, 1990. (audiotape)

MEDITATION

DEFINITION

There are a number of techniques for meditation, but they have in common the goal of focusing the mind inwardly and achieving a deeper level of consciousness. You can use meditation for stress reduction and relaxation, problem-solving, or for healing.

APPLICATIONS

Physiological: Hypertension, heart problems, insomnia, headache, chronic pain
Psychological: Stress, anxiety, procrastination, interpersonal relationships, mental acuity, depression, self-esteem, creativity

COLLATERAL CROSS-THERAPIES

Breathing exercises, yoga, t'ai chi, zen, Ayurveda, fasting, aromatherapy, biofeedback

CONTRAINDICATIONS

None

EQUIPMENT & MATERIALS

Although some people have learned to meditate *anywhere*, most beginners need a quiet room free from distractions and a comfortable chair, mat, or bed. You can also meditate outdoors anywhere that is comfortable and serene.

ORIGIN

Meditation in some form is associated with all the major religions of the world. Since ancient times, people have used moments of quiet contemplation to refocus their minds and to refresh and renew their spirits.

In some religions, meditation is practiced principally by the religious community, but in those of the East, meditation is part of everyday life for ordinary people. It is principally the meditation techniques of the Orient that have become popularized in the West, partly because of the introduction of Transcendental Meditation.

The specific technique of Transcendental Meditation (TM) became well-known throughout the world through the teachings of Maharishi Mahesh Yogi, who was a pupil of Indian religious leader Swami Brahmananda Saraswati in the 1940s. Later Maharishi Mahesh Yogi spent several years in seclusion in the Himalayan Mountains. When he returned to the world, he introduced Transcendental Meditation, a simple system of meditation that he believed anyone could follow.

Maharishi Mahesh Yogi might have remained an obscure guru had it not been for the Beatles rock group. They heard him speak in London, where he had begun an organization called the International Meditation Society. The Beatles were intrigued by the guru's teachings and soon became followers. Because of the rock group's immense popularity, TM got a great deal of publicity and quickly gained a following.

Shortly thereafter, Maharishi Mahesh Yogi introduced TM to the United States. The movement was widely publicized in the United States as it had been in England, and before long, thousands of people were using the Maharishi's method of meditation.

Throughout history, people have used the repetition of sounds or prayers to free their minds from the distractions of the outside world. Native Americans preparing to fight their enemies used hypnotic, sing-song war chants to prepare their minds for battle, and Buddhists focus using mantras.

There are so many approaches to meditation that nearly everyone can find a method with which he or she can be comfortable. Many of us already have a sense that the principles of meditation could be useful in today's fast-paced, stress-filled world. Whenever we say "get a grip on it" we're talking about focusing our minds inwardly to reduce stress and allow us to regroup. Scientific studies show that meditation *can* help reduce stress, lower blood pressure, and relax our entire nervous systems. Other studies have found that meditation can boost the immune response, so we can fight off disease more effectively.

INSTRUCTIONS

There are two basic approaches to meditation: One begins first with the body and then moves to the mind. The other concentrates primarily on the mind without reference to the body. Within these broad groups, there are further differentiations. In the start-with-the-body group, there is control versus relaxation.

In hatha yoga (see YOGA.), the practitioner first learns to control the body through various postures (*asanas*) and then works toward focusing consciousness through meditation. Before beginning to meditate, the yogic practitioner assumes an appropriate asana in which the spine is kept straight and the body is held still. The most famous meditative posture in yoga is the lotus position, sometimes called the Buddha pose, but there are other positions that are easier for Westerners to master.

Since the only essential components are a straight spine and a non-moving body, several yoga postures fill the bill. You can use Easy Posture, which is simply sitting cross-legged with your knees as low to the floor as possible. If even that is too difficult, try the Egyptian Posture by sitting in a straight-backed chair, feet flat on the floor and one palm on either thigh. Yogis discourage lying down for meditation because they believe it causes drowsiness.

Assume the posture, close your eyes, and breathe quietly and rhythmically through your nostrils. Then make your mind "one-pointed," that is, concentrate on a single object, concept, or word. The idea is to remove all extraneous thoughts from your mind. You can think of rushing water, peace, the color purple, or the middle of your forehead. It doesn't matter. Whatever works for you to drive all other thoughts from your mind. As your concentration deepens, your mind will move to subtler levels of consciousness where even this focus disappears. If you have a particular problem that's concerning you, you can think about your problem for a little while *before* you begin your meditation, but don't use the problem as the focus for emptying your mind of other thoughts. Achieving a meditative state is not about focusing your thinking; it is about not thinking of anything at all and letting your deeper levels of consciousness take over. Since most people find it very difficult not to think about something, the single-focus technique helps them to reach those deeper levels.

When you've finished meditating (yogis recommend twenty to thirty minutes twice a day), gradually return your mind to its normal level of consciousness. Sit quietly for a few minutes and allow your mind to wander a bit. Then open your eyes and blink several times. Stretch your legs out straight and your arms above your head. Lower your arms and then take two or three deep abdominal breaths. Massage your legs briefly, then stand up.

Yogis recommend that you meditate in solitude in a location completely free of outside distractions that would break your concentration.

Another method for arriving at a meditative state is through physically relaxing the entire body, rather than controlling it as in hatha yoga. To do this, concentrate on each part of your body in turn and let go of the tensions. Some people find it helpful to first tense the muscles and then relax them, while others simply concentrate on relaxation. You may repeat to yourself several times, "My toes are completely relaxed. They feel heavy and warm. They are very heavy and relaxed," and so on through your whole body.

Whether you start with the body or not, your principal goal in meditation is to do something with the mind. Some people find it helpful in focusing the mind to repeat a single syllable or word over and over. This is called a *mantra*; which is a Sanskrit term to describe a word or words that resonate with energy. The familiar "oom" is one example, but you can choose your own mantra.

A westernized variation of the mantra technique is called the Relaxation Response. Select a word (such as "peace"), a meaningful phrase, or a short prayer and repeat it each time you exhale while breathing naturally and sitting in a relaxed position in a comfortable chair.

Another technique is to concentrate on a single simple object, such as a geometric shape, until you've cleared your mind of distracting thoughts. In still another method, you use visualization to create a peaceful setting. You might, for example, envision a deserted beach where there is nothing but the warm sun, the sand, and gently lapping waves.

One of the simplest methods of focusing your mind in a one-pointed way is to concentrate on your own rhythmic breathing. Don't attempt to alter your breathing, simply observe its rhythm. Be sure to breathe through your nostrils and not your mouth. As you go deeper into the meditative state, you'll find that your breathing becomes slower and more relaxed.

Using the breathing method, you can even combine meditation with another proven stress-reducer: walking. Walk a little more slowly than usual and breathe normally. Walk for a few minutes, then begin counting the number of steps you take while inhaling and the number you take while exhaling. By linking your steps to your breathing, you can achieve a rhythm that is conducive to meditation.

All the meditative techniques we've discussed so far involve focusing your mind on a single subject or issue. These methods are all forms of *concentrative* meditation. There is another approach that is often called *mindfulness* meditation. With this technique, you allow your mind to wander at will, but you note each thought, feeling, and image that floats into your consciousness as if you were listening in on somebody else's conversation. Don't make any judgments about your thoughts, just observe them.

You can master any of the foregoing meditative techniques on your own with a little practice, but you have to take them seriously and approach them with the expectation that they will work. If you want further guidance, you can find plenty of books and tapes to guide you. Transcendental Meditation differs from the other methods in that it is not considered self-help. To learn TM, you will need to take a course from a qualified instructor.

FURTHER READING

Benson, Herbert M.D., and William Proctor. *Your Maximum Mind*. New York: Avon Books, 1989.

Chopra, Deepak. *Creating Health*. Boston: Houghton Mifflin, 1991.

————. *The Return of the Rishi*. Boston: Houghton Mifflin, 1988.

Denniston, Dennis, and Barry Geller. *The Transcendental Meditation*™ Book. Fairfield, Ia.: Fairfield Press, 1986.

Glassner, William. *Positive Addiction*. Harper & Row, 1985.

Goldsmith, Joel. *The Art of Meditation*. San Francisco: Harper & Row, 1990.

————. *The Invisible* Supply. San Francisco: Harper San Francisco, 1991.

Hanh, Thich Nhat. *A Guide to Walking Meditation*. Nyack, N.Y.: Fellowship Publications, 1985. (This book may not be available in stores or libraries, but you can order it from Fellowship of Reconciliation, PO Box 271, Nyack, NY 10960)

Mahesh Yogi, Maharishi. *The Science of Being and the Art of Living*. New York: Meridian, 1995.

Mason, Paul. *The Maharishi*. Rockport, Mass: Element, 1994. (biography)

Meditation (bimonthly magazine). Subscription information: 17211 Orozco St., Granada Hills, CA 91344-1132. Phone: 800/266-6624; Fax: 818/360-2059.

Roth, Robert. *Marharishi Mahesh Yogi's Transcendental Meditation*. New York: Primus, 1994.

Siegel, Bernie S., M.D., and Robert Gass. *Meditations for Finding the Key to Good Health*. Carson, Calif.: Hay House, 1992.

————. *Meditations for Overcoming Life's Stresses and Strains*. Carson, Calif.: Hay House, 1992. (audiotape)

RESOURCE GROUPS

Center for Spiritual Awareness
PO Box 7
Lake Rabun Rd.

Lakemont, GA 30552
Phone: 706/782-4723

Transcendental Meditation Executive Council
5000 14th St. NW
Washington, DC 20011
Phone: 202/785-5144

VISUALIZATION (ALSO CALLED CREATIVE VISUALIZATION OR GUIDED IMAGERY)

DEFINITION

Visualization is a technique that uses mental images to cause positive changes in a person's life. Visualization can incite the body's immune system to fight disease, and it can help solve emotional problems.

APPLICATIONS

Physiological: Asthma, cancer, headache, arthritis, chronic pain, other chronic conditions, overweight, premenstrual syndrome, vertigo, hypertension, temporomandibular joint disease (TMJ)
Psychological: Tension, stress, anger, substance addiction, insomnia, phobias

COLLATERAL CROSS-THERAPIES

Meditation, yoga, autogenics, biofeedback, affirmations

CONTRAINDICATIONS

None

EQUIPMENT & MATERIALS

You need only to be able to go to a quiet place, indoors or out, that is free from distraction.

ORIGIN

All societies throughout history have recognized the power of imagery and visualization to transform the circumstances of their lives. When we wish to compliment a person whose acts have brought changes to the world, we say, "He was a man of vision." It goes without saying that in order to change something, we first have to imagine the way the thing should be.

Nobody has any difficulty recognizing that external circumstances can be altered by first seeing what needs to be accomplished and then doing whatever is necessary to get it done. First-year Latin students will remember Caesar's remark about his experiences in Gaul—perhaps the ultimate in brevity for so vast an accomplishment—veni, vidi, vici. (I came, I saw, I conquered.)

Everyday life is all about envisioning what needs to be done and then doing it. Until fairly recently, most Western scientists believed that we could use our imaginations to apply to external circumstances, but they thought that the same process wouldn't work if we wanted to change something about the physiology of the body, because our minds were one thing and our bodies another. Over the past thirty or forty years, though, that perception has been changing. Research on the mind/body connection has shown that there is a link and we *can* use our minds to influence how our bodies behave.

INSTRUCTIONS

Visualization is not a passive activity. To use it, you must actively participate in the process of changing your body's responses. It is not necessary to have faith in a higher power to have visualization work for you, but you should approach the process with an open mind, expecting that the changes you want to accomplish *will* happen. (It doesn't matter if you have a few initial doubts as long as you work toward a more positive attitude each time you practice.)

Visualization is not just "positive thinking." With visualization, change is not superficial; it involves working at a much deeper level. At first you may practice visualization for a specific goal, but as you become more familiar with the process and learn to believe in its effectiveness, it can become an integral part of the way you view and react to life.

To practice visualization, go somewhere where you won't be disturbed and sit or lie in a comfortable position. Relax your body completely. Begin with your toes and move upward to your scalp, relaxing each muscle in turn. Let all your tension evaporate. (Don't rush this process; that can cause your tension to return.) Breathe deeply and slowly from the abdomen. See *The Breath of Life* for an abdominal breathing technique. When your body is relaxed, begin counting slowly backward from ten. Feel yourself sinking into a deeper level of consciousness with each count.

Now create a mental picture of the thing you want to have happen. For example, if you have headache pain, you might imagine that your headache is a little ball rolling around inside your skull. Picture yourself tilting your head and watching the ball roll out through your ear and keep on rolling till it's gone from sight. Have a skin rash? Imagine that each of those ugly little red blotches suddenly develops legs and trots off your body to disappear through a hole in the ground.

After you've banished your offenders, imagine that your head now feels wonderful or your body has clear and beautiful skin. Say to yourself (aloud if you like): "My head feels better than it ever has," "My skin is lovely," or whatever is appropriate.

Visualizations are entirely personal. You have to use what works for you, not what somebody else has found effective. If you have a disease and can imagine whole armies of policemen rushing into your body and carting off all the bad-guy germs, then go for it. Some people, however, prefer simply to see their problems as lumps that dissolve or liquids that float away through the fingertips.

One woman who had an aversion to birds successfully overcame her smoking habit by imagining each cigarette with feathers, a beak, and wings. Before long, she couldn't stand to have those ghastly, fluttery things anywhere near her face! (This image cured her cigarette problem, but of course, it did nothing for her bird phobia.)

Some people actually "see" vivid technicolor pictures in their minds when they visualize. For others, the visualizing experience is more like thinking about the image rather than having it appear fullblown before their eyes, so don't be distressed if your visualizations won't win any Oscars.

Try to practice visualizing at least once a day. Use the same image each time for the same problem unless you find it just doesn't work for you. Always end with some positive statements. I feel perfect; I am totally calm and relaxed; I am pain-free, etc. Such positive statements are called *affirmations*. You can find out more about AFFIRMATIONS in the section by that name.

You should always express affirmations in the present time. I *am* completely healthy, for example, not I *will* be completely healthy. Since we always decide in our minds to do something before we actually do it (even if the decision seems unconscious), you want your affirmation to indicate that you have already made the decision to be healthy.

You can use visualization to work on changing just about everything that is bothersome in your life. Some people like to imagine that there's a little all-wise guru living somewhere within their bodies. During visualization, they talk to the guru to find out how to solve their problems. Others picture a library where the books contain all the knowledge of the world. In the library, they can look up answers to their troubling questions. If you use this sort of visualization, you shouldn't expect that the guru will necessarily give you an answer on the spot, although that might happen once in a while, particularly if you've asked the same question before. More likely, though, you'll just realize one day that you know how to solve the problem or perhaps you may simply discover that it has disappeared.

You can combine visualization with relaxation techniques and with meditation. Visualization is not a panacea for all problems, but it can be very effective when traditional medicine has nothing further to offer. Some AIDS patients, for example, use visualization to relieve pain, to eliminate symptoms, and to give themselves a more positive outlook so that they can live satisfying and productive lives.

Skeptical that visualization can really change what's going on in your body? At Southern Methodist University, researchers asked thirty people to imagine a host of neutrophils and lymphocytes, two types of disease-fighting white blood cells, standing ready to do battle with invading germs. After six weeks of visualization, there was a measurable increase in the numbers of these cells in the bloodstreams of the participants.

If you need help getting visualizations to work for you, you might want to rent or buy an audio- or videotape to get you started. Many libraries stock these types of tapes. You can also check with one of the resource groups to see what they have available for purchase. Some healthcare practitioners also include visualization in their repertoires, but because of the individual nature of the therapy, there are few who specialize in it.

FURTHER READING

Barash, Marc. *The Healing Path*. New York: Putnam's Sons, 1993.

Fanning, Patrick. *Visualization for Change*. Oakland, Calif.: New Harbinger Publications, 1994.

———. *Visualization for Stress Reduction*. Oakland, Calif.: New Harbinger Publications, 1992. (audiotape)

Fanning, Patrick, and Jerry Landis. *Visualization for Treating Cancer*. Oakland, Calif.: New Harbinger Publications, 1992. (audiotape)

Gawain, Shakti. Creative Visualization. New York: Bantam Books, 1985

———. *Living in the Light*. San Rafael, Calif.: New World Library, 1991.

Healing Tape, The. Cos Cob, Conn.: Hartley Film Foundation, 1992. (videotape)

Little, Bill L. *Help Yourself Heal*. Minneapolis: CompCare Publications, 1990.

Naparstok, Belleruth. *Staying Well with Guided Imagery*. New York: Warner Books, 1994.

Siegel, Bernie, M.D. *Love, Medicine and Miracles*. New York: Mystic Fire Video, 1991. (videotape)

RESOURCE GROUPS

Academy for Guided Imagery
PO Box 2070

Mill Valley, CA 94942
Phone: 415/389-9324; Fax: 415-389-9342

　Autiotapes, self-help books, directory

American Imagery Institute
PO Box 13453
Milwaukee, WI 53213
Phone: 414/781-4045

　Audiotapes, books, workshops

HEALING "ARTS" AND HOBBIES

Perhaps you don't think of it as a therapeutic practice when you put your favorite symphony on the stereo, kick off your shoes, and lean back to let the music wash over you. You just like music, right? Well, think about it. Most music does have the power to change your mood, doesn't it? Music can make you feel happy, sad, refreshed and revitalized, or totally relaxed. Those are powerful effects, and they deserve to be called therapeutic.

Music can ratchet down stress and make you feel calm and relaxed, and the best part is, you don't have to do anything but listen. The other therapies in this section require a little more effort, but most are based on the premise that you enjoy doing them. In school, activities that add to a child's basic knowledge and pleasure in a subject are called "enrichment." Here we've outlined a few pursuits that have proved enriching to many people.

Art, music, and gardening are wonderful activities that you can lose yourself in and forget about the cares of the day, but only if you find pleasure in doing them. These are not activities you should take up because somebody tells you they're good for you. If you don't enjoy them, they'll only make you frustrated and angry that you're wasting your time. Find something else.

Any so-called hobby in which you can become absorbed will fight that major bugaboo of modern life—stress—and that's a giant step toward improved health. Stress isn't just about feeling tense and irritated; it's about soaring blood pressure, risk of heart disease and stroke, overeating, substance abuse, and a host of other problems. A stress-fighter that works for you is your big buddy, and you should cultivate the friendship.

ART THERAPY

DEFINITION

Art therapy is the therapeutic use of the visual arts to promote physical and emotional healing. Professional art therapists use the shapes and pictures that their clients make as a means of nonverbal communication that can lead to a better understanding of the client's behavior. This type of treatment is not a do-it-yourself project, however, and it is outside the scope of this book. Self-help with art therapy as described here refers simply to the emotional and/or physical benefit that a person can derive on his or her own from creating artistic projects.

APPLICATIONS

Physiological: Headache, stroke, arthritis, rheumatism
Psychological: Alcoholism, drug abuse, emotional problems, learning disabilities, tension, stress

COLLATERAL CROSS-THERAPIES

Music therapy, journaling, aromatherapy

RECOMMENDED ADJUNCT ACTIVITIES AND BEHAVIORS

Visiting art galleries and museums

CONTRAINDICATIONS

Allergies to paint, clay, or other art materials. Activities that require fine manual dexterity may not be appropriate for people with arthritis or rheumatism.

EQUIPMENT & MATERIALS

The equipment and materials you'll need depend upon the art medium you choose. Costs can range from a few dollars for a sketch pad and pencils or charcoal to a hefty outlay for a kiln, potter's wheel, clay, glazes, and other paraphernalia for ceramic work. If you want to try something that costs a lot for equipment and supplies, it's best to take a course first to see if you really like the activity before plunking down big bucks to outfit yourself.

ORIGIN

Long before there were written words, there was art. Humankind's desire for artistic expression goes back at least to the time of the cavemen. Throughout history, standards in beauty have changed with the times, but art remains a powerful means of self-expression that mirrors the artist's view of the world.

We can still appreciate the great works of art from earlier times because they have been lovingly preserved for their beauty and significance. But surely there was a caveman who was all thumbs, who nevertheless daubed away at the walls of his cave, uncaring that his bison was only a blob with legs. Some early Roman must have taken up hammer and chisel and hacked away at a piece of marble vainly attempting to carve out a recognizable human head. Great works of art end up in galleries and on public plazas; art works created by lesser mortals never meet the public eye.

Why then do people whose work falls woefully short of meeting current standards of beauty continue to carve, paint, sculpt, and throw clay against a wheel? Because it makes them feel good.

The origins of art therapy as a profession date back to the last century when some scholars began to take an interest in the psychological ramifications of art. As they pursued this line of thinking, they came to realize that creating art met some inner need in many people.

Later mental health professionals recognized that, although their patients often could not express their feelings in words, they could do so nonverbally through art. Art became a tool through which professionals could learn things about their patients.

INSTRUCTIONS

Professional art therapists are trained to recognize the significance of symbols and patterns, and they have a background in normal and abnormal behavior and skills in intervention methods. Professional art therapy is one form of psychological treatment, which is sometimes used alone but often in conjunction with other treatment methods. Obviously, you can't treat yourself with this kind of therapy; you have to consult a professional.

You can, however, use art to relax, reduce tension, vent hostility and aggression, and in some cases, improve motor skills. You don't have to have any talent, you only have to find what you do therapeutic and enjoyable. Think of it as a hobby with health benefits.

You don't even have to do art on a regular basis. Mad at your husband? Draw a picture of him with horns and a tail and big ugly fangs. Vent your anger on paper, and you may be surprised to find it melting away.

The form of art that you choose depends upon what appeals to you, your pocketbook, and the kinds of benefits that you'd like to get. Working with clay can provide needed exercise for arthritic hands. Painting big, bold designs on huge canvases can provide a sense of freedom for people who feel boxed in by too many responsibilities. Feel distracted and unable to concentrate? Try something detailed that demands close attention.

If you're intrigued by doing some kind of art but don't quite know what you'd like to try, you might want to experiment by taking some classes. In most communities, you can find classes in painting, drawing, and ceramics that are geared to amateurs. Try your local community college or high school. (Many high schools offer "lighted schoolhouse" programs where you can use the facilities of the art and ceramics departments after hours under the supervision of a professional.) Ceramic supply stores often offer classes too.

You may not become another Michelangelo or be discovered by a famous art critic, but that doesn't matter. If art provides therapeutic benefits for you, then never mind that one eye is higher than the other on that face you drew. Picasso's work looked funny to a lot of people too.

FURTHER READING

Adamson, Edward. *Art as Healing*. York Beach, Me.: Nicolas-Hays, 1984.

American Art Therapy Association, Inc. *Introduction, History, Organization, and Therapist (Of Art Therapy)*, Mundelein, Ill.: American Art Therapy Association, 1992.

Capacchione, Lucia. *The Picture of Health: Healing Your Life Through Art*. Santa Monica, Calif.: Hay House, 1990.

RESOURCE GROUPS

American Art Therapy Association
1202 Allanson Rd.
Mundelein, IL 60060
Phone: 708/949-6064

(This organization can provide referrals, books, and other information on the professional type of art therapy.)

GARDENING

DEFINITION

Gardening is gardening, but it can provide physical and mental fruits as well as the edible ones.

APPLICATIONS

Physiological: Flabby muscles, hypertension, headache
Psychological: Stress, anxiety, tension, insomnia

COLLATERAL CROSS-THERAPIES

Herbalism, healthful diet, vegetarianism

RECOMMENDED ADJUNCT ACTIVITIES AND BEHAVIORS

Visiting botanical gardens, reading gardening literature and seed catalogs

CONTRAINDICATIONS

None

EQUIPMENT & MATERIALS

What you'll need depends entirely upon the amount of space that you have and the type of gardening that you plan to do.

ORIGIN

Gardening began as a more efficient way of raising food crops than gathering them in the wild. Over the centuries, though, gardens have become more than utilitarian. The ancient civilizations of the Mediterranean were noted for their beautiful, well-designed gardens, which provided a feast for the eyes and nose as well as the palate. These gardens often featured herbs and other scented plants, and they were designed as places of repose and tranquility.

In more modern times, the English became justly famous for their formal, clipped, and well-tended country gardens attached to grand estates. Elaborate gardens like these and those of the Greeks and Romans, though, depended upon large staffs of free (slave) or cheap labor to keep them looking beautiful. The lord and lady of the manor could potter among the roses if they wished, but they didn't have to.

While the well-to-do fussed and fumed over whether it was appropriate to plant pink flowers next to red and debated the relative merits of the natural look versus the not-a-stem-out-of-place look, ordinary people went right on cultivating their hollyhocks and cabbages in whatever little plot of ground they could find.

In the beginning, people gardened because they had to raise their own vegetable food crops or go without. There was no supermarket down on the corner. Today, however, refrigeration and fast transportation make it possible for people in the industrialized world to buy vegetables, fruits, and flowers from all over the world right in their neighborhood store. Yet gardening is more popular than ever.

People today garden not because they have to but because they want to. There is something about the cycle of growth and change, of getting back to our roots (no pun intended), that is nurturing and fulfilling. People who love to garden may not think of it as therapy, but it is.

INSTRUCTIONS

Experts say that gardening is one of the great stress-relieving techniques. Gardening takes your mind off your daily problems, and it gives you work to do that produces results almost from day to day. Gardening is a pastime that is suitable for people of almost any age or degree of physical fitness. It provides exercise that ranges from mild to heavy-duty, depending upon your activities.

If you're older or have physical problems, you may want to investigate tools that make your work easier. You can buy long-handled trowels and weeders, for example, so you don't have to bend over, or you can get a seat that has handgrips to help you get up. Other tools have special grips that make them easier to hold. These are nice for people with arthritis and rheumatism.

Working in a garden is therapeutic in itself, but you can also design your garden as a healing retreat. The sounds of wind and water provide a soothing background that refreshes the spirit. Trees that rustle appealingly with the breezes include aspen, paper birch, and flowering dogwood. If you don't have room for rustling trees, bamboos and ornamental grasses give a similar, though more subdued, effect.

You can have water sounds even if your garden is small and your budget lean. All you need is a tub and a recirculating pump with a fountain attachment. If you have the space, a pond and a cascading waterfall are lovely to the eye as well as the ear.

Birds and insects can add "music" to your garden too. To attract them, add berry bushes for the birds and plants that are good sources of nectar and pollen for the insects. Thyme, lavender, and rosemary are irresistible to bees and they waft a heavenly scent throughout the garden.

Scent is another feature that adds to the charms of a therapeutic garden. Experts say that scent has strong psychological effects. Wonderful fragrances can be produced by the flowers or by crushing the leaves. Be aware though, that highly scented plants put their energies into producing the fragrance, so their colors are generally pale. In contrast, colorful flowers don't usually have much fragrance. A mix of the two will give you both scent and color.

Old-fashioned English roses are making a comeback because they smell wonderful, and they're very hardy. Nicotiana—the tobacco plant—has a marvelous fragrance if you plant the species *Nicotiana alata* or *N. sylvestris*. (Most of the hybrids are more colorful, but they don't have scent.)

To make your garden visually appealing, look at the textures of plants and the color of their foliage as well as the flowers. Interesting textures invite one to touch the plants, so think about mixing in plants with wooly, waxy, and/or velvety leaves.

If you would like a tranquil spot to relax and shed your tensions, but you don't have the time or the interest in tending plants, you might want to consider a Japanese garden. A Japanese garden has few plants, sometimes none at all. Instead, raked sand, pebbles, and rocks provide a serene retreat. Most Japanese gardens also include small bonsai specimens, but seldom are there flowers. The effect is stark but very peaceful.

FURTHER READING

Bayard, Tania. *Gardening for Fragrance*. Brooklyn: Brooklyn Botanic Garden, 1992.

Boner, Ann. *Fragrance*. New York: Canopy Books, 1993.

Cave, Phillip. *Creating Japanese Gardens*. Boston: C.E. Tuttle Co., 1993.

Glattstein, Judy. *Waterscaping*. Pownal, Vt.: Storey Communications, 1994.

Henry, Peggy, and Saxon Holt. *Gardening to Attract Birds and Butterflies*. New York: Avon Books, 1995.

Moody, Mary. *Creating Water Gardens*. Des Moines, Ia.: Better Homes and Gardens Books, 1994.

Restuccio, Jeffrey P. *Fitness the Dynamic Gardening Way*. Cordova, Tenn.: Balance of Nature Publications, 1992.

Oster, Maggie. *Reflections of the Spirit: Japanese Gardens in America*. New York: Dutton Studio Books, 1993.

JOURNALING (DIARY WRITING)

DEFINITION

Journaling is the writing of a personal journal (diary), not merely as a record of events, but as a means of gaining insight into one's own feelings and inner strengths.

APPLICATIONS

Physiological: Often establishes connection between mental and physical experiences

Psychological: Emotional problems, insights into personal strengths and weaknesses

COLLATERAL CROSS-THERAPIES

Music therapy, art therapy, meditation

RECOMMENDED ADJUNCT ACTIVITIES AND BEHAVIORS

Reading, especially other journals and biographies

CONTRAINDICATIONS

None

EQUIPMENT & MATERIALS

Blank notebooks, pens, and / or pencils. If you're devoted to technology (or have trouble with handwriting), you may, of course, write your journal on a typewriter or personal computer. You may also dictate your thoughts into a tape recorder for someone else to transcribe. If you can, though, it's nice to record your journal in your own handwriting.

ORIGIN

The tradition of journaling is as old as the first thought a human being ever had. Even before people had written language, they passed on their traditions and beliefs to their children and grandchildren through story-telling. Written language was a big milestone, though. Once people had a system of writing that others could understand, they could make permanent records of their lives and times that would last for generations more or less as the original writer intended, not filtered through years of interpretations by different tellers.

Some of our most fascinating and enduring works of literature are nothing more than the journals kept by authors who had a gift for making their experiences come alive for other people. In the beginning, people wrote mostly about what happened to them. Many early stories were about wars and triumphs in battle. The *Iliad* and the *Odyssey*, for example, were written by the Greek poet Homer in about 800 B.C., but they are thought to be based on war with Troy that actually occurred 300 years earlier. The stories were passed down by word of mouth until Homer wrote them down.

People have always been interested in *explaining* events, not just mentioning that they happened, and creative artists have struggled for centuries to give color and meaning to the lives they write about. Millions of perfectly ordinary people have kept diaries too, in which they've recorded their thoughts, feelings, and aspirations. Nearly every teenager has kept a diary, if only briefly. However, it was not until the advent of psychotherapy that journaling became recognized as a tool for helping us learn more about our lives and come to grips with our problems.

INSTRUCTIONS

Many people believe that only those who write well and easily can possibly get any therapeutic value from keeping a journal. Possibly this misconception arises from the supposition that the journal has to have merit for *other people*. Actually, most experts recommend that you keep a journal only for yourself. No one else ever need see it, so you don't have to worry if you can't spell or that you have only fragments of ideas, not complete sentences. Gradually, you'll begin to see a pattern to the things that you write that will help you to understand yourself better and possibly lead to solutions to inner problems.

If writing is difficult for you, but you want to try journaling, here's a good way to get started. Set aside fifteen minutes to a half hour every day, preferably at the same time each day. Pick up your journal and write continuously for the allotted time. Don't worry about what you're writing; it doesn't matter. Just keep writing, putting down any old thought that comes into your head. When your time is up, stop. Next day, do the same thing, but don't reread what you wrote the day before. At first, you may hate doing this, and it may seem silly, but it really does help you get started. Before long, you'll find you look forward to your daily writing, and you'll see that it's much easier to put down your thoughts.

There's no right or wrong to journaling, so you can peek at what you've written before any time you really want to. But if you can hold off for several weeks or even a month, you're likely to be very pleasantly surprised at how much progress you've made toward writing freely. It's a good idea to keep up this unstructured kind of writing indefinitely, but you may also want to develop a "dialogue" with yourself.

Having a conversation with yourself on paper is a technique that is sometimes called *guided* journaling. Its aim is to help you evaluate your life and work toward solutions to questions that trouble you. "Why don't I just solve the problem if I already have the answer," you may be thinking. Well, you probably *do* have the answer, but you don't know it yet. Let's suppose that your problem is that you dislike your job, but you need to work, and you really don't know what else you'd like to do. Here are a series of questions you might ask yourself:

1. What sort of an accomplishment would make me really proud?
2. What kinds of activities do I like to do best? (They don't have to be work-related.)
3. What do I absolutely detest doing?
4. Am I at my best in the morning or later in the day?
5. If I could have any job in the world, however farfetched it may seem, what would it be?
6. What reward for work is most important to me (money, prestige, feeling of helping others, short working hours, easy job, etc.)?
7. What reward for work is least important to me (same variables as above)?

There are a whole host of other questions you could ask yourself to help you define what sort of job you would like. Whatever your dilemma, if you keep asking questions and focusing in, you'll begin to gain insights into how you really feel about the situation.

It's important to write down both the questions and the answers so that you can review them as you work with the problem over time. Be as honest as you can with yourself, and take your time with your answers. It isn't important that you write well, but it is important you give careful thought to your inner dialogue.

Even if you haven't a care in the world, you may enjoy guided journaling. You can learn a lot about yourself by asking provocative questions. If you need help in getting started, you may be able to find a class in guided journaling. Otherwise, there are a number of excellent books available.

Many artists and writers use journaling to increase their powers of observation and to get their creative juices flowing. Often, they do not reread what they've written before, because it is the process and not the content that they find valuable. Other people with pent-up fears, anxieties, or hostilities find it therapeutic to vent these feelings on paper so they can get rid of them. These kind of entries usually aren't meant for rereading either. Whether or not you choose to look back at your previous entries depends upon your inclination as well as the type of journaling you've chosen. However, if you're keeping a journal to gain personal insights and to help solve problems, you'll probably want to reread the log from time to time to see how your thinking has changed. Don't judge by day-to-day progress, which may be almost imperceptible. Instead, look back several months or more. You may be pleasantly surprised at the positive changes you've made and the insights you've gained.

FURTHER READING

Adams, Kathleen. *Journal to the Self: 22 Paths to Personal Growth*. New York: Warner Books, 1990.

——. *Mightier than the Sword: The Journal as a Path to Men's Self-Discovery*. New York: Warner Books, 1994.

Aftof, Susan D. *Writing for Pleasure*. Oak Park, Calif.: The Center Press, 1992.

Baldwin, Christina. *Life's Companion: Journal Writing as a Spiritual Quest*. New York: Bantam, 1991.

Dahlstrom, Lorraine M. *Writing Down the Days: 365 Creative Journaling Ideas for Young People*. Minneapolis: Free Spirit Publishing, 1990. (for juveniles)

D'Encarnacao, Paul and Patricia W. D'Encarnacao. *The Joy of Journaling*. Memphis, Tenn.: Eagle Wing Books, 1991.

Hagan, Kay Leigh. *Internal Affairs*. San Francisco: Harper & Row, 1990.

Holzer, Burghild O. *A Walk Between Heaven and Earth*. New York: Bell Tower, 1994.

Progoff, Ira. *At a Journal Workshop*. Los Angeles: J.P. Tarcher, 1992.

Simons, George. *Keeping Your Personal Journal*. New York: Paulist Press, 1978.

RESOURCE GROUPS

Proprioceptive Writing Center
39 Deering St.
PO Box 8333
Portland, ME 0414
Phone: 207/772-1847

Seminars, writing classes, books, pamphlets

MUSIC THERAPY (MUSICOTHERAPY, MELODIOTHERAPY, RHYTHM PATTERNING)

DEFINITION

Music therapy involves either listening to music or playing an instrument for its therapeutic value.

APPLICATIONS

Physiological: Asthma, hypertension, migraine, intrauterine and postpartum infant growth stimulation, pain, trauma recovery, stroke recovery, senile dementia, Alzheimer's disease, physical movement limitations

Psychological: Insomnia, anxiety, depression, stress, hyperkinesis, autism, learning and communication disabilities

COLLATERAL CROSS-THERAPIES

Selective sensitization/desensitization, relaxation

RECOMMENDED ADJUNCT ACTIVITIES AND BEHAVIORS

Some may choose to heighten the effect of music listening by combining it with other sensory experiences: colored or flashing lights, aromas, indoor or outdoor settings, or touching textured materials.

CONTRAINDICATIONS

Although rare, there is some evidence of musicogenic seizure onset in epilepsy. Some rhythms, tonalities, and harmonies may adversely alter heart and metabolic rates, intensify emotional distress, or produce delusions in susceptible subjects.

EQUIPMENT & MATERIALS

Listening: Equipment for playing recorded music.
Playing: Musical instrument(s) of choice.

ORIGIN

Ancient. The first use of music was utilitarian, not aesthetic, and vocal, not instrumental. Early practitioners of magic sought to imitate sounds of nature, believing that "like affects like." That is, sounds approximating those of one's surroundings were avenues for communicating with and modifying forces thought to influence natural phenomena, physical and spiritual well-being, and behavior. Imitation led to organization, deliberate and purposeful repetition, and creation of sound messages meant to convey the wishes, direction, and power of the practitioner relative to his or her environment.

Unlike other arts, music was considered by early societies to be divine in origin. As such, it was an important intercessional tool for use as a palliative for simple discomfort, a potent curative for demonic possession, or an alternative "voice" for communicating directly with deities. The Greeks and Chinese found dinnertime melodies an effective aid to digestion. Native American and African shamans drummed and chanted away evil spirits. And the Christian church from its beginning regarded some music as divine, other music as evil or pagan. Just as David relieved the Israelite King Saul's melancholy and uncontrollable fits of rage with the playing of his harp, contemporary physicians and therapists use music in the treatment of chronic and acute mental, emotional, and physical disorders. The mathematical precision inherent in music lends itself well to therapeutic application.

INSTRUCTIONS

Self-directed music therapy is possible whenever and wherever you can establish a comfortable site free of interfering sensory distractions. Your own bed, an easy chair, or a grassy hillside—almost any location is suitable as long as it does not compete with the music. Of greater importance than setting, however, is the selection of music for listening. Although taste in music is highly subjective, there are certain guidelines that are helpful in creating specific therapeutic environments.

Technique for Listening: Set aside a time block of approximately an hour when you know you will not be disturbed. Choose a comfortable site for sitting or reclining. Whether you use a headset or conventional speakers is a matter of choice; again, your comfort is the most important consideration. Wear loose clothing. If it suits your mood, dim or cover any bright light sources, including the sun. It is best to use a continuous loop tape or an automatic changer for your recordings so that you can keep the music playing and not break the mood created by the music.

A normal heartbeat ranges from sixty to eighty beats per minute. You might want to check your pulse before and after your listening sessions, perhaps even chart it, in order to monitor the effectiveness of your therapy. It is possible to slow your heartbeat and actually lower your blood pressure, at least temporarily, by quietly listening to music with a beat somewhat slower than your heartbeat. Because popular music usually has a beat considerably faster than sixty beats per minute, you will have to choose your selections carefully. Try the *Venus* portion of Holst's *The Planets*, the first movement of Ravel's *Mother Goose Suite*, or Bach's Brandenburg Concerto No. 4.

On the other hand, just as music can be effective in slowing bodily functions, it is also very useful for setting a pace for physical activity. For instance, if you are doing aerobic exercises, walking, or taking part in some other conditioning regimen, some selections of march music or other spirited music will help you maintain an even, steady pattern for your repetitive movements. Music is effective in teaching rhythm, particularly with children who may require patterning exercises or autistic persons who seem most comfortable in a regulated environment.

Those persons who have difficulty with motor skills may find the fingering of guitar strings, flute fingerholes, or piano keys beneficial.

The ability of music to create a therapeutic atmosphere is well known. Some musical selections have a calming effect while others may be useful for mood elevating. Recognition of personal taste is essential in choosing music intended for psychological reaction. The piped-in "elevator music" so prevalent in office buildings is intended to produce a restful, pleasant ambiance. To some listeners, however, it has exactly the opposite effect, setting their teeth on edge and making them irritable.

If you enjoy playing a musical instrument, this can also be therapeutic. Try soothing melodies to relax, lively ones to lighten your mood. Something rousing or difficult to play can drain away anger. Do you play an instrument that you can attack with vigor, like the piano or drums? By all means, give it a workout and let your tensions go. Learning a new piece can help you temporarily forget a vexing problem, but it's probably the wrong choice if you're playing to calm down. In that case, it's better to choose something that you can play effortlessly so you can let the flow of the music work its magic.

Some people make music part of their daily lives. If you're one of those who listens appreciatively and often throughout the day, you're probably already getting an incidental therapeutic benefit, but you may want to set aside a time just for listening (or playing).

Most people who seldom listen to music don't dislike it; they just don't think about it much. If you're one of these, try adding music to your life. It's just a radio-click away, and you may find it's just the ticket to get rid of a pounding headache or lull you to sleep at the end of a busy day.

FURTHER READING

Alvin, Juliette. *Music Therapy*. New York: Basic Books, 1966.

Alvin, Juliette, and Auriel Warwick. *Music for the Autistic Child*. New York: Oxford University Press, 1992.

Drury, Nevill. *Music for Inner Space: Techniques for Meditation and Visualization*. San Leandro, Calif.: Prism Press, 1985.

Friedman, Robert. *Sound Techniques for Healing Arthritis*. Santa Fe: Brain Sync, 1993. (audiocassette)

Friedman, Robert, and Kelly Howell. *Sound Techniques for Healing High Blood Pressure*. Santa Fe: Brain Sync, 1993. (audiocassette)

Garfield, L. Maggie. *Sound Medicine*. Berkeley, Calif.: CelestialArts, 1987.

National Center for Music Therapy, Inc. *Music Therapy Makes a Difference*. Silver Spring, Md.

Schulberg, Cecilia H. *The Music Therapy Sourcebook: A Collection of Activities*. New York: Human Sciences Press, 1981.

Strauss, Sally. *Inner Rhythm*. San Francisco: Chase Publications, 1984.

Watson, Andrew, and Nevill Drury. *Healing Music: The Harmonic Path to Inner Wholeness*. Garden City, N.Y.: Prism Press, 1987.

Woods, Alana. *The Sound of Healing*. Santa Fe: Open Sky Music, 1992. (video)

RESOURCE GROUPS

American Association for Music Therapy
PO Box 27177
Philadelphia, PA 19118
Phone: 215/242-4450

Newsletter *Tuning In*, journal *Music Therapy*; membership directory; convention

National Association for Music Therapy
505 11th St. SE
Washington, DC 20003
Phone: 202/543-6864

Newsletter, journals, handbook, directory. Annual conference.

PET THERAPY

DEFINITION

Pet therapy uses contact with a pet to promote emotional and psychological healing.

APPLICATIONS

Physiological:　Hypertension, overweight, cardiovascular benefits (e.g. from walking a dog)
Psychological:　Depression, stress, tension, insomnia, feelings of isolation

COLLATERAL CROSS-THERAPIES

Exercise

RECOMMENDED ADJUNCT ACTIVITIES AND BEHAVIORS

Reading about pets; attending dog and / or cat shows

CONTRAINDICATIONS

People with allergies often have trouble keeping dogs or cats. Some allergic people successfully keep cats by bathing them frequently, and there are at least two breeds of dog (soft-coated wheaten terrier and poodle) that shed little and have almost no dander, so they generally make suitable pets for people with allergies. Check with your allergist, though, before getting even these pets.

EQUIPMENT & MATERIALS

The equipment you need depends upon the type of pet you choose. Most pet needs are obvious, but if you're uncertain as to what you might need to keep a given type of pet, check with a veterinarian.

ORIGIN

Wolves became the first domestic dogs, when early people decided they could tame these animals to help them with their work. In the beginning, dogs were not pets as we know them today; they worked for a living, principally as herders and hunters. However, through close contact, people and animals grew to trust and have affection for one another.

Cats have had a rocky road throughout history. In ancient Egypt, they were pampered and revered, but later, during the Middle Ages, when people got hysterical about witchcraft, cats were thought to be witches' "familiars," and they were often tortured and burned.

Since ancient times, people have kept birds in cages to enjoy their colorful plumage and cheerful songs. Medieval hunters often trained falcons to hunt prey. Although falcons weren't pets, there was close contact between man and bird.

Over the years, people began to keep more and more animals simply as pets. Today, in the United States alone, people own roughly sixty million dogs, fifty million cats, forty-five million fish, and eight million birds, not to mention all the rats, hamsters, lizards, turtles, and other creatures that people might call pets.

Most pets are cherished members of the family, but it is only recently that researchers have discovered that pets provide health benefits for their owners. In an important study, investigators interviewed ninety-six people who were hospitalized for serious heart problems. One of the questions on the survey was whether or not they had pets. In a followup a year later, eighteen people had died. Twenty-eight percent of those who didn't have pets had died, whereas only six percent of those who did have pets had died. So Fido or Fluffy may be more than a friend; your pet could be a lifesaver.

Today pet therapy is a recognized form of treatment. Pets are often brought into nursing homes, hospitals, and even prisons for their healing effect.

INSTRUCTIONS

If you feel lonely, depressed, or stressed out, you might want to consider a pet. Bonding with a dog or cat can help you feel less isolated, especially if you live alone. Remember, though, that a pet requires care, so don't get one unless you're willing to devote the time necessary.

When deciding what type of pet to get, consider your circumstances. A large dog, for example, might make you feel secure, but if you live in an apartment, a sheepdog probably isn't the pet for you. Big dogs require plenty of exercise, whereas, a few turns around the block may be enough for a Chihuahua.

Cats make good pets for city dwellers, but you might also want to consider birds or fish. Watching fish swim lazily about their aquarium can be a very relaxing experience.

On the other hand, if you have the space and need to get more exercise, a big dog can be just the ticket. Dogs give you a reason to walk, and you and your pet can spend many pleasurable hours exploring your neighborhood on foot.

Before you get any pet, check with a veterinarian to find out the requirements of the particular animal you're considering. Some dogs get terribly lonely when left alone all day. If you work, take that into consideration. You might want to think about a cat instead or even a dog *and* a cat to keep each other company. Unless you have very little room, two pets aren't much more trouble than one, and you'll have twice as much companionship.

Remember that having a pet is only good therapy if you're fond of animals. If you don't like them, you're likely to have *more* stress by acquiring a pet, but if cozying up to a kitty sounds like just what the doctor ordered, it may truly be.

FURTHER READING

Axelrod, Herbert R. *Tropical Fish for Those Who Care*. Neptune City, N.J.: T.F.H. Publications, 1994.

Barish, Eileen. *Vacationing with your Pet!* Scottsdale, Ariz.: Pet-Friendly Publications, 1994.

Barrie, Anmarie. *Hamsters for those Who Care*. Neptune City, N.J.: T.F.H. Publications, 1994.

Coborn, John. *The Proper Care of Reptiles*. Neptune City, N.J.: T.F.H. Publications, 1993.

Cutts, Paddy. *Caring for Your Cat*. New York: Smithmark, 1994.

Fogle, Bruce. *ASPCA Complete Dog Training Manual*. New York: Dorling Kindersley, 1993.

Freshwater Aquarium Basics. Charlotte, N.C.: Lotus Land Pictures, 1994. (videotape)

Gallerstein, Gary A., and Heather Acker. *The Complete Bird Owner's Handbook*. New York: Howell Book House, 1994.

Hawcroft, Tim. *First Aid for Dogs* (also *First Aid for Cats and First Aid for Birds*). New York: Howell Book House, 1994.

Kilcommons, Brian, and Sarah Wilson. *Childproofing your Dog*. New York: Warner Books, 1994.

Marder, Amy. *Your Healthy Pet*. Emmaus, Pa.: Rodale Press, 1994. (dogs and cats)

McHattie, Grace. *The Cat Lover's Dictionary*. New York: Carroll & Graf Publishers, 1994.

Morton, E. Lynn; Chuck Morton; and Matthew M. Vriends. *Ferrets*. Hauppauge, N.Y.: Barron's, 1995.

Rees, Yvonne. *The Complete Book of Cats*. New York: Crescent Books, 1993.

Sandford, Gina. *Tropical Fish Identifier*. Philadelphia: Courage Books, 1994.

Taylor, Michael. *Pot-bellied Pigs as a Family Pet*. Neptune City, N.J.: T.F.H. Publications, 1993.

Whiteley, H. Ellen. *Understanding and Training Your Cat or Kitten*. New York: Crown Publishers, 1994.

Wrede, Barbara. *Before You Buy That Puppy*. Hauppauge, N.Y.: Barron's, 1994.

RESOURCE GROUPS

A local shelter or chapter of the American Society for the Prevention of Cruelty to Animals (ASPCA) is an excellent place to get a furry pet and save a life at the same time. Be sure to have your animal neutered; there are too many unwanted pets as it is.

ALTERNATIVE HEALING SYSTEMS AND PRACTICES

Western medicine doesn't take a back seat to any other healthcare system when it comes to technological sophistication, advanced surgical techniques, and the variety of drugs available to treat illness and disease. Nevertheless, more and more people are investigating alternative therapies and healthcare systems, and it is partly because of the very sophistication of medicine in the West today.

Early in this century, the family doctor would stop by the house to visit the sick. In those days, treatment might include a pot of herb tea or a homeopathic remedy. With the rise of the pharmaceutical industry, that changed. Today you are much more likely to get a prescription for a potent drug. Many people today are concerned both about the effects of drugs—particularly for long-term use—and their cost.

Also, people don't just want to be treated; they want to know what's going on, and they want to take an active part in the management of their health. Many Western physicians have been slow to realize this, although changes are underway, and so people have begun to take a serious look at alternatives that seem to offer a more natural way of healing.

Another attractive feature of the alternatives is that many emphasize wellness, not just cures when you get sick. Also, there's a growing suspicion among many patients that their physician may view them as another case of hives or the third broken arm today. People want their doctors to recognize that there's a whole person attached to that broken arm or that face with the rash on it. Alternative practitioners seem to do that. In fact, the principles behind many alternative systems insist upon a recognition of the mind/body connection and a perception of the person as a total being.

This is a self-help book, not a medical text. The descriptions of the alternative systems are not meant to encourage you to become your own healthcare practitioner but rather to give you a brief idea of what these systems are all about.

Many mainstream physicians have learned new techniques from alternative practitioners, and there's a growing respect among M.D.s for practices they once frowned upon. Alternative medicine and traditional medicine seem to be moving closer together, but for now, you might find the optimum in healthcare by recognizing that each system has its strengths and choosing accordingly.

AYURVEDA (AYURVEDIC MEDICINE; ALSO SPELLED AYUR-VEDA)

DEFINITION

Ayurveda (pronounced i-er-vay-dah) is a system of preventive medicine and healthcare based on ancient Indian precepts.

APPLICATIONS

Physiological: Ayurvedic medicine is applicable to the same range of disease prevention and cure as western medicine.
Psychological: Nervousness, agitation, insomnia, depression; promotes sense of well-being and "perfect health"

COLLATERAL CROSS-THERAPIES

Aromatherapy, music therapy, yoga, transcendental meditation, pranayama, herbalism, walking, other exercises for specific body types, massage

RECOMMENDED ADJUNCT ACTIVITIES AND BEHAVIORS

Moderation and balance in all things

CONTRAINDICATIONS

None

EQUIPMENT & MATERIALS

Exercise mat or rug (for performing yoga), herbs, massage oils, aromatherapy oils

ORIGIN

Like other oriental healing practices, Ayurveda's beginnings are shrouded in antiquity. The name *Ayurveda* is taken from two Sanskrit words: *ayus* meaning "life" and *veda* meaning "science." Thus Ayurveda literally means "the science of life." We know that Ayurveda dates back at least 5,000 years in India, but it is undoubtedly much older than that. Ayurvedic medicine is rooted in the Vedas, the most ancient of Hindu scriptures, and in later sacred texts. The basic tenets of Ayurveda derive from the collected wisdom of sages, who tuned in to the subtle vibrations of nature to develop their methodology. In this respect, Ayurveda differs from Western medicine, which is based on the scientific method of observing, forming a hypothesis, and then testing that hypothesis to see if it holds true.

Ayurveda is not only a complete system for healing and the prevention of disease, it is a method for living one's life. The Ayurvedic philosophy is to teach a person about the powers of nature to keep us healthy, and then help him or her to use these powers in daily living.

INSTRUCTIONS

Ayurveda teaches that the five basic elements are Earth, Water, Fire, Air, and Ether. In the human body, these elements manifest themselves as three principles (humors) known as the *tridosha*. The tridosha govern all aspects of the body, mind, and consciousness (spirituality). The humors that make up the tridosha are the *vata dosha* (air and ether), the *pitta dosha* (fire and water), and the *kapha dosha* (earth and water). In any individual, one (or two) of these doshas is usually dominant, although an occasional person has equal amounts of all three. Good health comes from keeping the doshas in balance.

In order to balance the doshas, you must first determine what type of constitution you have from the seven possibilities: vata, pitta, kapha, vata-pitta, pitta-kapha, vata-kapha, and vata-pitta-kapha. (Everyone has some of all three doshas within himself or herself; the concept refers to those that are dominant.) You cannot change your basic constitution—that is genetically predetermined—so you must learn to balance your dominant dosha with the other doshas. The following chart describes some of the characteristics of each dosha.

CHARACTERISTIC	DOSHA		
	VATA	PITTA	KAPHA
Body type	Thin; very tall or very short	Medium height; slender	Well-developed; tend to overweight
Hair	Curly and scanty	Thin, silky, reddish, or brown	Thick, dark, soft, and wavy

Appetite	Variable appetite; crave sweet, sour, salty tastes; like hot drinks	Strong metabolism and appetite, good digestion; crave sweet, bitter and astringent tastes, cold drinks	Regular appetite; slow digestion; crave pungent, bitter, and astringent foods
Characteristics	Creative, active, alert, restless; talk and walk fast, but tire easily	Poor tolerance for sunlight, heat, or hard work; moderately active	Move slowly; good stamina; generally healthy, peaceful, and happy
Psychological characteristics	Quick understanding but short memory; little willpower, tolerance, confidence, or boldness; nervous, fearful, anxious; poor reasoning power	Good comprehension, intelligent, sharp; good speaker; tendency toward hate, anger, and jealousy; ambitious; like to be leaders	Tolerant, calm, forgiving, and loving, but also greedy, possesssive, and envious; slow comprehension, but good memory
Sleep habits	Sleep little	Moderate sleep	Sleep soundly and long
External interactions	Make and spend money quickly; tend to remain poor	Like luxuries; usually moderately well-off	Earn money and hold on to it; tend to be wealthy

The chart above is very simplified; if you want to learn more about what type you are, consult one of the books in the *Further Reading* section following.

Ayurveda teaches that health is order and disease disorder. By keeping the doshas in equilibrium, the body, mind, and consciousness work in harmony and thus keep disease at bay. If a person does develop a disease, healing comes through nature, but a person cannot hope to experience healing if his or her everyday life is out of whack.

The Ayurvedic lifestyle is one of moderation. A healthful (largely vegetarian) diet, yoga, the chanting of a mantra, and meditation are part of daily practice. Herbal medications, purges and other cleansing practices, color therapy, and gemstone therapy are all treatments that might be used for the person who does become ill.

Below is an example of a daily routine that a follower of Ayurveda might practice to maintain good health:

- Rise before dawn.
- Excrete waste products and clean the mouth and teeth.
- Examine the tongue for signs of illness; then clean it by scraping with a silver scraper to massage not only the tongue, but the internal organs it affects.
- Massage the body with warm sesame oil and then bathe.
- Exercise (including breathing) and meditate.
- Eat breakfast (the previous part of this routine should always be accomplished before 8 A.M. because breakfast is not supposed to be eaten after 8).
- Work or other routine morning activities.
- Have lunch before noon if possible.
- Eat dinner before sundown.
- Go to sleep before 10 P.M.

Ayurvedic practitioners also recommend a short walk about fifteen minutes after each meal. One may also choose to meditate or perform yoga at other times during the day.

Even if you don't want to follow a complete Ayurvedic routine, you might want to incorporate some of its components into your lifestyle. The warm sesame oil massage in the morning before your bath or shower, for example, is surprisingly pleasant and invigorating. Store the sesame oil in a plastic bottle so you don't have to worry about broken glass and bare feet. Then warm the oil by putting the bottle in a wash-bowl of hot water. Massage with long, firm strokes. Be sure to include your face and head (but wash the oil from the bottoms of your feet before you step into the tub so you don't slip). Then follow with a brisk invigorating shower or a nice bath.

Because Ayurveda is a complete way of living, we can only describe a few of the details in this volume. If you're intrigued by what you've read here, there are many books and videotapes available to help you learn more.

FURTHER READING

American Association of Ayurvedic Medicine. *Maharishi Ayur-Veda: Review of Scientific Research,* 1990.

Chopra, Deepak, M.D. *Creating Health,* Boston: Houghton Mifflin Co., 1987

———.*Perfect Health. The Complete Mind/Body Guide,* New York: Harmony Books, c1991.

———. *Quantum Healing: Exploring the Frontiers of Mind/Body Medicine.* New York: Bantam Books, 1989.

———. *Quantum Healing Workshop.* South Burlington, Vt.: Mystic Fire Audio, 1990. (audio)

──────. *Return of the Rishi: A Doctor's Search for the Ultimate Healer*, Boston: Houghton Mifflin Co., 1988.

Douillard, John. *Body, Mind, and Sport.* New York: Harmony Books, 1994.

Lad, Vasant. *Ayurveda: The Science of Self-Healing*, Santa Fe: Lotus Press, 1985.

Lele, R.D. *Ayurveda and Modern Science*, Bombay: Bharatiya Vidya Bhavan, 1986.

Maharishi Ayurveda Medical Center. *Maharishi Ayurveda: Natural Health Care for the Rejuvenation of Mind and Body.* Maharishi Ayurveda Corporation of America.

──────. *Patient Education Program.* Washington, D.C.: Maharishi Ayurveda Corporation of America, 1987.

Murthy, N. Anjneya, and D.P. Pandy. *Ayurvedic Cure for Common Diseases.* New Delhi: Orient Paperbacks, 1982.

Rhyner, Hans A. *Ayurveda: The Gentle Health System.* New York: Sterling Publishing Co., 1994.

Svoboda, Robert E. *Parkruti: Your Ayurvedic Constitution.* Albuquerque: Geocom, Ltd., 1989.

RESOURCE GROUPS

American Association of Ayurvedic Medicine
1115 Elkton Dr., Ste. 401
Colorado Springs, CO 80907
Phone: 800/532-8332

Ayurvedic Institute
PO Box 23445
Albuquerque, NM 87192-1445
Phone: 505/291-9698

The Institute for Human Potential and Mind/Body Medicine
8010 Frost St. Ste. 300
San Diego, CA 92123
Phone: 800/827-4277

Deepak Chopra, M.D., is executive director. The institute offers educational and other programs.

Maharishi Ayurveda Health Center
679 George Hill Rd.
Lancaster, MA 01523
Phone: 617/365-4549

Maharishi Ayur-Veda Health Center
PO Box 282

Fairfield, IA 52556
Phone: 515/472-5886 or 800/248-9050

Information, referrals to Ayurvedic physicians in your area.

Maharishi Ayurveda Health Center
17308 Sunset Blvd.
Pacific Palisades, CA 90272
Phone: 213/454-5531

Maharishi Ayurveda Health Center
2112 F St. NW
Washington, DC 20037
Phone: 202/785-2700

Quantum Publications
PO Box 598
South Lancaster, MA 01561
Phone: 800/858-1808

This is a source for information on books, audiotapes, and videotapes, by Dr. Deepak Chopra and for herbal products used in Ayurvedic practice.

COLON THERAPY (COLONIC IRRIGATION, COLON HYDROTHERAPY, COLONIC LAVAGE, COLONICS)

DEFINITION

Colon therapy is purported to cleanse and detoxify the colon (large intestine) by removing accumulated waste material through irrigation with water (colon hydrotherapy) to which various other substances, including herbs, might be added.

APPLICATIONS

Physiological: Constipation, diarrhea, flatulence, colitis, parasitic infection, diverticulitis, other gastrointestinal problems, skin disruptions
Psychological: Depression, stress

COLLATERAL CROSS-THERAPIES

Vegetarian diet, healing diets, fasting, hydrotherapy, yoga, meditation, aerobic exercise, breathing exercises

RECOMMENDED ADJUNCT ACTIVITIES AND BEHAVIORS

Change in dietary habits; diet should be higher in fiber, fresh fruits, and vegetables and lower in meat and dairy products.

CONTRAINDICATIONS

Physicians generally either disapprove of colonic therapy or think it is useless. They say there is no medical reason to irrigate the colon and that the colon, if left alone, naturally cleanses itself. Some medical practitioners say that colonic lavage is actually harmful. They suggest that frequent use can cause chronic constipation by distending the colon and causing it to be unresponsive to the normal stimulation of dietary bulk. They also say that repeated use can deplete the body of vital nutrients and cause dangerous electrolytic imbalance. Other hazards physicians cite are infection from improperly sterilized equipment, the possibility of perforating the colon and/or pushing fecal matter higher up with forceful streams of water. Coffee enemas, which are recommended by some alternative practitioners, are believed by many mainstream practitioners to cause diarrhea, dehydration, and anxiety. Most of the concerns about infection stem from an infamous event in 1981, when health authorities traced six deaths and a number of other cases of amebic dysentery to a single colonic irrigation machine that had been improperly cleansed. Improvements in sterilization procedures and the development of disposable syringes and tubes seem to have largely eliminated this problem because there have been no such incidents in recent years. In truth, neither proponents nor detractors of colonic therapy have much scientific evidence to back up their claims. Still, colonic irrigation is controversial therapy, and you would be wise to discuss it with your healthcare practitioner before you try it.

EQUIPMENT & MATERIALS

Enema bag with fountain syringe, sea salt, baking soda, and lubricant, which can be hand lotion, vegetable oil, or surgical lubricant. You can also use a hot water bottle with a syringe attachment.

ORIGIN

The enema is the predecessor to colonic therapy. Introduction of liquids into the colon for cleansing dates at least as far back as the Egyptians. Their famous medical work, the Ebers Papyrus, written in about 1500 B.C., recounts that physicians used a reed to insert watery substances into the rectum. In Greece, Hippocrates and later Galen reported on using enemas, particularly to reduce fevers. The Romans, too, used enemas for internal cleansing.

We know of at least one early Christian aesthetic community that used colonic irrigation in conjunction with their religious beliefs. They viewed the body as the temple of the soul, and they wanted to keep it pure, so they used enemas to flush out uncleanliness and diseases that defiled the temple.

By and large, though, the history of colonics is relatively sparse. This is probably due in part to the nature of the subject, which does not lend itself gracefully to public conversation.

In the latter part of the nineteenth century and the early part of the twentieth, some physicians used colonics to treat high blood pressure, heart disease, and depression. In his sanitorium in Battle Creek, Michigan, physician and cereal mogul Dr. John H. Kellogg used enemas extensively in his treatments. However, when synthetic drugs came along, most mainstream physicians began prescribing them and stopped using colon therapy except for chronic constipation.

Colon therapists and traditional medical practitioners agree that a diet high in fiber, plenty of liquids, exercise, and regular evacuation habits are key to keeping the colon functioning properly. Beyond this point, however, they differ. Colon therapists point out that carnivores in the animal world have much shorter colons than do humans, so food (meat) passes through relatively quickly. They contend that because "transit time" (the medical term for the time it takes food to be digested and pass out of our bodies) in humans is much longer, meats and other fatty foods form a sort of sludge that sticks to the walls of the colon and putrefies.

Toxins produced by the putrefying sludge enter the bloodstream and cause a variety of diseases. Colonic irrigation flushes out the sludge and removes the toxins so the body can heal itself. (Medical doctors don't buy this theory. They say that there is no sludge buildup and that the colon is self-cleansing.) Colon therapists cite these reasons for waste buildup:

- Low-fiber, high-fat foods
- Poor food combinations that compete for digestive enzymes (e.g., meat and potatoes)
- Eating too much or too fast
- Drinking large quantities of liquids at meals that dilute digestive enzymes
- *Not* drinking enough liquids in general
- Stress and other negative emotions
- Illness and/or medications that slow down bodily functions
- Toilet habits based on convenience rather than the natural urge

Today most people who practice colonic therapy professionally are chiropractors, naturopaths, and other alternative healthcare practitioners. The American Colon Therapy Association maintains its own National Certification Panel, but only one state—Florida—licenses colon therapists. There the procedure is a subspecialty of massage therapy, and the practitioner must complete a 100-hour course and a written examination.

Most other states take a less benign view of colonics. In California a few years ago, physicians lobbied for a bill that would have prevented anyone who was not a physician from giving an enema. Public ridicule—"give an enema, go to jail"—probably helped defeat the bill. Florida and California remain principal centers for colonic therapy.

INSTRUCTIONS

What can you expect from a session with a professional colon therapist? First, you can expect the premises to be hygienic and clean. (If they're not, run, don't walk, out the nearest exit.) Professional colon therapists usually use purified water and disposable tubes to guard against infection. Large amounts of water (anywhere from five to twenty gallons) are introduced via a tube inserted into the anus. Another tube takes away the waste material and deposits it into a tank. The water may be warm or cool, or the therapist may alternate warm and cool flushes. The therapist may massage the abdomen to dislodge sludge adhering to the colon walls. The whole process is repeated a number of times until the colon is completely flushed out. A typical session lasts from forty-five minutes to an hour.

Sometimes oxygen, friendly bacteria, aloe vera, wheatgrass juice, or other nutrients are added to the water to feed the body through the colon. This is known as a nutrient colonic. Psyllium seeds might be added too, to "brush" the colon.

You can try colonic irrigation for yourself in the privacy of your own home using an ordinary enema bag with a fountain syringe. (Enema bags are available at most pharmacies.) Prepare the enema solution by adding one tablespoon of sea salt and one tablespoon of baking soda per quart of water. The water temperature should be about 98° F. Fill the enema bag with the solution. Since this will be a messy procedure, you'll want to do it in the bathroom while sitting on the appropriate appliance. Lubricate both the anus and the tube with vegetable oil, hand lotion, or surgical lubricant. Professional machines use gentle water pressure, but you'll have to make do with gravity feed, so hang the enema bag about three feet above you (a nearby towel rack high on the wall might do the trick). Insert the tube just past the inner sphincter muscle (approximately an inch and a half). Hold the tube in place and open the valve to allow about a pint of the liquid to flow into the colon. Hold briefly, then remove the tube and allow the solution to drain out. Repeat as many times as is necessary. (Don't introduce too much water at one time because this can stretch the colon.)

Some people believe that slightly warmer water (101°F.) helps reduce bowel spasm, while cooler water (75°–80°F.) tightens up a sluggish colon. Never use colonic therapy if you have rectal bleeding.

How can you tell whether colonic therapy will help you with your problems? According to colon therapists, the treatment helps those with chronic constipation, diarrhea, flatulence, and skin disruptions, but the person must also adopt healthful eating habits for the treatments to have any long-lasting value.

Oral Cleansing: If colonic irrigation isn't to your liking, you may be more interested in colon-cleansing products that can be taken by mouth. Internal cleansers taken orally usually consist of a bulking agent plus various herbs. These cleansers purport to loosen gooey matter stuck to the sides of the colon and to reduce harmful bacteria as well as to promote the absorption of water-soluble vitamins and protein. There are at least a half dozen such products on the market. Check your local herbal shop or health-food store.

Many colon therapists recommend that when you take an oral cleanser you also brush your skin daily to stimulate the lymphatic system. Use a dry long-handled bath brush and "sweep" your body from the extremities toward your abdomen. Then sweep your torso, front and back, from the neck downward. Use the same sweeping strokes on your face, starting from the center and stroking outward. Then sweep up your neck and the sides of your face. (On your face, you'll want to use a softer brush, such as a cosmetic brush.)

We realize that colon therapy is not a practice that everyone will want to try, but this book is about offering choices so that you can select your own methods of self-care. Colon therapy does not have as large a following as do some of the other measures we've discussed, but its adherents are enthusiastic and truly believe it's helpful. Because the traditional medical community almost uniformly condemns the practice, please do not undertake colon therapy without discussing it thoroughly with your healthcare practitioner. If used improperly, even proponents admit that it can be dangerous.

If you decide to visit a professional colon therapist, it's important to check credentials. Since Florida is the only state that has licensing procedures, be sure that the therapist you consult is certified by the American Colon Therapy Association. You might also want to check with others who've visited the practitioner to see what their experiences were. And, as we said earlier, if the premises are not clean and hygienic, do *not* undergo the treatment.

FURTHER READING

Walker, Norman W., D.Sc., Ph.D. *Colon Health: The Key to Vibrant Life*. Phoenix: O'Sullivan Woodside, 1979.

Weinberger, Stanley. *Healing Within: The Complete Colon Health Guide.* Larkspur, Calif.: Colon Health Center, 1988.

RESOURCE GROUPS

American Colon Therapy Association
11739 Washington Blvd.
Los Angeles, CA 90066
Phone: 310/390-5424

Pamphlets, seminars

California Colon Hygienists' Society
209 Morning Sun Ave.
Mill Valley, CA 94941
Phone: 415/383-7224

Pamphlets; referrals to therapists in your area

International Association of Colon Therapy
2204 N.W. Loop #410
San Antonio, TX 78230
Phone: 210/366-2888

Dr. Robert A. Wood Institute
PO Box 530
Valparaiso, IN 46384

Source for self-use colonic products and programs

HOMEOPATHY

DEFINITION

Homeopathy works on the principal that the same substance that causes symptoms of illness will, if taken in minute doses, cure that illness by triggering the immune system.

APPLICATIONS

Physiological: Arthritis, headache, earache, allergies, autoimmune diseases, colds, insomnia, rheumatism, indigestion, constipation, chronic conditions for which the long-term use of more potent drugs would be undesirable
Psychological: Insomnia, depression, stress, irritability

COLLATERAL CROSS-THERAPIES

None specifically

CONTRAINDICATIONS

Homeopathy is not a treatment for emergencies; consult your healthcare practitioner before using homeopathic remedies for serious illness, broken bones, or end-stage disease of any sort.

EQUIPMENT & MATERIALS

Purchased homeopathic remedies; for self-care, you will probably also want a book detailing the remedies and their uses.

ORIGIN

In the fifth century B.C., the Greek physician Hippocrates believed in the principle that "like is treated with like." That belief has come down through history in various folk remedies, such as taking "a hair of the dog that bit you" as a hangover cure after a wild night. (For anyone who has not heard that expression, it means having another drink, and it is not a recommended therapy.) Treating like with like is also the cornerstone of homeopathy, but it was not until the latter part of the eighteenth century that Western physicians began to develop the system that is known today as homeopathy. Homeopathy was not an invention nor was it a sudden discovery. It evolved over a forty-five-year period, from about 1790 to 1835.

Dr. (Christian Friedrich) Samuel Hahnemann was a German physician and the most accomplished translator of medical texts of his era. During his translation of English physician William Cullen's important work, *Materia Medica*, Hahnemann read the material avidly. He was impressed with Cullen's detailed description of the use of Peruvian (cinchona) bark to treat chills and fever (probably this was malaria). Cullen knew what cinchona bark would do for someone who was ill. What effect would it have on a person who was perfectly well? Hahnemann wondered. He decided to try it on a healthy specimen: himself. Somewhat to his surprise, he found that the "cure" gave him the very symptoms it was designed to treat. Intrigued, he decided to try the same experiment with other drugs. (Hahnemann's friends and family apparently were a trusting lot, for they all served as guinea pigs in his research.) Drug after drug provoked the symptoms of the disease it was supposed to cure and sometimes other symptoms as well.

Hahnemann then set about researching the literature to find other instances where the cure and the disease evoked similar symptoms. Since he was an accomplished linguist, his reading ranged through the texts of many countries. Hahnemann was able to document sixty-three drugs that met the criteria of like curing like.

From his findings Hahnemann deduced that the specific chemical properties of a drug were unimportant. What mattered was the drug's effect upon the symptoms of the disease. He also believed that signs and symptoms were the only useful clues a physician could rely on (as opposed to various "theories" of disease). When he spoke of "signs and symptoms," however, Hahnemann referred to the total person, not just to the manifestations of disease.

Hahnemann called his belief that like cures like the Law of Similars. Its corollary, the Law of Infinitesimals, derives from the belief that the drugs used to treat illnesses should be given in very diluted doses. Diluted doses were necessary, Hahnemann and his followers felt, because the patient was already suffering from symptoms like those that would be produced by the drug, and a strong dose might be more than the patient could tolerate. Hahnemann's theories dictated that only a single remedy be used for a given disease. Combinations of drugs were ruled out.

In 1796, Hahnemann published his "Essay on a New Principle for Ascertaining the Curative Powers of Drugs." In it he criticized the current state of medical practice (which at the time relied heavily on leeches, bloodletting, and the like) and outlined his theory of "homeopathy." (He coined the term *homeopathy* from the Greek word *homoios* meaning "like." Traditional medicine is called "allopathic" meaning medicine, which in simplified terms means the use of a counteracting agent to alleviate disease effects: "A pill for an ill." By 1810, Hahnemann had fully developed his theory of homeopathy, and he published *The Organon of the Rational Art of Healing* outlining it in detail.

Homeopathy was not an overnight sensation in the medical profession, although Hahnemann did attract something of a following, and he established a medical school. In 1820, Hahnemann was forced to leave Leipzig, where he had been practicing, because of a dispute with the local apothecaries. He refused to purchase their medications, preferring to make his own according to his exacting standards. The government sided with the apothecaries and forbade him to dispense his homemade homeopathic remedies. Hahnemann went to Köthen where he had a patron who convinced the local authorities to allow him to practice medicine.

His theories might never have gotten a wider exposure had it not been for the cholera epidemic that swept through Europe in 1831. Traditional medicines proved ineffective, and physicians stood by helplessly while thousands died. Hahnemann alone deduced that the disease was caused by some form of tiny organism that could be checked by antiseptic practices. His work during the epidemic brought Hahnemann international acclaim. Later when a similar epidemic invaded England in 1840, people who took a homeopathic remedy had a better survival rate than those who took conventional medications, and this added to a growing acceptance of this form of medicine.

Hahnemann moved to Paris in 1833. There he found a very receptive audience for his homeopathic theories, and the monarchy itself issued a royal decree authorizing him to practice homeopathy.

In 1825, a Danish physician named Hans B. Gram introduced homeopathy into the United States. At first its practice spread rapidly. In the early part of the twentieth century, there were homeopathic medical societies in forty-six of the forty-eight states, 286 homeopathic hospitals and related institutions, twenty homeopathic medical colleges, and thirty-two medical journals.

However, partly due to opposition from the American Medical Association, homeopathy fell out of favor, and by mid-century, there were few practitioners. Homeopathy emerged from dormancy in the 1970s, and today homeopathic remedies are used by a growing number of traditional and alternative healthcare professionals.

Homeopathic remedies are manufactured from natural plant, mineral, and animal substances and are prepared in accordance with the *Homeopathic Pharmacopoeia of the United States*, the official manual. A specific quantity of a pulverized substance is mixed with either alcohol or water to form a solution. Then the solution is diluted to a ratio of 1:100. This dosage is known as 1c. One drop of 1c may be further diluted by the same ratio. This makes a 2c dosage. At the 3c level, the original substance is only one part in one million, and the amounts given are often even more diluted than that. Homeopaths believe, however, that the more a remedy is diluted, the more potent it becomes.

Critics acknowledge that such low concentrations of curative ingredients in homeopathic remedies are safe even when the ingredient is potentially toxic at a higher concentration, though they do not believe that increasing the dilution strengthens the medication. In fact, detractors question whether such minute amounts can do any good at all. A number of scientific studies suggest that they can. In 1991, the *British Medical Journal* reported that eighty-one of 105 controlled studies worldwide found "positive" results for homeopathic treatments. The report took issue with the methodology of some of the studies, but nevertheless found the results promising enough to warrant further study. In a more recent report in the December 10, 1994, issue of *Lancet*, another highly regarded British medical journal, a research team led by Dr. David Reilly at the University of Glasgow found "more than a placebo effect" in three randomized, double-blind studies of homeopathic remedies.

Homeopathy is well respected in many parts of the world, including Europe, Latin America, and Asia. Members of the British royal family are said to be adherents. Homeopathic practitioners who also have medical or osteopathic degrees often take a mix-and-match approach, prescribing homeopathic remedies for some ailments, but relying on traditional treatments for others.

INSTRUCTIONS

There are so many comprehensive books on homeopathic remedies available today that it is easy to study up and learn how to treat common ailments on your own. Homeopathic medicines are considered over-the-counter drugs by the Food and Drug Administration, so you do not need a prescription to try the remedies.

However, bear in mind that homeopathic treatments are designed for individual people, not individual diseases. The appropriate remedy for a specific illness is based on the patient's complete physical, mental, and emotional profile as well as the diagnosis of the problem. So you might have a cold and your neighbor might have a cold, but you wouldn't necessarily take the same homeopathic remedy.

If you visit a homeopath, the case history is likely to involve much more than just what seems to be ailing you and what has ailed you in the past. The homeopath may ask about moods and emotions, what makes you happy, what depresses you, what foods you like, how you get on at your job, and a host of other questions designed to get a complete picture of your life. Many people who use homeopathic remedies for self-care start out with this kind of professional workup and then move on from there.

If you want to treat yourself with homeopathic remedies without benefit of professional advice, you should develop a total profile on yourself just as the practitioner would. The more you learn about yourself and the remedies, the better able you will be to make intelligent choices.

One way to learn more about homeopathic self-care is to join a homeopathic study group of other nonprofessionals. There are many such groups throughout the country. Contact the National Center for Homeopathy to see if there's one in your area.

With or without a study group, you'll probably have to do some experimenting to find remedies that work for you. Obviously if you have a serious illness, you should consult a professional, but for everyday ailments like colds and headaches, you'll do no harm to try several remedies until you find the one that's right. And, after all, it's the remedies for these common conditions that you're likely to need most often.

For a cold, for example, you can choose from belladonna, aconite, euphrasia, allium, bryonia, and several others. The one that you choose would depend upon how you got your cold, the type of symptoms, whether it's a head cold or a chest cold, and what makes the symptoms better or worse. Bryonia might be just the ticket for a cold lodged in your chest, a dry cough, and dry lips. If the cold made you thirsty and irritable, then all the more reason to try bryonia. On the other hand, aconite might be your answer if the cold came on suddenly just after you'd spent an afternoon trudging about in a biting wind. Constant sneezing, raw throat, restlessness, and feeling worse at night are other symptoms that would point to aconite as the possible treatment of choice.

The names of plant-derived homeopathic remedies differ somewhat from the botanical names of the plants and are often completely different from the common names. Rhus toxicodendron, for example, is the name of a homeopathic remedy for arthritis and rheumatism, among other things. The plant's botanical name is *Toxicodendron radicans*, but we know it as plain poison ivy.

This example demonstrates the difference between herbal remedies and homeopathic ones. You obviously wouldn't boil up a bunch of poison ivy and make a poultice or drink a tea made from it, but in the extremely diluted form in which you purchase homeopathic remedies, rhus toxicodendron won't cause you to break out in a rash. A number of remedies are of this nature: toxic unless prepared homeopathically. It goes without saying that, while you can treat yourself homeopathically, you should not try to prepare your own homeopathic remedies. They are readily available at herbal shops, health-food stores, and homeopathic pharmacies.

Homeopathy is a complete healthcare system just as allopathic medicine is, so we can't possibly do it justice within these pages. The foregoing discussion gives you a brief overview, but if you're considering choosing a homeopathic physician as your principal healthcare practitioner, you'll want to learn more. Although you don't have to know more to experiment with various homeopathic remedies on your own—they're harmless even when they don't help—common sense suggests that the more you know, the sooner you'll find remedies that work for you. (Conversely, you may decide that homeopathy isn't for you at all.)

If you're fortunate enough to have a homeopathic pharmacy nearby, use it as a resource. Ask your friends who use homeopathic remedies what works for them. Read, or perhaps join a study group. If you like what you learn, you may want to get a complete workup from a homeopathic physician. He or she can help you zero in on the proper medications, not just for your ailments but for you as an individual with those ailments.

FURTHER READING

Bilological Therapy (quarterly scientific journal; $10), Menaco, PO Box 11280, Albuquerque, NM 87192

Grossinger, Richard. *Homeopathy: An Introduction for Skeptics and Beginners*. Berkeley, Calif.: North Atlantic Books, 1993.

Hersen, Paul. *The Homeopathic Treatment of Children*. Berkeley, Calif.: North Atlantic Books, 1991.

Homeopathy: Natural Medicine for the 21st Century. Alexandria, Va.: National Center for Homeopathy, 1990.

Lockie, Andrew, M.D. *The Family Guide to Homeopathy*. New York: Simon & Schuster, 1993.

Lockie, Andrew, M.D., and Nicola Geddes. *The Women's Guide to Homeopathy*. New York: St. Martin's Press, 1993.

MacEoin, Beth. *Homeopathy*. New York: HarperPaperbacks, 1994.

Meyer, Eric, and J.P. LeGrand, *The Family Encyclopedia of Homeopathic Medicine*. New York: Instant Improvement, 1993.

Nyholt, Dave. *The Complete Natural Health Encyclopedia*. Tofield, Alberta, Canada: Global Health, 1993.

Rose, Barry, M.D. *The Family Health Guide to Homeopathy*. Berkeley, Calif.: Celestial Arts, 1993.

Ullman Dana. *Discovering Homeopathy*. Berkeley, Calif.: North Atlantic Books, 1991.

RESOURCE GROUPS

Homeopathic Academy of Naturopathic Physicians
14653 Graves Rd.
Mulino, OR 97042
Phone: 503/829-7326

Referrals to naturopaths who use homeopathic remedies

Homeopathic Educational Services
2124 Kittridge St.
Berkeley, CA 94704
Phone: 510/649-0294

International Foundation for Homeopathy
2366 Eastlake Ave. E., Ste. 301
Seattle, WA 98102
Phone: 206/324-8230

Membership $25; national directory of homeopaths; *Resonance*, bimonthly magazine; referrals to local practitioners

National Center for Homeopathy
801 N. Fairfax St., Ste. 306
Alexandria, VA 22314
Phone: 703/548–7790

Membership $40; monthly newsletter, *Homeopathy Today*; also books, homeopathic kits; referrals to local practitioners

NATURAL HYGIENE (LIFE SCIENCE)

DEFINITION

Natural hygiene is a philosophy of health that postulates that the body heals itself if a person lives according to the way that nature intended. Natural hygiene emphasizes vegetarian diet, periodic fasting, and food combinations to promote good health.

APPLICATIONS

Physiological: Proponents of natural hygiene believe that the human body is completely self-sufficient and self-healing, so that no diseases will develop when the body is treated properly. However, an overweight person may shed pounds if he or she follows the program.
Psychological: See above.

COLLATERAL CROSS-THERAPIES

Vegetarianism, fasting, exercise

RECOMMENDED ADJUNCT ACTIVITIES AND BEHAVIORS

None

CONTRAINDICATIONS

The diet recommended by proponents of natural hygiene contains only healthful foods, but it is fairly restrictive. Although followers don't believe in consulting healthcare practitioners, we recommend that you do (before undertaking the diet) if you have food allergies, serious medical conditions, or are pregnant.

EQUIPMENT & MATERIALS

You may want to purchase a juicer or blender for making your own fresh fruit and vegetable juices.

ORIGIN

For many of us, the word *hygiene* has lost its original meaning. We think of hygiene as referring principally to cleanliness: brushing our teeth and washing our hands. However, broadly speaking hygiene is the science and art of preserving and improving health. As such, some of its most important precepts formed a part of the wisdom of the Egyptians at least as long ago as 1500 B.C., but it is to the Greek physician Hippocrates that practitioners of Natural Hygiene trace their roots. Hippocrates stated that "Thy food shall be thy remedy," and this is the philosophy that Natural Hygienists espouse today.

People from many cultures historically practiced certain dietary habits, both for reasons of health and for religious purposes. Among these are the Greeks, Romans, Jews, Christians, Indians, and Chinese. The idea that diet can influence overall health is certainly not a new one, nor is the contention that the body will heal itself (or not fall into disrepair in the first place) if a person lives the proper lifestyle.

The premises behind natural hygiene are ancient ones, but its development as a specific practice is less than 200 years old in the United States. In 1830, a group formed an organization called the American Physiological Society, which espoused natural foods as the key to good health. Within a few years, the APS established a library and store in Boston. The store, which sold natural foods, was the forerunner of the modern health-food store.

About 1850, four physicians, Isaac Jennings, Mary Gove, William Alcott, and Sylvester Graham began the Natural Hygiene movement in earnest. They advocated lifestyle and dietary changes to promote more healthful living. One of Dr. Graham's principal goals was to get people to eat whole-wheat bread, rather than bread made from refined flour. Hence, whole-wheat flour became known as *graham* flour, and from this we get our modern-day graham cracker.

Other physicians who wanted a more naturalistic approach to medicine soon joined the ranks. The philosophy, which was first known simply as *Hygiene*, evolved slowly over time. Contributors to its development included Dr. Russell Trall, who formed a national hygienic association in 1862. In 1872, Dr. Trall wrote a book called *The Hygienic System* that further spread the word about Natural Hygiene.

Proponents of Hygiene advocated a strictly vegetarian diet, consisting principally of raw foods, such as vegetables, nuts, and seeds. They felt that such a diet would prevent people from getting sick.

Hygiene had a fair number of followers for about fifty years, but when Louis Pasteur proposed the "germ theory" as the cause of disease around the turn of the century, Hygiene slipped from favor. It never died out completely, but it had few followers until Dr. Herbert M. Shelton published *The Science and Fine Art of Food and Nutrition* and other books on the Hygiene concepts of diet and nutrition. From 1928 to 1981, Dr. Shelton operated a "health school" in San Antonio that included a laboratory, clinic, and teaching program. Advocates consider Shelton's work the backbone of the Natural Hygiene movement. More recently, T.C. Fry has been a prominent spokesperson for Natural Hygiene.

When the American Natural Hygiene Society was founded in 1948, the word "Natural" was added to the name to differentiate it from the general practice of hygiene as most people view it. Some followers of Natural Hygiene call the system Life Science, but the principles are basically the same.

INSTRUCTIONS

The premise behind Natural Hygiene is that the body is always striving for health and that it achieves this by continuously cleansing itself of deleterious waste material. Practitioners believe that the human body is completely self-sufficient and that it will keep itself disease-free and in proper working order if a person adheres to the natural laws of life.

By following a diet of raw foods, principally vegetables, fruits, seeds, and nuts and by eating foods in certain combinations, a person can ensure that the digestive (cleansing) process works properly. A few cooked foods are allowed but only in small amounts. Periodic fasting is also part of the regimen.

Natural Hygiene stresses the importance of maintaining proper weight for good health, but "dieting" is not part of the program. People naturally achieve their optimum weight if they eat the right foods at the proper times.

In their book *Fit for Life*, Harvey and Marilyn Diamond suggest that the body has three daily natural cycles:

- noon to 8 P.M.—appropriation (eating and digestion)
- 8 P.M. to 4 A.M.—assimilation (absorption and use of food)
- 4 A.M. to noon—elimination (getting rid of body wastes and food debris)

By eating mostly processed and cooked foods, we make it difficult for the body to assimilate food and eliminate wastes properly. The buildup of toxic waste leads to overweight.

The Diamonds present three principles of healthful eating. The first is that foods with a high-water content are all-important to the body. Since the body itself is composed of 70% water, people should eat foods that have a 70% water content. Only raw fruits and vegetables contain that much water, so fruits and vegetables should make up about 70% of the diet. The remaining 30% can be divided among other more "concentrated" foods.

Natural hygienists maintain that just drinking lots of water won't do the trick because we need the nutrients contained in the water content of fruits and vegetables to properly cleanse the inside of the body. In fact, they say you won't need to drink so much water if you eat foods with a high water content. They discourage drinking water with meals, and they recommend drinking only distilled water.

The second principle is that eating foods in appropriate combinations will increase energy. Digestion of food requires more energy than anything else the body does, but certain combinations of foods make digestion easier and more efficient. Natural hygienists believe that the human body is not designed to digest more than one so-called *concentrated* food (anything that is not a fruit or a vegetable) at once. Therefore, you should eat only one type of concentrated food at each meal.

The third principle involves the proper consumption of fruit. According to natural hygienists, fruit is the most important food we can eat. Fruit has the highest water content of any food, and it requires the least energy to digest. To get the benefits from fruit, however, you should eat it when the stomach is empty, and you should not eat any other foods along with it. The fruit should always be fresh, never canned or cooked, but it can be in the form of juice if it isn't processed.

What will your diet be like if you follow a natural hygiene plan? First, you'll have only fresh fruit or juice until noon (no coffee or tea), but you can have as much of that as you like. (This is to avoid eating anything that requires a lot of energy to digest during the elimination cycle.) If you want to feel you're eating a meal, make a fruit salad. When you're especially hungry, try bananas, which are more filling.

From noon to 8 P.M., during the eating cycle, you can have lunch and dinner (or several small meals) composed primarily of fresh vegetables plus one form of concentrated food, such as starch. (Natural hygienists discourage eating either meat or dairy products, but if you do eat them, wait until dinner time, when your workday is nearly over.) The general premise is that fresh fruits and vegetables should be eaten early in the day when energy requirements are highest. As the day progresses, you can add steamed vegetables, raw nuts, and seeds. Then grains, breads, potatoes, and legumes. Because meat, fish, chicken, and dairy are hardest to digest, they should be eaten only sparingly and only late in the day. (Remember that, overall, concentrated foods should make up only 30 percent of your total daily diet.) Midnight snacking is out because after 8 P.M. your body has begun its assimilation cycle.

Natural hygienists recommend having an all-fruit day from time to time. Eating nothing but fruit and fruit juice is supposed to be energizing, and it contributes to maximum weight loss if that is a problem.

Devotees emphasize that the Natural Hygiene diet is part of a lifestyle and not a reducing diet *per se*, but because the calorie count is low, overweight people will undoubtedly lose weight. However, remember that proper diet is only part of the Natural Hygiene philosophy. In addition, one should exercise regularly; get plenty of rest, fresh air, and sunshine; learn to handle stress; and avoid negative influences. Natural hygienists believe that good health is normal and is as simple to achieve as living in harmony with nature. Health and disease are a continuum. The same physiological laws govern the body in sickness and in health. Therefore—except for extraordinary circumstances—healing results from actions undertaken by the body on its own behalf. If you want to follow the Natural Hygiene program, there are a number of books that offer recipes and further details. See the *Further Reading* section that follows.

FURTHER READING

Altman, Nathaniel. *Eating for Life*. Wheaton, Ill.: Theosophical Publishers, 1974.

Carrington, Hereward, Ph.D. *The History of Natural Hygiene*. Mokelhumne Hill, Calif.: Health Research, 1964.

Diamond, Harvey. *Your Heart, Your Planet*. Santa Monica, Calif.: Hay House, 1990.

Diamond, Harvey, and Marilyn Diamond. *Fit for Life*. New York: Warner Books, 1987.

———. *Fit for Life*. Burbank, Calif.: Warner Home Video, 1987. (video)

———. *Fit for Life II*. New York: Warner Books, 1988.

———. *A New Way of Eating*. New York: Warner Books, 1993.

Fry, T.C. *Superior Foods, Diet Principles and Practices for Perfect Health*. Austin, Tex.: Life Science, 1983.

Gewanter, Vera. *A Passion for Vegetables*. New York: Viking Press, 1980.

Shelton, Herbert M., Ph.D. *Natural Hygiene, Man's Pristine Way of Life*. San Antonio, Tex.: Dr. Shelton's Health School, 1968.

RESOURCE GROUPS

American Natural Hygiene Society
PO Box 30630
Tampa, FL 33630
Phone: 813/855-6607

Membership $25; magazine *Health Science*; conferences, seminars; local referrals

Bionomics Health Research Institute
PO Box 36107
Tucson, AZ 85740
Phone: 602/297-0798

Newsletter *Health-O-Gram* (10 issues $13.50); also books

International Association of Professional Natural Hygienists
2000 S. Ocean Dr.
Hallandale, FL 33009
Phone: 305/454-2220

Quarterly newsletter $12; referrals to local practitioners

Life Science Institute
1108 Regal Row
PO Box 609
Manchaca, TX 78652
Phone: 512/280-5566

Audio- and videotapes, books; newsletters: *The Healthway Advisor* and *The Health Science Newsletter*; bimonthly magazine *Healthful Living* (subscription $18); also home study course

Natural Hygiene, Inc.
PO Box 2132
Huntington Station, Shelton, CT 06484
Phone: 203/929-1557

Membership $15; bimonthly magazine *Journal of Natural Hygiene*; books, audio- and videotapes

NATUROPATHY (NATUROPATHIC MEDICINE)

DEFINITION

Naturopathy (natural medicine) is a system of healthcare that emphasizes prevention of disease and the use of natural treatments to assist the body's own healing power. Naturopaths use all forms of alternative medicine, including hydrotherapy, nutrition, Ayurveda, acupuncture, homeopathy, exercise, massage, counseling, and herbalism.

APPLICATIONS

Physiological: Broad application for diseases and illnesses not requiring surgery, radiation, chemotherapy, or the like; particularly applicable to chronic problems where the long-term use of pharmaceuticals is not desirable (e.g., arthritis, chronic pain); natural childbirth; obesity
Psychological: Stress, tension, insomnia, substance dependency

RECOMMENDED ADJUNCT ACTIVITIES AND BEHAVIORS

Lifestyle changes where appropriate

CONTRAINDICATIONS

Naturopathic treatments are safe and gentle, but medical emergencies, traumatic injuries, and life-threatening illnesses require more aggressive measures.

ORIGIN

Like the alternative healing systems upon which it relies, naturopathic medicine traces its roots to the philosophical principles of Hippocrates, a Greek physician who lived several centuries before the birth of Christ. Before Hippocrates, most people believed that illness was caused either by magic or by angry gods who were displeased with the sufferer. To cure the disease, one had to restore the god's good humor, often by some sort of sacrifice. Hippocrates taught that disease and illness had rational causes that could be found in nature, so he looked for their cures in nature as well. Hippocrates and his followers also believed that the body has its own power to heal.

Although the principles of naturopathy have been known for 2,000 years, in its modern form, naturopathy grew out of alternative medicine practiced in eighteenth- and nineteenth-century Europe and America. The term *naturopathy* was coined by a German immigrant, Dr. John Scheel, who practiced medicine in New York City in the late 1800s. He used the term to describe a system of healing that emphasized treating the whole person using natural methods. Early on, naturopathic physicians were greatly influenced by the teachings of Father Sebastian Kneipp, who popularized hydrotherapy in Europe, and hydrotherapy became one of their principal cures. The chief U.S. proponent of Kneipp's theories was Benedict Lust. Lust and others broadened the scope of treatments, so that shortly after the turn of the century, naturopaths included diet, exercise, nutritional therapy, herbs, homeopathic remedies, electrotherapy, manipulative treatments (such as chiropractic), and other natural cures in their lexicon.

Lust started a school in New York City—the American School of Naturopathy—which graduated its first class in 1902. Lust's program emphasized eliminating harmful habits, introducing healthful habits, and then developing a new and more healthful lifestyle. "Harmful" habits included the use of alcohol and nicotine, immoderate sleeping and eating patterns, and eating meat. These were to be replaced by a moderate regimen featuring exercise, proper breathing, appropriate choice of food, and a positive mental attitude. Treatments included baths of nearly every description: Turkish, air, light, mud, steam, and sitz. Fasting and skeletal manipulation were also important parts of the protocol.

Naturopathy flourished. At one time, there were at least twenty naturopathic schools throughout the United States, and naturopathic physicians were licensed to practice in nearly every state.

Until the mid-1930s, naturopathy and traditional medicine coexisted quite amiably, and many mainstream physicians incorporated forms of naturopathic healing into their practices. For example, traditional practitioners commonly prescribed herbal remedies and baths, often as their first line of treatment. However, the disciplines gradually began to go off in quite different directions. When man-made drugs came along, traditional practitioners began prescribing them instead of homeopathic or herbal remedies. Also, during the two world wars, there were tremendous advances in surgical techniques. Mainstream medicine adopted a more technological approach to treatment, and aided by the influence of powerful pharmaceutical companies, was able to convince both the government and the public that theirs was a superior approach to healthcare. If traditional medicine was good, then other healthcare systems must be bad, or so reasoned the politicians. Accordingly, state legislatures throughout the United States passed legislation that often severely curtailed the practice of alternative forms of healing.

With the passage of time, however, people have come to realize that surgery and drugs are not always the best answers to medical problems, and today there is renewed interest in more natural, and often less toxic, forms of treatment. Naturopathy, with its emphasis on prevention and healthful lifestyle, is once again receiving favorable attention from both the public and some mainstream medical practitioners.

Naturopathy is not one system of alternative healing but a combination of many. Some naturopathic physicians specialize in a specific type of therapy, while others draw on a wide variety of disciplines, which include: herbal medicine, exercise therapy, physical therapy, nutrition, homeopathy, acupuncture, acupressure, hydrotherapy, natural childbirth, and lifestyle counseling.

Although naturopathic medicine encompasses a variety of therapies, all naturopathic practices follow certain basic tenets. One is that preventing disease is better than treating it after the fact. A naturopathic physician will guide a patient toward a healthful lifestyle, but the patient must also take an active role, both in maintaining wellness and in the healing process, should illness occur.

The naturopath treats the whole person, not just the symptoms of a particular disease. Health or illness results from a complicated interaction of hereditary, dietary, physical, environmental, and emotional factors that are unique to any given individual. The naturopathic practitioner considers all aspects of a person's life when prescribing treatment.

Perhaps the most important principal of naturopathy is the assumption that nature is the greatest healer. Naturopathic practitioners use treatments and medicines that support the natural processes of recovery. Because they do not use artificial drugs, their treatments tend to be gentler and have fewer side effects. Noninvasive measures take precedence wherever possible. Overall, naturopathy is a more conservative approach to health care than traditional medicine. The aim is not the quick cure, but the safe cure. (Naturopaths do not perform major surgery, prescribe pharmaceutical drugs, or deliver radiation therapy. When a patient requires these treatments, he or she will be referred to a medical doctor.)

INSTRUCTIONS

How does naturopathy fit into the lives of ordinary people? Whether or not you choose a naturopath as your healthcare practitioner, you can follow some of the practices on your own. For example, when you have a headache, what do you usually do? Swallow a couple of aspirin? Instead, you might sip a cup of rosemary, peppermint, or sage tea. Or take a nap. Or a walk. Massaging the back of the neck relieves some headaches. In other words, if you want to follow naturopathic practices, you will first turn to something totally safe and natural.

Then you'll want to consider why you had the headache in the first place. Remember that part of the natural method of healing is that you discover the cause of the problem and eliminate it, so that it won't happen again. Obviously, an occasional headache is nothing to worry about, but if you have persistent headaches or *always* get a headache when your sister Lil comes to visit, then you have some ongoing problems that need attention.

Headaches can have physical causes, and you'll want to visit your healthcare practitioner if you can't pinpoint the cause of persistent headaches (and get rid of them) yourself. However, a large percentage of headaches are stress-related. The naturopathic way of healing supports many stress-diffusing techniques. Instead of waiting until stress builds up to where a troop of tom-tom players takes up residence behind your eyes, try to pinpoint the major tension builders in your life and eliminate the ones that you can. Then build in some safe, natural stress reducers as part of your daily routine. Exercise, self-massage, hot baths, herbal teas, and mental relaxation techniques are all naturopathic methods for keeping stress in check.

The point is that it's up to you to pay closer attention to your body, your lifestyle, and your interactions with the environment and other people so that you can take charge of your own health. Because you're in charge, naturopathy doesn't categorically tell you to do this or that to cure illness or keep well. There are many roads to good health, and naturopathic philosophy teaches that when you're in tune with your own mind and body, you will be able to determine the appropriate safe and natural treatment for yourself. There are plenty of books and videos available to help you learn more about keeping well using naturopathic principles.

FURTHER READING

Bricklin, Mark. *The Practical Encyclopedia of Natural Healingd*. New York: Penguin Books, 1990.

Gordon, Jay. *Alternative Medicine: Natural Home Remedies*. Puyallup, Wash.: Future Medicine Publishing Co., 1994. (video)

Healthy and Wise, free quarterly newsletter, published by John Bastyr College Clinic, 1408 NE 45th St., Seattle, WA 98105. Phone: 206-632-0354

Kusick, James. *A Treasury of Natural First Aid Remedies from A-Z*. West Nyack, N.Y.: Parker Publishing Co., 1995.

Lobay, Douglas G. *21st Century: Natural Medicine*. Kelowna, B.C., Canada: Apple Communications, c1992.

Murray, Michael T. *Natural Alternatives to Over-the-Counter and Prescription Drugs*, New York: William Morrow, 1994.

Murray, Michael T., and J.E. Pizzorno. *Encyclopedia of Natural Medicine*. Rocklin, Calif.: Prima Publishing, 1991.

Naturopath, The, monthly newspaper on natural healthcare. Order information: 1920 N. Kilpatrick, Portland, OR 97217. Phone: 503/285-3807

Polunin, Miriam, and Christopher Robbins. *The Natural Pharmacy*. New York: Collier Books, 1992.

RESOURCE GROUPS

American Association of Naturopathic Physicians
2366 Eastlake Ave. E., Ste. 322
Seattle, WA 98102
Phone: 206/323-7610

(Ten states currently license naturopaths, and seventeen others are considering doing so. In states without licensing, virtually anyone can set up a practice whether or not he or she is properly trained. Contact the association above for names of practitioners in your area who meet licensing standards. If your state does grant licenses, you can also call your state board of naturopathic examiners.)

National College of Naturopathic Medicine
11231 SE Market St.

Portland, OR 97216
Phone: 503/255-4860

Ontario College of Naturopathic Medicine
60 Berl Ave.
Toronto, ON M8Y3C7, Canada

Prima Publishing
PO Box 1260MP
Rocklin, CA 95677
Phone: 916/786-0426

Encyclopedia of Natural Medicine can be ordered directly from here.

NUTRITIONAL SUPPLEMENT THERAPY (INCLUDING VITAMIN THERAPY, AMINO-ACID THERAPY, ORTHOMOLECULAR NUTRITION, AND LIFE EXTENSION THERAPY)

DEFINITION

Nutritional supplement therapy is the use of nutritional supplements, including vitamins, minerals, amino acids, and enzymes, to treat physical and psychological problems. For therapeutic purposes, nutritional supplements are generally taken in doses exceeding the recommended daily allowances (RDAs).

APPLICATIONS

Physiological: Acne, allergies, body odor, burns, cancer, carpal tunnel syndrome, elevated cholesterol, colds, diabetes, dry skin, eczema, glucose intolerance, heart arrhythmias, heart disease, high blood pressure, infertility, kidney stones, leukoplakia, measles, menstrual cramps, muscle cramps and spasms, osteoporosis, Parkinson's disease, periodontal disease, premenstrual syndrome (PMS), rickets, scurvy, stroke, ulcers, wounds
Psychological: Depression, schizophrenia, stress

COLLATERAL CROSS-THERAPIES

Healing diets, vegetarianism, herbalism

RECOMMENDED ADJUNCT ACTIVITIES AND BEHAVIORS

Healthful, balanced diet

CONTRAINDICATIONS

Some nutritional supplements can build up to toxic levels in the body if taken in excessive amounts. Do not undertake to cure yourself of specific conditions with nutritional supplements without first checking with your healthcare practitioner. He or she can tell you whether the supplements you propose to take are likely to help and, more importantly, whether they might do you any harm.

EQUIPMENT & MATERIALS

Nutritional supplements of choice

ORIGIN

Although nutritional supplements as such are of fairly recent origin, the theory that certain foods can cure diseases goes back to ancient times. Physicians in earlier civilizations might not have known what the specific component of the food was that did the trick, but—no doubt by empirical evidence—they learned that foods could heal.

Hippocrates noticed that Greek armies on the march suffered from bleeding gums. Although he didn't know the true cause—vitamin C deficiency—he correctly associated the problem with eating only dried foods. Later during the age of discovery when sailors were on the high seas for long periods of time, they experienced the same symptoms. The disease is called *scurvy*, and it can occur whenever people are deprived of fresh foods over extended periods.

James Lind, a Scottish physician attached to the British navy, described scurvy in 1753 and introduced a cure: citrus fruits. Thereafter British sailors became known as "lime-juicers," later shortened to "limeys," which is still a nickname for the British, although it no longer applies just to sailors.

The term *vitamin* was coined by a Polish biochemist, Casimir Funk, in 1911. For many years, the disease called *beriberi* had puzzled scientists. Beriberi was common among rice-eating populations in the Orient, but the odd thing was that beriberi had not always been a problem. Funk discovered that beriberi only came into the picture after people began to eat *polished* rice, and he proved that a substance in rice polishings—the part that is discarded when rice is polished—would prevent the disease. He named this substance *vitamin* from the words *vita* meaning life and *amine* meaning a nitrogen compound. (The vitamin that prevents beriberi is thiamine or vitamin B_1.)

Before long, scientists had discovered a whole host of other vitamins. Even today we are not certain as to how—or even whether—all vitamins impact on human nutrition, but there are thirteen that are considered essential. They are: carotene (vitamin A), thiamine (vitamin B_1), riboflavin (vitamin B_2), niacin (vitamin B_3), pantothenic acid, pyridoxine (vitamin B_6), biotin, folic acid, vitamin B_{12}, ascorbic acid (vitamin C), vitamin D, vitamin E, and vitamin K. All but two of these vitamins are synthesized by plants and will be present in a diet of vegetables, fruits, and unrefined carbohydrates. Vitamin D is actually a hormone that requires sunlight to be synthesized in the skin. Vitamin B_{12} is synthesized by microorganisms.

Vitamins don't provide energy like proteins and carbohydrates, but they are necessary for the body to properly metabolize other foods. Vitamins A, D, E, and K are called fat-soluble vitamins because they mix with and dissolve in fat. The other essential vitamins are water-soluble.

Unlike vitamins, minerals aren't synthesized by plants. Minerals are found in the soil and water, from which they are taken up by plants. Mineral deficiencies can cause some diseases, but so can excesses of certain minerals. A deficiency of iron, for example, results in iron-deficiency anemia, but excesses of iron can cause damage to the liver, including cirrhosis.

Amino acids are other important nutrients. Amino acids are known as the "building blocks of protein" because various combinations of amino acids form the proteins in all living creatures. At one time, scientists thought that the amino-acid combinations in meat were the perfect source of protein in the human diet. They thought proteins from vegetable sources were inferior, but today we know that vegetable protein can give humans all the essential amino acids they need, without the excess fat found in meat. There are twenty amino acids, which are all found in unprocessed foods of all sorts, but in varying amounts.

Amino acids are classified as essential and nonessential. Essential amino acids are not manufactured by the body, so a person must include them in the diet. Nonessential amino acids are manufactured by the body, and therefore, we don't need to eat foods that contain them. Essential amino acids include tryptophan, threonine, valine, lysine, isoleucine, leucine, phenylalanine, and methionine. Some authorities include arginine and histadine on this list.

We still have a great deal to learn about nutrition and the role that various nutrients play in health. Only a few years ago, many nutritionists advocated a diet high in protein. Today people are told they eat much too much animal protein and that a strictly vegetarian diet is more healthful. Now new research has linked various foods to a decreased risk of cancer, heart disease, high blood pressure, and various other diseases.

Many healthcare practitioners believe that people can get all the nutrients that they need—and in the right combinations—from a healthful diet rich in complex carbohydrates, vegetables, and fruits. Others believe that supplements of vitamins, minerals, and/or amino acids can help cure certain conditions. This schism is just as evident in alternative circles as it is in mainstream medicine. The controversy is not likely to be resolved in the near future, but with each new research study, scientists seem to find an additional piece of the puzzle.

INSTRUCTIONS

If you are interested in vitamin and mineral supplementation, you may want to check the chart below to see if you have a condition that might be helped by a supplement. Remember to check with your healthcare practitioner first, though.

HEALTH PROBLEM	NUTRITIONAL THERAPY
Acne	Zinc
Allergies	Vitamin B complex, vitamin C, pantothenic acid
Body odor	Zinc
Burns	Vitamin A
Cancer	Antioxidants; vitamins A and C
Carpal tunnel syndrome	Vitamin B_6 (pyridoxine)
Cholesterol (elevated)	Niacin, potassium
Colds	Vitamin C
Depression	Folic acid
Diabetes	Chromium
Dry skin	Vitamin A
Eczema	Vitamin B complex, vitamin E
Glucose intolerance	Chromium
Heart arrhythmias	Magnesium
Heart disease	Magnesium, niacin
High blod pressure	Vitamin C, calcium, magnesium, potassium
Infertility	Vitamin C
Kidney stones	Vitamin B_6 (pyridoxine), magnesium
Leukoplakia	Vitamin A
Measles	Vitamin A
Menstrual cramps	Magnesium

Muscle cramps and spasms	Magnesium, potassium
Osteoporosis	Calcium
Parkinson's disease	Vitamin E
Periodontal disease	Calcium, magnesium, zinc
Premenstrual syndrome	Vitamin E, calcium
Rickets	Calcium, vitamin D
Schizophrenia	Folic acid, niacin, vitamin C, vitamin B_6
Scurvy	Vitamin C
Stress	Pantothenate
Stroke	Potassium
Ulcers	Zinc
Wounds	Vitamin A, vitamin C

Amino-acid supplementation did not become practical until the early 1960s when free-form amino acids became widely available. Advocates of amino-acid therapy believe that, because many diseases and emotional problems are biochemical in origin, amino acids can be used to treat them.

In her book *The Way Up From Down*, psychiatrist Priscilla Slagle detailed her use of amino-acid therapy to overcome years of depression that had resisted any other form of treatment. One of the key elements in Dr. Slagle's book, however, is L-tryptophan, which is no longer sold in the United States. Because a single contaminated batch of tryptophan caused several deaths, the FDA took the supplement off the market and has never seen fit to allow it to be sold again. (Elsewhere in the world tryptophan is widely available.) The chart below lists some uses for amino-acid supplements.

CONDITION	AMINO ACID SUPPLEMENT
Alcohol dependence	L-glutamine
Chronic pain	DL-phenylalanine
Depression	L-tryptophan, L-tyrosine, and phenylalanine
Herpes	L-lysine
Insomnia	L-tryptophan
Overweight	DL-phenylalanine

In the 1980s, Durk Pearson and Sandy Shaw developed a program called "Life Extension" that uses nutritional supplements, including amino acids, vitamins, and minerals. The goal of Life Extension is to retard the effects of aging.

Another program that uses nutritional supplements as treatments is called *orthomolecular therapy*. The word "orthomolecular" was coined by chemist and Nobel prize winner Linus Pauling. The orthomolecular approach maintains that each person has unique nutritional needs based on heredity, environmental factors, and metabolism. Research in orthomolecular therapy is particularly concerned with a nutritional approach to treating schizophrenia, hypoglycemia, learning disabilities in children, substance abuse, depression, cancer, and a number of other diseases. Orthomolecular therapy is not for the do-it-yourselfer, but you can find out more about it by contacting the Huxley Institute for Biosocial Research.

If you are interested in any of the programs that use nutritional supplements to cure diseases or promote health, you might want to read one of the books listed in the *Further Reading* section.

FURTHER READING

Braverman, Eric R., and Carl Curt Pfeiffer. *The Healing Nutrients Within*. New Canaan, Conn.: Keats Publishing, c1987.

Chaiton, Leon. *Amino Acids in Therapy*. New York: Thorsons, 1985.

Cott, Allan; Jerome Agel; and Eugene Boe. *Dr. Cott's Help for your Learning Disabled Child*. New York: Time Books, 1985.

Erdmann, Robert, and Meirion Jones. *The Amino Revolution*. New York: Simon & Schuster, 1989.

Hendler, Sheldon Saul. *The Purification Prescription*. New York: William Morrow and Co., 1991.

Jochems, Ruth. *Dr. Moerman's Anti-Cancer Diet*. Garden City Park, N.Y.: Avery Publishing Group, 1990.

Newbold, H.L. *Mega-Nutrients: A Prescription for Total Health*. Los Angeles: Body Press, 1987.

Newstrom, Harvey. *Nutrients Catalog*. Jefferson, N.C.: McFarland and Co., 1993.

Pauling, Linus. *How to Live Longer and Feel Better*. New York: W.H. Freeman, 1986.

Pearson, Durk, and Sandy Shaw, *Life Extension: A Practical Scientific Approach*. New York: Warner Books, 1983.

Prasad, Kedar N. *Vitamins Against Cancer*. Rochester, Vt.: Healing Arts Press, 1989.

Quillan, Patrick, and Noreen Quillan. *Beating Cancer With Nutrition*. Tulsa, Okla.: Nutrition Times Press, 1994.

Sessions, John L. *Coping With Cancer*. Greenwich, Conn.: Devin-Adair, 1985.

Sheffrey, Stephen. *Vitamin C: The Pros and Cons*. Ann Arbor, Mich.: Prion Books, 1991.

Slagle, Priscilla, M.D. *The Way Up From Down*. New York: St. Martin's Press, 1992.

Somer, Elizabeth. *Vitamins, Minerals, and Nutrition: The Top 100 Questions and Answers*. Danbury, Conn.: Grolier Educational Corporation, 1988.

Zisk, Gary, M.D. *The Amino Acid Super Diet*. New York: G.P. Putnam's Sons, 1988.

RESOURCE GROUPS

Canadian Schizophrenia Foundation
7375 Kingsway
Burnaby, B.C. V3N 3B5, Canada
Phone: 604/521-1728

Orthomolecular nutrition; membership $25, quarterly newsletter; books, pamphlets, articles

Durk Pearson & Sandy Shaw's *Life Extension Newsletter*
PO Box 92996
Los Angeles, CA 90009

Monthly newsletter; subscription $34.95

Huxley Institute for Biosocial Research, Inc.
900 North Federal Highway, Ste., 300
Boca Raton, FL 33432
Phone: 800/783-3801 or 407/393-6167

Orthomolecular therapy; membership $25; newsletter; books, pamphlets, audiotapes; referrals to physicians practicing orthomolecular nutrition

Life Extension Foundation
2490 Griffin Rd.
Fort Lauderdale, FL 33312
Phone: 800/841-5433

Membership includes *Life Extension Report* and *Life Extension Update* (monthly newsletters), discount on mail-order supplements; also books and audiotapes

Linus Pauling Institute of Science and Medicine
440 Page Mill Rd.

Palo Alto, CA 94306
Phone: 415/327-4064; Fax: 415/327-8564

Research into use of vitamin C and other nutrients for treatment of cancer, heart disease, and other diseases; books, reprints of lecture series

Princeton BioCenter
862 Route 518
Skillman, NJ 08558
Phone: 609/924-8607

Clinic specializing in orthomolecular nutrition; also research center; extensive list of low-cost publications

AFTERWORD

We hope you've enjoyed your tour through *The Self-Health Handbook*. Now that you've read the book, why not sit down and develop a plan for achieving and maintaining vibrant good health? The first step is to recognize that your mind, body, and spirit are not separate entities but fully integrated parts of a whole that forms a unique being: *you*. If you neglect one part, the rest won't work as well. (You wouldn't drive on a flat tire even though the motor was humming along, would you?) That's what holistic health is all about: treating the whole person. So as you develop your program for a healthy life, keep that in mind.

Although these pages contain many treatments for common ailments, your new plan will help you the most if it emphasizes *preventing* problems through a more healthful lifestyle. Of course you won't become a perfect person, so you will have illnesses from time to time. We hope they will all be minor ones that you can treat safely with natural methods. Most natural methods are just as good as (and sometimes better than) costlier, more potent traditional medicines, but there are problems that must be treated by healthcare professionals. Your program should include consultation with a healthcare professional for any serious illness or injury. High-tech equipment, surgical procedures, drugs, and laboratory tests can be lifesaving in some situations.

Consulting a professional doesn't mean that you need to abdicate responsibility for your health, though. You should discuss your diagnosis and the treatment options with your practitioner. Ask questions if you don't understand something. Find out if there is a safer, more natural treatment that you can try before resorting to stronger measures. If your practitioner is unwilling to discuss your case, find someone else who is. It's *your* health, and only you can make the final judgment about how to enhance it. To do this, you must make informed choices. We hope *The Self-Health Handbook* has helped you do that.

INDEX